CLINICAL ANATOMY
& PHYSIOLOGY
of the
Swallow Mechanism

Kim Corbin-Lewis, PhD, CCC-SLP
Associate Professor
Department of Communicative Disorders and Deaf Education
Utah State University

Julie M. Liss, PhD, CCC-SLP
Associate Professor
Department of Speech Sciences
Arizona State University

Kellie L. Sciortino, PhD, CCC-SLP
Montgomery, Alabama

THOMSON
DELMAR LEARNING   Australia Canada Mexico Singapore Spain United Kingdom United States

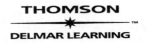

THOMSON

━━━━━★━━━━━ ™

DELMAR LEARNING

Clinical Anatomy and Physiology of the Swallow Mechanism

by Kim Corbin-Lewis, PhD, CCC-SLP, Julie M. Liss, PhD, CCC-SLP, and Kellie L. Sciortino, PhD, CCC-SLP

**Vice President,
Health Care Business Unit:**
William Brottmiller

Editorial Director:
Cathy L. Esperti

Acquisitions Editor:
Kalen Conerly

Developmental Editor:
Juliet Steiner

Marketing Director:
Jennifer McAvey

Marketing Coordinator:
Chris Manion

Editorial Assistant:
Molly Belmont

Art and Design Coordinator:
Christi DiNinni

Production Coordinator:
Jessica McNavich

Library of Congress Cataloging-in-Publication Data:
ISBN: 1-5659-3967-0

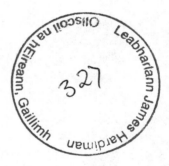

NOTICE TO THE READER

Publisher does not warrant or guarantee any of the products described herein or perform any independent analysis in connection with any of the product information contained herein. Publisher does not assume, and expressly disclaims, any obligation to obtain and include information other than that provided to it by the manufacturer.

The reader is expressly warned to consider and adopt all safety precautions that might be indicated by the activities described herein and to avoid all potential hazards. By following the instructions contained herein, the reader willingly assumes all risks in connection with such instructions.

The publisher makes no representations or warranties of any kind, including but not limited to, the warranties of fitness for particular purpose or merchantability, nor are any such representations implied with respect to the material set forth herein, and the publisher takes no responsibility with respect to such material. The publisher shall not be liable for any special, consequential, or exemplary damages resulting, in whole or part, from the readers' use of, or reliance upon, this material.

CONTENTS

FOREWORD   VII
PREFACE   IX
ACKNOWLEDGMENTS   XIII

CHAPTER 1 Examination of the Oral Swallow Component   1

Stages of Deglutition   2
Structural Framework for the Swallow Mechanism   2
Visual Inspection of Structures in the Oral Cavity   9
Sensory Receptors   37

CHAPTER 2 Examination of the Pharyngeal Swallow Component   41

A Description of the Pharyngeal Phase   42
Pharyngeal Anatomy   44
Triggering the Pharyngeal Swallow Response   48
Swallowing and Respiration   62

CHAPTER 3 Examination of the Esophageal Swallow Component   67

Esophageal Structure   68
Esophageal Innervation   73
Esophageal Blood Supply   78
Esophageal Physiology   80
Esophageal Pressure Measurement Using Manometry   87

CHAPTER 4 Control of the Normal Swallow   93

Modeling Swallowing and Dysphagia   94

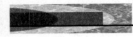

CHAPTER 5 Direct and Indirect Oropharyngeal and Esophageal Imaging 109

Anatomical Planes of View 110
Diagnostic Imaging Methodologies 122
Manometry and pH Studies 145

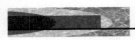

CHAPTER 6 Physiological Bases of Neurogenic Dysphagia and Treatment Strategies 151

Neurological Pathology 152
Neural Regulation of Swallowing 152
Neurogenic Dysphagia 152
Clinical Presentation of Neurogenic Dysphagia 162

CHAPTER 7 Physiological Bases of Structural Etiologies of Dysphagia and Treatment Strategies 187

Acute Structural Changes 188
Progressive Transformations 202
Head and Neck Cancer 210
Pharyngeal Cancer 217
Laryngeal Cancer 217
Esophageal Neoplasms 223
Radiation Treatment for Head and Neck Cancer 224

EPILOGUE: FUTURE DIRECTIONS 235
APPENDIX A 241
APPENDIX B 245
GLOSSARY 251
INDEX 267

FOREWORD

When the Dysphagia Series was nascent, I hoped for an anatomy and physiology book. The reason was simple: speech books were being used and every clinician and every researcher knew that speech anatomy and physiology, while important and complex, was different from swallowing anatomy and physiology. Sometimes the differences were small, more often they were large. Now *Clinical Anatomy and Physiology of the Swallow Mechanism* joins the Dysphagia Series, and what an addition it is. The authors, Kim Corbin-Lewis, Julie M. Liss, and Kellie L. Sciortino, have written a classic book. This book delivers on its title. The authors discuss clinical anatomy and physiology. They do it so well that this book could become the text for a dysphagia course, not just the text for an anatomy and physiology class nor a supplementary text for an overview course.

How did they do this? Readers will be able to answer this question for themselves by reading any chapter. Here are a few of my answers.

Clearly these authors know the struggles of swallowing-impaired persons, and they know the evaluative and treatment approaches clinicians take to them. They know students as well. As a result, the discussions of structures and muscles and movements are put into a clinical context. All of us in the speech-language pathology profession are familiar with the usual idealized views, often artfully and realistically rendered, of the structures of the head and neck. These authors give us these and other images as well. These other images are taken from the clinical, endoscopic, and videofluoroscopic examinations used to evaluate dysphagia. These are trenchant images and they make memorizing muscles and structures easier. Indeed I do not know a more richly and intelligently illustrated book in speech-language pathology. Want to see a PEG insertion? Look in Chapter 3 at Figure 10. Want to see the real, rather than stylized, relationship of trachea and esophagus? Look in the same chapter at Figure 1. Such figures abound.

The authors also know the issues confronting scientists and clinicians. They discuss the esophagus as well as the oropharynx. As a result, this book will serve the profession in the next decade as it comes to grips with the interaction of oropharyngeal and esophageal mechanisms and with its place in the evaluation and management of both. They discuss the physiologic bases of all the extant behavioral, medical, and surgical treatments. I bet someone, sometime, told them such an emphasis was too broad. If so, they ignored this advice and readers are the beneficiaries. Leading clinicians over two decades have been beseeching clinicians to base treatment decisions on physiologic and pathophysiologic principles. Clinicians want to do what is best, but they have had to struggle to relate patterns of swallowing difficulty to specific treatments. These three authors show the way. Clinicians who discover this book will put it within arm's reach of their clinical suites. Table 6–5 may well be worth the book's price.

These authors know students. The text is leavened with figures, anecdotes, clinical cases, and inviting language. I can imagine pulling an all-nighter not because a test is looming but because the story of normal and abnormal swallowing these authors tell is so engaging.

This book cost these authors lost weekends, sleep, and pounds. They persevered. They could have taken shortcuts but they did not. Instead they prevailed. The result is a book of admirable scholarship and amazing grace. The Dysphagia Series and dysphagia clinicians, scientists, and students are the benefactors.

John C. Rosenbek, PhD
Series Editor

PREFACE

Clinical Anatomy and Physiology of the Swallow Mechanism grew from a need for instructional materials that addressed anatomy and physiology of the swallow mechanism *specifically* and considered factors not relevant to speech production but crucial in the understanding of normal and abnormal swallow performance. Anatomy and physiology textbooks have not been written from the perspective of normal and disordered swallow function. While most of the structures used in speech and swallowing are the same, the sequence of activation, relative amount of participation, and integration with other organ systems is not. For example, the role of the respiratory system during the swallow cycle is critical in a manner far different from that found in speech production. Rather than providing the raw material for sound generation, during deglutition protection of the airway from foreign material (food) and temporary arrest of function is essential. The coordination between swallowing and breathing becomes a complex but essential component in evaluation and management of dysphagia. Likewise, the relationship between bolus consistency and duration of upper esophageal sphincter (UES) opening is irrelevant to speech production and not included in anatomy and physiology texts used in clinical training programs for speech-language pathologists. Bolus characteristics and effect on swallow efficiency becomes critical to the speech-language pathologist managing caloric needs and successful eating in a patient with dysphagia. These structures and their functions for swallow need their own forum. While the material in this text is not *new,* the perspective from the role of a speech-language pathologist addressing dysphagia is.

Speech-language pathologists have a thorough grounding in anatomy and physiology for voice and speech production provided during coursework in communicative sciences and disorders. Structures and function of the respiratory, phonatory, articulatory, resonatory, and neural systems are all covered at both the undergraduate and graduate levels of training. The digestive system typically is not covered in depth and complex interactions with other organ system functions are rarely addressed. Many graduate programs, at the time of this writing, do not have dedicated courses to the study of dysphagia. This clinically-focused textbook is designed to assist speech-language pathologists and students in applying and extending their knowledge base to the study of anatomy and physiology of normal deglutition and dysphagia in the adult population. For seasoned clinicians, the textbook is designed to further their ability to recognize and articulate physiology-based problem solving during the clinical examination. It is not our intent to completely rewrite a general anatomy textbook by including detailed description of all structures and functions in speech and language production. Rather, we have attempted to focus on those structures relevant to swallow function.

This book focuses on the mature mechanism because, while we view adult and pediatric feeding and swallowing as related, they are clearly separate fields given the myriad of developmental factors at play in pediatric problems. The developmental sequence of sensory and motor-skill development and structure maturation crucial to pediatric feeding issues would require a different focus.

We also hope that the material presented in this book will have a broader appeal to members of trans-disciplinary dysphagia teams by providing common ground in the description of structure and function of the swallow mechanism across specialty areas. Medical terminology is used throughout the text in an effort to provide a core vocabulary needed in a medical setting. Wherever possible, multiple common terms for the same structure are provided. These most often represent terms coined by different specialty areas such as neurology, radiology, otolaryngology, gastroenterology, or speech-language pathology. A glossary has been provided to assist the new clinician or student unfamiliar with basic medical terminology.

A secondary goal of this textbook is to provide a clinical framework for students and clinicians in which to identify the necessary clinical questions to be answered for each individual patient. Accurate, effective, and efficient diagnosis and management of dysphagia has its foundation in a clear and comprehensive grasp of normal anatomy and physiology of the aerodigestive systems. Anatomy, physiology, and clinical management are not separate entities. Clinical management must be informed by an individual's anatomy and physiology. Cookbook approaches to management decisions and techniques can have devastating results in individuals with dysphagia. Poor outcomes may range from minimal harm (such as no change in swallow function) to increased risk or presence of pneumonia to a catastrophic result (such as death). Careful attention to each individual's idiosyncratic anatomy and physiology during swallow function is an absolute necessity for successful management.

We have liberally incorporated appropriate primary research findings and references as they relate to normal and abnormal physiology. Often research from medicine and fields outside of speech-language pathology is not directly incorporated into teaching materials. This is a double-edged sword—in this rapidly progressing field of dysphagia diagnosis and management, primary research uncovers past misconceptions as well as creates new ones. The evolution of the field is such that today's beliefs are often proven incorrect tomorrow. Recognizing this fact, but feeling a strong need for inclusion of clinically-relevant primary research into the theoretical foundation for practicing clinicians, we have attempted to provide a current view of aerodigestive physiology. We anticipate, and hope for, continued advancement in the understanding of this complex topic. The clinician or student will not go wrong if they allow the knowledge base in aerodigestive physiology to guide their practice. This allows for change and adaptation of methods and techniques throughout a career.

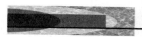 ## HOW TO USE THIS TEXT

Since our primary focus of this book is clinical, the format of the book was designed to lead the student/clinician through structures as they would be encountered in a diagnostic evaluation. We begin with the oral cavity (Chapter 1), which might be assessed visually, and follow with chapters on the pharynx (Chapter 2) and esophagus (Chapter 3), which should be assessed radiographically and/or endoscopically. Chapter 4 explores issues related to normal control and variation of deglutition and the external influences to the swallow sequence that must be accounted for in clinical practice. Chapter 5 provides a detailed overview of common clinical measurement and imaging techniques of the swallow mechanism. Chapters 6 and 7 address common abnormal findings in adults and the underlying physiology of the disturbance to swallow function. Neurogenic and structural abnormalities that may lead to dysphagia are covered separately. We have also included the theory-based rationale for clinical management strategies in current use. We feel strongly that research should drive clinical techniques and involve all practitioners in exploring treatment outcome.

To further our goal of making this text clinically relevant, we have incorporated *Clinical Notes* in boxes throughout the chapters to highlight common (or uncommon) clinical information useful to the clinician working with dysphagia. To help focus readers on the key points in each chapter, *Learning Objectives* are included and can be incorporated in classroom instruction or in self-study. We have also provided *Study Questions* designed to encourage clinicians and students to address anatomical and physiological factors in their clinical decision-making. The answers to these study questions can be found in Appendix B. Hopefully, this will encourage self-directed learning.

We hope that you find the information timely, relevant, and thought-provoking as you develop and hone your dysphagia diagnosis and management skills.

Kim Corbin-Lewis
Julie M. Liss
Kellie L. Sciortino

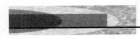

ABOUT THE AUTHORS

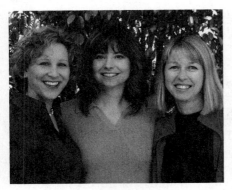

From left to right: **Kellie L. Sciortino, Julie M. Liss, and Kim Corbin-Lewis.**

Kim Corbin-Lewis, PhD, CCC-SLP, is an Associate Professor at Utah State University in the Department of Communicative Disorders and Deaf Education. She earned her PhD from the University of Wisconsin-Madison. She teaches in the areas of dysphagia, motor speech disorders, voice, speech science, and anatomy and physiology. Kim has been a practicing speech-language pathologist for 24 years.

Julie M. Liss, PhD, CCC-SLP, is an Associate Professor at Arizona State University in the Department of Speech and Hearing Sciences. She was awarded her PhD from the University of Wisconsin-Madison. She teaches in the areas of dysphagia, motor speech disorders, neuroscience, and anatomy and physiology.

Kellie Sciortino, PhD, CCC-SLP, is in private practice in Montgomery, AL. She received her PhD from Arizona State University. She has taught in the areas of dysphagia, voice, and craniofacial anomalies.

ACKNOWLEDGMENTS

Many have shared their time, knowledge, and experience to support the writing of this textbook. We acknowledge the generous assistance of V. Duane Bowman, MD, for outstanding clinical endoscopic photos, Douglas Child, MD, for assistance with radiologic terminology and images, Bryan Larsen, MD, for his critical reading, Austin Spitzer, MD, for sharing radiographic images, and LeAnn Chlarson, MS, CCC-SLP, for fluoroscopic images. Special thanks to Andy Anderson of the Utah State University Biology Department for access to the human dissection lab. James Jones provided invaluable assistance with the dissections.

We extend our gratitude to Laura Parsons, Annie-Karine Lamoreaux, Danna Huntzinger, and Eric Okelberry for their much-appreciated contributions to figure and glossary preparation and text editing. Special thanks to Brynne Davies for assistance with image preparation.

We have had help and support along the way from multiple editors whom we would like to thank—Juliet Steiner, Debra Flis, and Marie Linville. Special thanks to Juliet Steiner who saw this project through to completion.

Our deepest thanks to the series editor, Jay Rosenbek, PhD, who invited us to be a part of the Dysphagia Series, and challenged us to conceive of an anatomy book that has clinical roots.

And thanks to our patient and supportive families—David, Danica, and Alexandra Lewis; John, John Justin, Vanessa, and Donald Caviness; Ned, Nicolette, and Gianna Maria Sciortino; Maynard and Judy Filter. They have shared the long journey which began while at least five of them were yet to join the world.

CHAPTER 1

Examination of the Oral Swallow Component

LEARNING OBJECTIVES

After completing the chapter and reviewing the study questions, you should be able to:

- Understand the overlaid functions of the oral component of the aerodigestive tract

- Understand the anatomy and physiology relevant to the oral stage of swallowing

- Describe the primary bony framework and muscles used for bolus formation and oral transport

- Understand the role of sensation in the oral phase of swallow

- Appreciate the normal variation in oral anatomy and physiology.

INTRODUCTION

Consider this twist of fate: the evolutionary changes of the human vocal tract that permit us to produce the rich and varied sounds of speech are the very same changes that predispose us for risk of **aspiration** and choking. The culprit is the large supralaryngeal space created by the rather low position of the adult human larynx in the neck. This space serves as the common pathway for breathing, **deglutition** (the act of swallowing), and the shaping of sound waves for speech production. Further, this space distinguishes us from most other mammals, which possess largely separate respiratory and digestive pathways because of larynges that rest high in the neck (Laitman & Reidenberg, 1993). Respiration, swallowing, and speech can, therefore, be viewed as overlaid functions in the human aerodigestive tract. It is no small coincidence, then, that the practitioners of speech-language pathology have embraced the study, assessment, and treatment of swallowing disorders. Speech-language pathologists are, after all, uniquely poised to understand and appreciate the highly complex functioning of the upper aerodigestive tract.

1

In studying the anatomy of the speech mechanism you have, in essence, studied the anatomy of the swallow mechanism. Although the effectors are the same—the lips, cheeks, tongue, velum, and so forth—the functions are substantially different. Throughout the chapters, you will see familiar structures in a new light. We will present the anatomy as it relates specifically to the function of swallowing.

STAGES OF DEGLUTITION

Classically, deglutition has been divided into four consecutive stages: oral preparatory, oral, pharyngeal, and esophageal (Logemann, 1983). In the first stage, food is taken into the mouth, manipulated into a cohesive bolus, and held there momentarily as it is prepared for transport. Preparation may include chewing (incorporating saliva into the bolus to form a smooth and cohesive mass), breaking the bolus into small parcels, and channeling it into a depression formed on the surface of the tongue. The bolus will be compressed by the tongue against the hard palate prior to the next stage. In the oral stage, the bolus is propelled posteriorly toward the oropharynx. As the bolus reaches the oropharynx, a pharyngeal swallow response is initiated, setting into motion a series of airway-protective and bolus-propulsive events associated with the pharyngeal stage. The esophageal phase is initiated by relaxation of the **upper esophageal sphincter (UES)** at the top of the esophagus that allows the bolus to begin its descent toward the stomach. This four-stage model is highly intuitive and appears to be quite straightforward. However, the more we study the act of swallowing, the more we learn that it is a highly adaptive function whose details vary considerably with what is being swallowed (e.g., bolus size, consistency, viscosity, temperature, taste, and mode of delivery), and the characteristics of who is doing the swallowing (e.g., age, sex, variations in anatomy, and idiosyncratic behaviors). It is from this vantage point that we explore the anatomy and physiology associated with the various stages of the **swallow**.

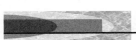

STRUCTURAL FRAMEWORK FOR THE SWALLOW MECHANISM

Orofacial anatomy for deglutition begins with a description of the structural framework for the soft tissues of the orofacial structures. Coverage is restricted to bones that serve as attachment sites for the muscles of facial movement integral to swallow and mastication, specifically the maxillae, palatine bones, zygomatic bones, mandible, and temporo-mandibular joint (Figure 1-1). A comprehensive description of other structures in this region can be found in any general anatomy text.

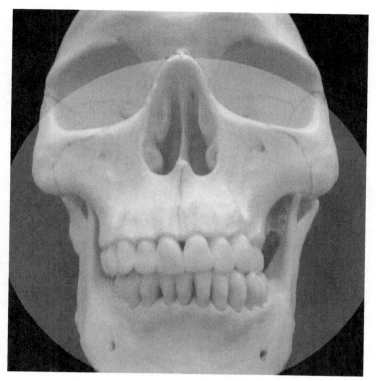

Figure 1-1. Anterior view of skull with location of interest highlighted.

Cranium

The human skull is comprised of 22 bones that articulate through immovable joints called **sutures**. Of these bones, several are of particular importance for the study of swallowing because they serve as points of attachment for muscles associated with the preparation or propulsion of the bolus. These include the temporal bone, the sphenoid bone, the palatine bone, and the maxillae. The mandible, the most moveable part of the facial skeleton, will be described in the next section.

The irregularly shaped **temporal bones** (Figure 1-2) form the lateral sides of the cranium. These bones not only house the organs of hearing and balance within their inner petrous portions, they also form the footing for the temporomandibular joint. Three processes are evident on the external surface of the temporal bones that are important attachment sites for muscles used during swallow. The **mastoid process** is large and prominent, and it can be felt by palpating the cranium just behind the ear lobe. It is the attachment site for the large sternocleido-mastoid muscle, and the medially placed mastoid notch is the insertion point for the **digastric muscle**, which contributes to the floor of the

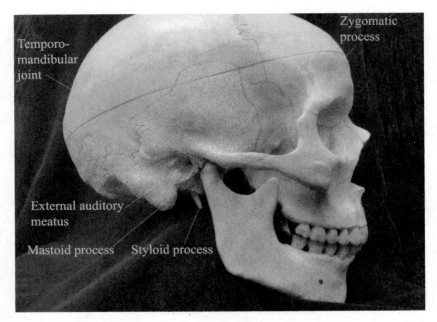

Figure 1-2. Lateral view of cranium and facial skeleton.

mouth. The **styloid process**, a hook-like projection of bone, cannot be easily palpated. It lies medially and posteriorly to the mastoid process and is the origin for three muscles involved in deglutition: the styloglossus, stylopharyngeus, and the stylohyoid muscle. The **zygomatic process** extends anteriorly to form a suture with the zygomatic bone of the face. It, along with the zygomatic bone, serves as an attachment site for various muscles of facial expression.

The **sphenoid bone** is located deep within the cranium and its various processes serve as attachment sites for several muscles associated with swallowing. Figure 1-3 shows a schematic of the location of this bat-shaped bone that is hidden within the facial skeleton. Peering through the orbits in Figure 1-3, we can see the **lesser wings** and part of the **greater wings** of the sphenoid. The **lateral** and **medial pterygoid plates** extend inferiorly from the greater wings. A hook-like extension, called the **hamulus**, descends from the medial pterygoid plate. We will learn more about these important attachment sites in the following sections.

Facial Skeleton

The bony framework of the oral cavity is visually evident—the maxillae provide structure to the upper face while the mandible provides the

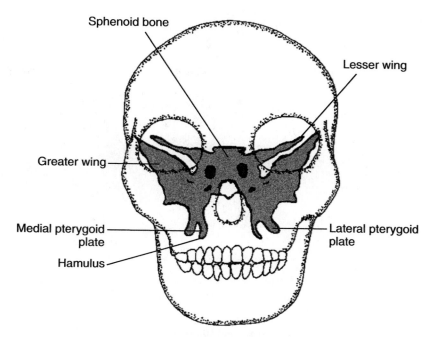

Figure 1-3. Sphenoid bone in situ.

hinged-action lower portion of the face (Figure 1-4). These bones serve as anchor sites for dentition, as well as for the muscles of facial expression and mastication. Mediated at the temporomandibular joint, these bones play a vital role in the oral preparatory stage and, to a lesser degree, the oral stage of the swallow sequence. The complex act of mastication relies on a mandibular dental arch that fits within the maxillary arch. Muscular attachments to the mandible allow a three-dimensional rotary movement pattern integral to the grinding of food and bolus formation. Mandibular opening with a labial/lingual seal assists in oral pressure generation necessary for the oral transport phase of the swallow sequence.

Maxillae and Palatine Bones

The maxillae are paired, multidimensional bones that form the framework for four surfaces: the anterior aspect of the **midface**, the initial portion of the **hard palate** (along the horizontal plane), the inferior surface of the **orbital cavity** (superolaterally), and the lateral sides of the **nasal cavity** (medially) (Figure 1-5).

The maxillae can be thought of as having a central horizontal section flanked by a U-shaped raised ridge of bone (Figure 1-6). The raised ridge is known as the **alveolar process** or **ridge** and contains spongy (cancellous) bone with sockets for the eight teeth in the two upper

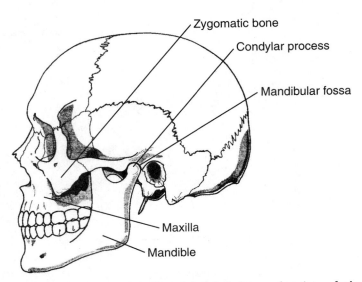

Figure 1-4. Lateral view of skull and facial skeleton, showing relationship between maxilla and mandible.

quadrants of the mouth. In addition to housing the maxillary dentition, it is an important contact point for the tongue during the oral phase of swallowing. The central horizontal section is formed by the merging of two plates of bone that meet at midline to form the **intermaxillary suture**. However, this is not formed by two single plates meeting at midline. The majority is formed by the **palatine processes** of the maxillae. It accounts for three-quarters of the hard palate and, on its superior surface, the floor of the nasal cavity. The posterior one-quarter of the hard palate is formed by the **palatine bones**. These are the points of attachment for the **palatal aponeurosis**, a thin sheet of connective tissue that gives rise to the muscles of the soft palate. The initial segment of the horizontal section of the maxillae is formed by the **premaxilla**. Though rarely visible in adults, sutures delineating the premaxilla radiate from the intermaxillary suture to the space between the lateral incisors, on each side, and the cuspid teeth.

Zygomatic Bones

The small, paired zygomatic bones form the cheekbones as they articulate with processes from the frontal, maxillae, and temporal bones (Figure 1-7). Some of the fibers of the **masseter muscle** originate from the zygomatic bone.

Mandible

The mandible in an adult is considered to be a single, U-shaped bone with a **ramus** on each side projecting superiorly and posteriorly (Figure

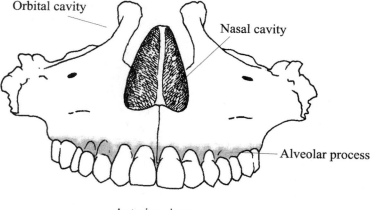

Anterior view

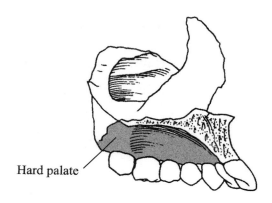

Medial view

Figure 1-5. Anterior and medial views of the maxillae.

1-8). The **mental symphysis**, oriented vertically at the anterior midline, is where the two halves of the mandible fuse and ossify in the first year of life. The primary landmarks on the anterior surface of the body include bilateral **mental foramen** where the mental nerve and blood vessels exit to the frontal surface of the bone. The mandible is prominent in radiographic images of the head. The **angle of the mandible**, where the body ends and the ramus begins, is frequently used as a landmark for bolus movement from the oral cavity to the pharyngeal cavity. When the bolus passes this point, the pharyngeal stage of swallow is considered to have begun. The ramus of the mandible divides into an anterior projection, the **coronoid process**, and a posterior projection, the **condylar process**. The coronoid process is the attachment site for

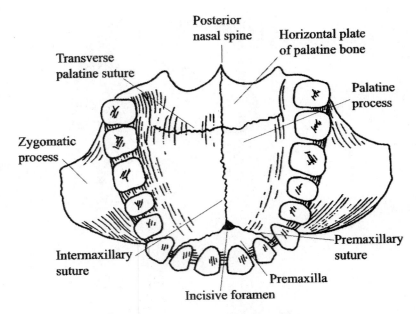

Figure 1-6. Inferior view of hard palate.

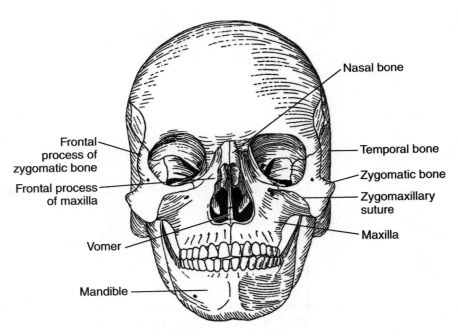

Figure 1-7. Anterior view of skull and facial skeleton.

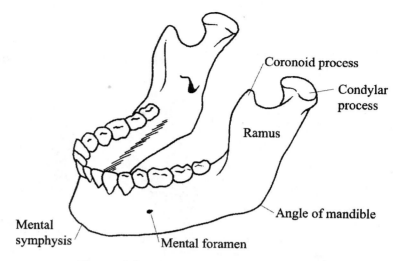

Figure 1-8. Anterolateral view of the mandible.

the **temporalis muscle**. The head of the condylar process articulates with the temporal bone at the **mandibular fossa** and forms the **temporomandibular joint (TMJ)**.

Temporomandibular Joint

The temporomandibular joint (TMJ) is formed by the articulation of the condylar process of the mandible at the mandibular fossa of the temporal bone (Figure 1-9). This unique joint allows for movement in three planes to produce jaw depression and elevation, jaw protrusion and retraction, and jaw lateralization. Unlike requirements for speech, chewing often involves movement in all of these planes, resulting in a rotary pattern of mandibular displacement (Moore, Smith, & Ringel, 1988; Komiyama, Asano, Suzuki, Kawara, Wada, Kobayashi, & Ohtake, 2003). A series of ligaments, such as the temporomandibular, sphenomandibular, and stylomandibular ligaments, attach to the joint and prevent overextension of movement resulting in dislocation of the joint.

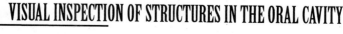

VISUAL INSPECTION OF STRUCTURES IN THE ORAL CAVITY

Now that we have covered the bony framework, let us consider the structures relevant to swallowing that can be seen on visual inspection of the face and oral cavity. The oral cavity can be thought of as a box, consisting of a top and bottom with four walls. The top is the hard and soft palates, the bottom is the tongue and mouth floor, the anterior wall is comprised of the lips and teeth, and the cheeks and teeth create the

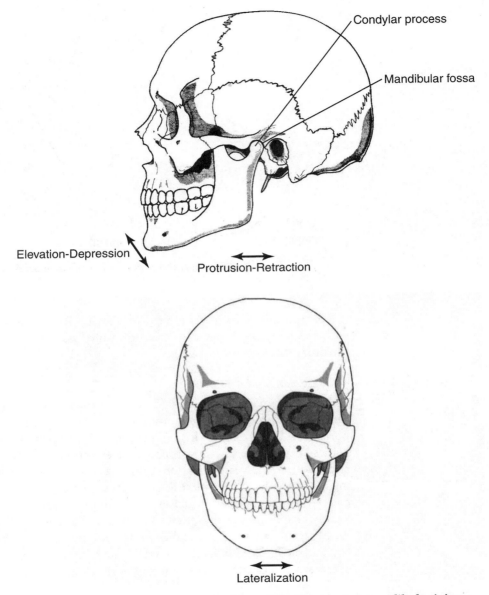

Figure 1-9. Movement planes about the temporomandibular joint.

lateral walls (Figure 1-10). The posterior wall of this box has two potential configurations. The back of the pharynx (the oropharynx) is one wall, and it is what you see on visual inspection of the oral cavity. There is a potential wall, however, that is created by contact of the tongue dorsum with the relaxed soft palate. This configuration is common during the oral preparatory stage when food is being chewed. The tongue-

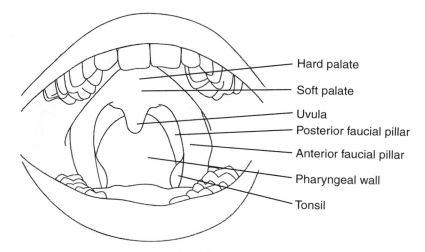

Figure 1-10. Schematic of the oral cavity.

velum contact discourages food from slipping into the pharynx while normal breathing is occurring through the nose (Figure 1-11a). When the tongue dorsum is lowered and the velum is elevated, the posterior pharyngeal wall serves as the back of the box (Figure 1-11b). This is the configuration that occurs at the onset of the pharyngeal stage of the swallow, which will be discussed in the next chapter.

Anatomical Landmarks of Orofacial Structures

The structures that comprise the boundaries of this imaginary box do not normally vary from person to person. That is, the lips and teeth always form the anterior wall, the cheeks and teeth form the lateral walls, and so forth. However, the appearance of the inside of the oral cavity is as unique as the face in which it resides. This normal variation in structure and function should come as no surprise. It creates a difficult task for the clinician, however, who is striving to understand the range of "normal" and distinguish it from abnormal. In this section, we review the landmarks of the face, oral cavity, and oropharynx that are most pertinent to mastication and swallowing.

Lips

The anterior wall of the imaginary box is composed of the lips (Figure 1-12), which overlie the anterior dentition. The external lips are comprised of epithelium that is distinguished from the surrounding face by its high pigmentation. This difference in color creates a zone called the

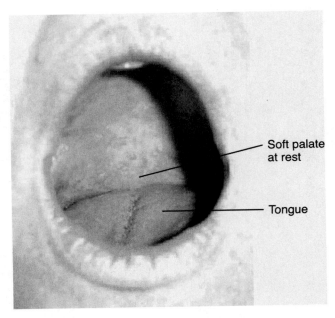

Soft palate
at rest

Tongue

Figure 1-11a. Anterior view of soft palate at rest against the posterior tongue.

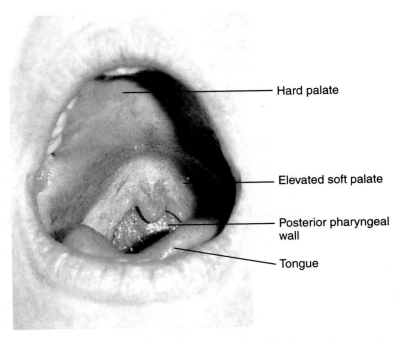

Hard palate

Elevated soft palate

Posterior pharyngeal wall

Tongue

Figure 1-11b. Anterior view of the elevated soft palate.

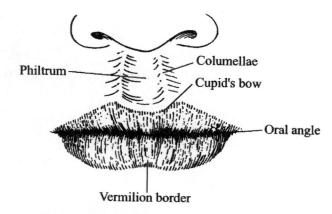

Figure 1-12. Anterior view of face and lips.

vermilion border. A notch on the upper lip at the vermilion border, sometimes called **Cupid's bow**, forms the base of two columns, called **collumellae**, that extend superiorly to the base of the nose. The groove formed between the collumellae is called the **philtrum**. The upper and lower lips meet laterally, forming the corners of the mouth, or the **oral angles**. The oral angles are important landmarks because they serve as attachments for many muscles associated with lip movement.

Sulci

If the lips were transparent, we would see the space, or sulcus, that exists behind them as they rest against the teeth and gum (alveolar ridges of the maxilla and mandible). This space is called the **labial** or **anterior sulcus**)—the superior labial sulcus is between the upper lip and gums, and the inferior labial sulcus is between the lower lip and gums (Figure 1-13a). In each of these sulci, we also would be able to see a strand of skin, or **frenulum**, that extends from the inside of both the upper and lower lips and attaches to the gum area adjacent to the central incisors. These are called the upper and lower **labial frenula**, and they are visible by retracting the upper and lower lips.

The lateral walls of the imaginary box form another set of sulci (Figure 1-13b). These **buccal** or **lateral sulci** reside between the inner aspects of the cheeks and the adjacent teeth, and they are frequently the site of *pocketed* food. This pocketing is common when the muscles of the cheek have insufficient tone to keep the bolus between the occlusal surfaces of the teeth. The food then slips into these sulci and accumulates, usually without the patient recognizing the problem. Buccal sulci can be visualized by retracting the cheeks adjacent to the teeth and alveolar ridges.

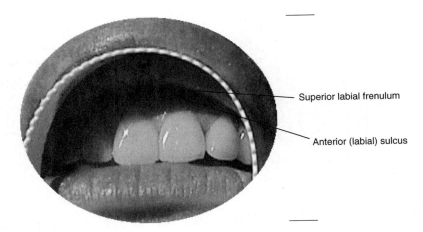

Superior labial frenulum

Anterior (labial) sulcus

Figure 1-13a. Anterior sulcus and superior labial frenulum.

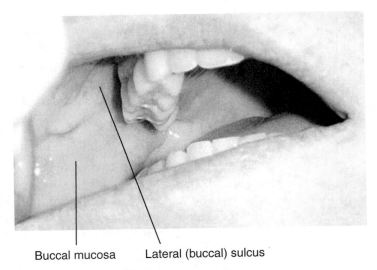

Buccal mucosa

Lateral (buccal) sulcus

Figure 1-13b. Lateral (buccal) sulcus.

CLINICAL NOTE

1-1

Squirreling

Appropriate tone in the labial and cheek muscles prevents food from accumulating in the anterior and lateral sulci during the oral stages of deglutition. Any decrease in tone or sensation may result in a clinical phenomenon known as *pocketing* or *squirreling*. This is frequently seen among patients who have paralysis or weakness of facial muscles due to involvement of the facial nerve (CN VII). Patients can be instructed to clear the accumulated material with their finger or tongue periodically during the meal. Food that is not cleared presents a serious choking hazard.

Faucial Pillars

The lateral aspects of the oral cavity also contain other landmarks that do not involve the cheek tissue, per se, but that are still part of the lateral boundaries of the imaginary box. These are thin bands of skin that extend from the top to the bottom of the oral cavity and form two sets of curved arches, called the **anterior** and **posterior faucial arches** or **pillars** (Figure 1-14). These arches are actually formed by underlying muscle tissue, **palatoglossus** and **palatopharyngeus muscles**, respectively, which we will discuss later. The space between the two faucial arches is the location of the **palatine tonsils**. The amount of tonsilar tissue varies widely from person to person. When a person has had a tonsillectomy, the space between these two faucial arches is empty.

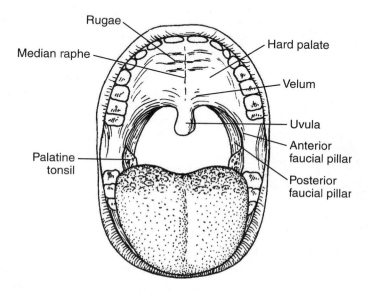

Figure 1-14. Anterior view of faucial pillars and oral cavity landmarks.

Palate

The top of the oral cavity consists of the hard and soft palates, and is therefore fixed anteriorly and flexible posteriorly. Again, referring to Figure 1-14, the hard palate is rimmed by the upper dentition, which is embedded in the alveolar ridge of the maxillae. The mucosal surface covering the hard palate (which is contiguous with the rest of the mucosal surface in the oral cavity) is not smooth. A few strokes of the hard palate with your tongue will reveal a series of raised ridges, or **rugae**, immediately behind the central incisors. At midline there is a groove that extends the length of the hard palate. This groove, called the midline or **median raphe**, is created by the underlying suture where the two halves of the palatine bones fused during fetal development. The soft palate, or **velum**, extends posteriorly from its attachment to the hard palate. The attachment site consists of a broad, flat sheet of connective tissue called the palatal aponeurosis. Although this transition area may be palpated, there are no distinct visual landmarks on the mucosal surface to demarcate the boundary between the hard and soft palates. At the termination of the soft palate is the **uvula**, which hangs at midline in the oropharynx.

Normal variations in the configuration of the top of the oral cavity are abundant. First, there is a range of normal variation in **palatal vault** height and width. Second, a **torus palatinus** (bony palate) is sometimes present at the anterior end of the midline raphe. This appears as a bulge or pad that presumably occurs during fusion of the palatine bones in fetal development. It has no known functional significance or consequence. Other variations include uvular size and orientation, and oropharyngeal cavity depth. **Bifid uvulae** may indicate the presence of a submucosal cleft of the soft palate, or they may be isolated and benign.

CLINICAL NOTE 1-2

Clefts and Defects of the Hard and Soft Palates

The hard and soft palates form the structural boundary between the oral and nasal cavities. Any defect of this boundary has serious implications for deglutition, particularly for the oral phases. Structural defects may occur congenitally, as in the case of cleft palate, or they may result from surgery or trauma to the palate. Clinically, patients may exhibit nasal regurgitation. Infants, who rely on the palate for extraction of milk from a breast or bottle, may have significant difficulty feeding.

Tongue

The bottom of the imaginary box is the tongue, which is formed by the mandible and soft tissue structures and rests on the floor of the mouth. The floor is rimmed by the alveolar ridge of the mandible and its asso-

ciated dentition. The tongue actually is much larger than we can appreciate on a visual oral examination. Even with the tongue protruded as far as possible, we can see only to a V-shaped region of bumps called the **circumvallate papillae** (Figure 1-15a). Beyond this region, the tongue takes a nearly 90-degree turn into the pharynx where the **root** of the tongue attaches to the hyoid bone (Figure 1-15b). The surface of the tongue is divided obviously into right and left halves by a **central sulcus**, which runs its length. This sulcus is created by the underlying muscle pairs that blend at midline as they meet their mates. The tongue is tethered, anteriorly, to the floor of the mouth by way of the **lingual frenulum**.

The tongue (as well as portions of the palate, pharynx, larynx, and esophagus) is covered with nearly 10,000 taste buds. These taste buds contain taste receptor cells that tend to respond most strongly to a certain primary flavor (sour, sweet, salty, bitter), and less strongly to the others. Although not visually distinguishable, the taste buds most sensitive to sweet and salty flavors are clustered on the front of the tongue. Sour flavors are transduced most readily on the sides of the tongue, and bitterness is sensed most strongly at the back of the tongue at the area of the **fungiform papillae**.

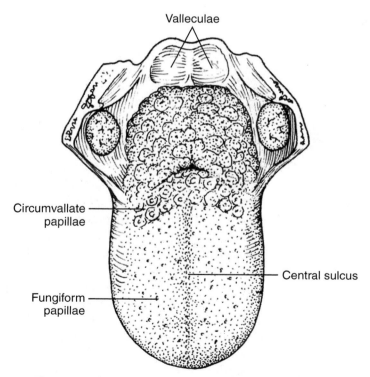

Figure 1-15a. Superior view of extended tongue in situ.

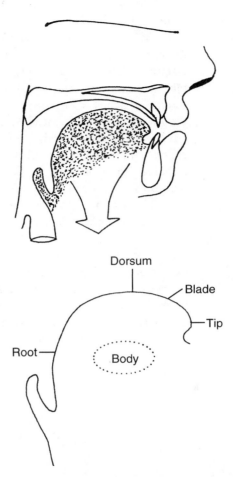

Figure 1-15b. Lateral view of tongue.

Dentition

You have likely learned a great deal about teeth in your previous courses on speech anatomy and craniofacial anomalies. Because teeth are potentially speech articulators, we pay special attention on oral examination to their presence, health, and configuration. We take into account the relationship between maxillary and mandibular dentition as we determine the adequacy of dental occlusion.

Despite the importance of teeth for speech production, the very names of the teeth themselves—incisors, canines—reveal the importance of dentition in the preparation of food for swallowing. But the importance of teeth goes way beyond allowing you to negotiate a raw carrot or a well-done steak. The prolonged absence of any teeth can result in bone resorption, which effectively changes the configuration of the alveolar ridge. Further, teeth provide, by way of the trigeminal nerve, crucial sensory information about the nature of the bolus. This sensory information helps to modulate chewing force, speed, duration, and jaw excursions. It is also thought to influence the type and amount of salivary secretion. Thus, teeth are major players in the oral preparatory phase of deglutition.

The first set of teeth, called **deciduous**, begins erupting in a child's first year of life. The full set of 20, which includes upper and lower sets of **central** and **lateral incisors**, **canine** teeth, and **molars**, is typically complete by a child's third birthday (Figure 1-16). These primary teeth then shed over the course of about seven years and are replaced by **permanent dentition**. In the adult maxillae, the four incisors are flanked by one set of canine teeth, two sets of **bicuspids**, and two or three sets of molars. This configuration is mirrored on the alveolar ridge of the mandible, for a full complement of 32 teeth (Figure 1-17). In a normal occlusion, the maxillary teeth, especially the incisors and canines, slightly overlap the corresponding mandibular teeth (Figure 1-18). The cusps of the first mandibular molars fall just ahead and inside of the cusps of their maxillary mates (Angle's Class I neutrocclusion). Disturbances of this relationship result in the appearance of an overjet or overbite (Angle's Class II malocclusion), an underbite or prognathic jaw (Angle's Class III malocclusion), or a crossbite when the dental arches are displaced laterally. Severe cases of malocclusion may affect bolus preparation in the oral stage. Similarly, the absence, destruction, or misalignment of individual teeth may also negatively impact deglutition.

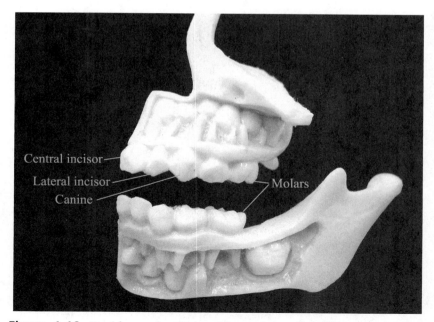

Figure 1-16. Deciduous dentition with portions of maxilla and mandible cut away to reveal embedded teeth roots and permanent dentition.

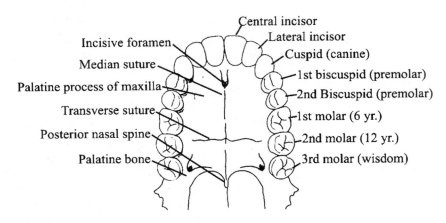

Figure 1-17. Inferior view of adult hard palate with permanent dentition.

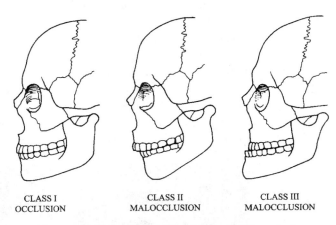

CLASS I OCCLUSION
CLASS II MALOCCLUSION
CLASS III MALOCCLUSION

Figure 1-18. Angle's Class I, II, and III occlusions.

CLINICAL NOTE 1-3

Dentures

Dentures, particularly full plates, cover significant portions of the oral mucosa and alveolar ridges, thereby reducing the quantity and quality of sensory feedback in the oral phase of eating. Veyrune and Mioche (2000) used electromyography to show that denture wearers had difficulty adapting to differences in bolus textures. The study revealed that people without dentures used relatively less muscle activity than the denture wearers to chew various textures of beef. Also, the chewing patterns of the edentulous persons were related to beef tenderness. The chewing patterns of the denture wearers were less dependent on the beef texture. Although this study did not include persons with dysphagia, it is conceivable that dentures in such patients would present an array of mechanical and sensory deficits that would exacerbate their eating problems.

Posterior Pharyngeal Wall

Now to mention briefly the last wall of our imaginary box formed by the oral cavity: the posterior pharyngeal wall. This can be visualized best when the velum is elevated and the posterior tongue is depressed. There are no specific landmarks on the posterior wall at the level of the oropharynx, but we will discuss this region in great detail in the next section.

Salivary Glands

A smooth, moist layer of epithelial tissue covers the entire surface of the oral cavity and aerodigestive tract. This is commonly known as the **mucosal surface**. In the oral cavity, glandular tissue located beneath the mucosal surface excretes **saliva** through tiny openings called **salivary ducts**. Saliva consists of a watery **serous** component, a thicker **mucous** component, and an **enzyme** responsible for breaking down starch. The importance of saliva to the health of the oral cavity and the function of swallowing cannot be overemphasized. Because of its antibacterial and antacid properties, saliva helps to prevent tooth decay and infections of the oral mucosa. It is a critical component in swallowing for two reasons. First, incorporating saliva into dry or sticky foods through chewing results in the formation of a manageable bolus. Second, saliva keeps the oral mucosa moist, which reduces friction along the path of the bolus and thus aids in deglutition. Reductions in salivary flow or impairments in its viscosity can have serious implications for swallowing. Dry mouth, or **xerostomia**, can result from medications, radiation treatment, neural damage, and even the normal aging process.

CLINICAL NOTE 1-4

Sicca

Sicca sydrome is an autoimmune disease characterized by xerostomia (dry mouth) and dry eyes, and may be associated with another autoimmune disease called Sjögren syndrome. Dryness of mucosal tissue is central to the sicca syndrome. In the mouth, dryness results from abnormal salivary output, and can lead to difficulty in swallowing and an oral-pharyngeal dysphagia. The absence of saliva also can create problems for dental hygiene, resulting in tooth decay. Saliva provides an antibacterial function in the oral cavity and keeps growth of organisms in check. Saliva also has antacid properties that can neutralize acids in foods and reflux. There is no cure for the xerostomia of sicca syndrome; however, patients may obtain temporary relief from over-the-counter mouth moisteners, or cholinergic drugs, such as pilocarpine, that may stimulate salivary or lacrimal flow. Diet modifications to avoid dry and sticky foods may be beneficial.

There are three major sets of salivary glands in the oral cavity: the **parotid, sublingual**, and **submandibular glands**. These glands together produce saliva at a rate of 0.1 ml/min during rest and up to 4 ml/min during active secretion. Salivary volume and flow rate appear to account for the majority of individual variation in swallowing frequency (Rudney, Ji, & Larson, 1995). The submandibular glands are responsible for most of the oral secretions, up to 70%. The parotid and sublingual glands produce the remaining 25% and 5%, respectively. Each of the sets of glands is comprised of different types of secretory cells. The parotid glands produce only serous fluid and the sublingual glands produce mainly mucus. The submandibular glands contain both serous and mucous cells. Thus, the composition of saliva at any given time depends on the relative contributions of the various glands.

In contrast to striated muscle, salivary glands are innervated by the autonomic nervous system through autonomic fibers of cranial nerves. Interestingly, both parasympathetic and sympathetic stimulation results in facilitation of salivary flow. The sympathetic system does so directly, with activation of the salivary glands. The parasympathetic system does so indirectly by providing sustained blood flow to the glandular tissue. Not only can stimuli such as the presence of food in the mouth promote salivation, but so can the sight and smell of food. Even the thought of food can influence the amount and rate of salivary flow. To demonstrate, imagine yourself right now biting into a big, juicy lemon wedge.

Parotid Salivary Glands

The parotid glands are the largest set of glands and they are located in the posterior and inferior cheeks (Figure 1-19). The bulk of the superficial parotid gland overlies the ramus of the mandible. Some people can stimulate salivary flow from the parotid glands by massaging the jaw area just below the earlobe. The bony boundaries of the space occupied by parotid glands include the ramus of the mandible anteriorly, the mastoid process posteriorly, and the styloid process medially. Therefore, the glandular tissue is adjacent to all of the muscles that attach to these bones (including the masseter and medial pterygoid muscles at the mandible; the sternocleidomastoid and posterior belly of the digastric at the mastoid process; and the stylohyoid, styloglossus, and stylopharyngeus muscles at the styloid process). Additionally, branches of the facial nerve (CN VII) run through the parotid, as does the upper end of the external carotid artery. We can estimate the location of the parotid ducts by drawing an imaginary line across the cheek from the tragus of the ear to the middle of the philtrum. If we divide this line into thirds, the parotid duct would be located beneath the middle third of this line. Parotid gland secretion through these ducts is mediated by the glos-

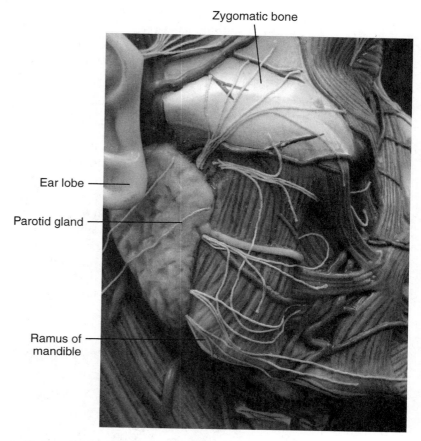

Figure 1-19. Lateral view of mandibular region and parotid gland.

sopharyngeal nerve (CN IX) from the **inferior salivary nucleus** located in the pons in the brainstem.

Sublingual Salivary Glands

The second set of salivary glands is located immediately beneath the mucosal surface of the floor of the mouth, along the internal surface of the jaw. Because of their position beneath the tongue, they are called sublingual glands. You can estimate the location of the sublingual glands by finding the floor of the mouth beneath the back molars and tongue with your fingers. Move your finger anteriorly, keeping it at the base of the interior mandible and the floor of the mouth, to trace the course of the gland. This glandular tissue rests on the mylohyoid muscle and is sandwiched between the genioglossus muscle medially and the mandible laterally. The two halves of the gland meet anteriorly at the midline of the jaw. Unlike the parotid, which has one major duct per gland, the sublingual glands have up to 20 small ducts that secrete saliva onto the floor of the mouth. The secretion is mediated by facial nerve fibers (CN VII) that originate in the **superior salivary nucleus** located in the pons in the brainstem.

Submandibular Salivary Glands

The final set of salivary glands is housed under the mandible and is therefore called the submandibular glands (Figure 1-20). Recall that the sublingual glands are located along the internal surface of the mandible. Most of the submandibular gland tissue also is located along the internal surface of the mandible; however, it is deep to the mylohyoid muscle. There also is a smaller portion of gland that is deep and rests on the hyoglossus muscle. The submandibular duct emerges from the larger portion of glandular tissue and travels about 5 cm to open on the floor of the mouth at the side of the lingual frenulum. Like the sublingual gland, secretions are mediated by facial nerve fibers (CN VII) that originate in the superior salivary nucleus.

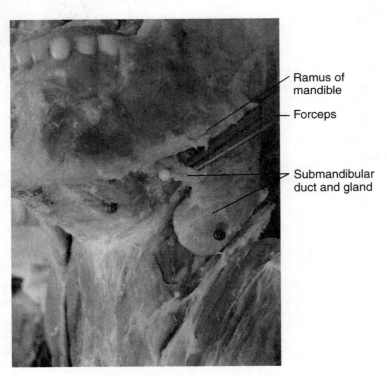

Ramus of mandible

Forceps

Submandibular duct and gland

Figure 1-20. Submandibular gland.

Muscles of Orofacial Structures

The facial, lingual, mandibular, and velar muscles involved in the formation of speech sounds are the very same muscles recruited for bolus preparation and transport. However, the actions of these muscles are quite different for speech and deglutition. In this section, we examine these muscles within the context of swallow function, specifically, how these muscles act to accomplish the goals of the oral stage of deglutition. Bolus preparation, and transport to the oropharynx, requires the smooth and coordinated movements of the lips, jaw, cheeks, tongue, and velum. The precise combination of muscles activated to accomplish bolus preparation and transport is strongly related to the nature of the bolus (size, temperature, viscosity, and so forth) and the nature of the swallower (such as age, sex, oral configuration, and idiosyncratic behaviors).

Lips

The muscles of the lips serve two primary functions in the oral stage of deglutition. The first is a prehensile, or grasping, function, and the second is the creation of an anterior seal of the oral cavity. Both of these functions involve approximation, or closure, of the lips with varying degrees of force and protrusion. As you can imagine, these muscles must be synergistically coordinated with those of the jaw to accommodate mom's plea to *chew with your mouth closed*. The muscles that are activated to accomplish this task fall in the domain of **muscles of facial expression**. The muscles of facial expression are so named because of their apparent association with the betrayal of emotion—such as smiling, frowning, furrowing the brow, and pursing the lips. All of these muscles are innervated by the facial nerve (CN VII), and differ from most other muscles because they often arise from and insert into muscle or skin rather than bone. The muscles of facial expression are illustrated in the two panels of Figure 1-21.

Lip closure is accomplished largely by contraction of the superior and inferior **orbicularis oris muscles** (*orbicularis* means orbiting or circular and *oris* means mouth). This closure is critical for containing a liquid bolus in the mouth, especially while the liquid is in the anterior portion of the oral cavity. It is also critical during the oral transport stage when the bolus is being moved posteriorly. The superior and inferior orbicularis ring the periphery of the lips, permitting an almost sphincter-like action when they co-contract. Because their fibers arise from other muscles in the area, there are no definite origins or insertions. However, the superior and inferior muscles do meet laterally to form the oral angles. Strong contraction of these muscles is responsible

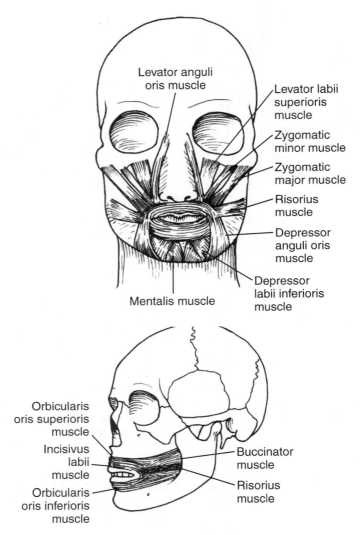

Figure 1-21. Muscles of facial expression.

for lip puckering or pursing. The smaller superior and inferior **inci-sivus labii muscles** run parallel to the orbicularis oris muscles and assist them in puckering the lips.

Simply looking in the mirror while you eat a piece of sticky candy will convince you that lip closure and protrusion does not adequately characterize lip movement during the oral preparatory stage of swallowing. The lips also may part, retract, and press. The upper and lower lips may move toward or away from each other. The left and right halves of the lips may mirror each other or move asymmetrically. Such movements require the activation of other muscles that insert into the orbicularis oris muscles. Contraction of these muscles, singularly or in combination, serves to displace the lips from their neutral, or lightly closed, position.

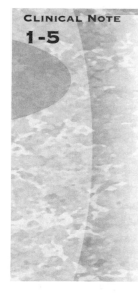

CLINICAL NOTE

1-5

Lip Strength and Task Requirements

Murray, Larson, and Logemann (1998) conducted an electromyographic study of the perioral muscle activity associated with liquid swallows from a spoon, a straw, and a cup. They reported several important findings. First, it takes very little, if any, perioral muscle activity to contain a small amount of liquid in the mouth. However, it may be the case that as bolus size increases, so too does the muscle activation needed to create an adequate anterior seal. Second, simple lip contact with the spoon or the cup was accomplished with little or no perioral muscle activation. In contrast, lip contact with the straw was associated with more activation, perhaps in anticipation of the pucker. Perhaps the most interesting finding of this investigation was the extremely high levels of perioral muscle activation associated with sucking liquid from a straw. These values exceeded those of maximal lip compression by 35%. Thus, sucking from straws may prove to be a fruitful therapeutic technique to build labial strength for cases in which labial weakness interferes with the oral stages of the swallow.

These other muscles can be conceptualized as occurring in sets that nearly mirror each other on the upper and lower lip. The names of these muscles often indicate both the attachment sites and the direction of movement the lip takes when the muscle is contracted. Thus, the terms levator and depressor indicate upward and downward movement, respectively. The term **anguli** refers to the oral angles, and the term **labii** refers to lip. Moreover, all of these muscles are paired, such that they occur on both the right and left halves of the lips. Now you should be able to appreciate how the following four muscles are essentially analogous pairs.

levator anguli oris—depressor anguli oris

levator labii superioris—depressor labii inferioris

The anguli oris muscles either raise the oral angles (levator) or depress them (depressor). The labii muscles either raise the upper lip (levator superioris) or depress the lower lip (depressor inferioris).

Other muscles are not mirrored on the upper and lower lips. The upper lip can move up and back because of the **zygomatic muscle**. This muscle originates at the zygomatic bone and inserts into the upper lip and oral angle. The lower lip, alone, enjoys the ability to *pout* because of the **mentalis muscle**. This muscle originates at the mandible and inserts into the skin of the lower lip. When this muscle contracts it causes the lower lip to protrude and the chin to wrinkle.

Cheeks

The primary function of the cheeks in the oral stages of swallowing is to offer a flexible, lateral boundary for bolus containment and manipulation. A lax cheek permits food to enter the lateral sulci for temporary storage during mastication or bolus formation. The generation of cheek tension assists in moving food out of the lateral sulci and onto the tongue or between the occlusal surfaces of the teeth, and this is presumably accomplished by the dynamic coordination of cheek muscle activity, tongue activity, and chewing pattern (see Casas, Kenny, & Macmillan, 2003). Tense cheeks minimize the area of the lateral sulci and prevent food from pocketing there. Take a sip of water and notice how tense your cheeks become (and how tightly your lips press together) as the liquid bolus is transported back toward the oropharynx. Cheek tension is created primarily by the contraction of two muscles of facial expression, the **buccinator** and the **risorius muscles**. The buccinator muscle originates at the **pterygomandibular ligament** (where it blends with fibers from the **superior pharyngeal constrictor muscle** to create the **pterygomandibular raphe**) and courses horizontally to, in essence, form the cheeks. The upper and lower portions of the muscle split as it reaches the mouth, where it inserts into the superior and inferior orbicularis oris muscle at the oral angles. Contraction of the buccinator tenses the cheeks and also draws the corners of the mouth laterally. A smaller and more superficial muscle, the risorius, runs parallel to the buccinator and assists in drawing the corners of the mouth laterally. Both of these muscles are innervated by the facial nerve (CN VII).

Tongue

The tongue is perhaps the most important structure in the oral stage of swallowing. It serves to hold and manipulate the bolus within the oral cavity and to transport the bolus posteriorly to initiate the pharyngeal stage of the swallow. This is accomplished by two general categories of muscles, intrinsic and extrinsic. Intrinsic tongue muscles are housed entirely within the tongue. When they contract, they cause changes in the shape of the tongue (making it longer, shorter, fatter, flatter, pointier, or blunter). The extrinsic tongue muscles originate on structures outside the tongue and insert into it. They are responsible for changing the position of the tongue relative to the mandible (elevation, protrusion, retraction, and depression). The intrinsic and extrinsic muscles of the tongue exhibit coordinated contraction patterns that permit an almost infinite number of tongue configurations and positions.

Intrinsic Tongue Muscles. There are four sets of intrinsic tongue muscles that make up the body of the tongue (Figure 1-22). They are ori-

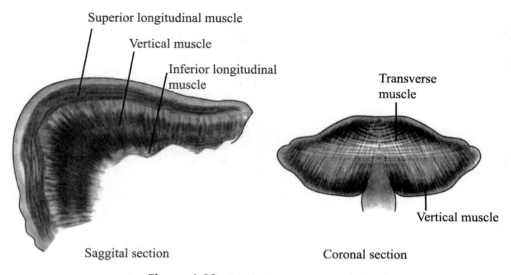

Superior longitudinal muscle

Vertical muscle

Inferior longitudinal muscle

Transverse muscle

Vertical muscle

Saggital section

Coronal section

Figure 1-22. Intrinsic tongue muscles.

ented in three directions: two in the longitudinal direction, and one each in the horizontal and vertical planes. The longitudinal fibers course along both the superior and inferior surfaces of the tongue. The **inferior longitudinal** fibers originate at the hyoid bone and tongue root and terminate in the tongue tip. When the inferior longitudinal lingual muscle contracts, it serves to shorten the tongue and depress the tip. The **superior longitudinal** fibers originate near the tongue root, travel primarily in the middle section of the tongue, and terminate short of the tongue tip. Some of the fibers insert into the lateral margins as they course anteriorly. Contraction of the superior longitudinal muscle shortens the superior aspect of the tongue, thereby turning the tip upward. Other fibers of this muscle—specifically, those that insert laterally—can create a concave depression on the tongue surface when they contract. This is important for creating a channel in the midline of the tongue to hold, in particular, a liquid bolus. Between these two layers of longitudinal fibers are the **transverse** fibers. These fibers arise from the lingual **septum** and insert into the lateral edges of the tongue. Contraction of the transverse fibers causes the tongue to elongate and narrow. Short **vertical** fibers, found mostly near the apex of the tongue, course from the underside to the top of the tongue. Contraction of the vertical muscles flattens the tongue. All of the intrinsic tongue muscles are innervated by the hypoglossal nerve (CN XII).

Extrinsic Tongue Muscles. There are three primary pairs and one secondary pair of extrinsic tongue muscles (Figure 1-23). Before we discuss each pair in some detail, we can guess about their primary functions

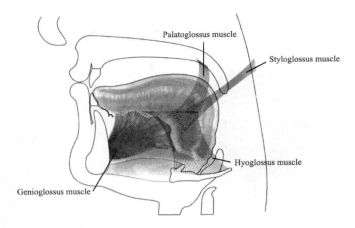

Figure 1-23. Extrinsic tongue muscles.

simply by knowing the location of the non-tongue attachment sites. When the muscle originates at sites above the tongue, the muscle's contraction serves to elevate the tongue. When the muscle originates below the tongue, its contraction serves to depress the tongue. With the same intuitive simplicity, muscles with attachments anterior to the tongue serve to protrude it (pull tongue forward) and posterior attachment sites are associated with tongue retraction (pull tongue backward). These general principles hold true for all of the extrinsic tongue muscles, though their precise actions are somewhat more complicated.

The **styloglossus muscle** originates at the styloid process of the temporal bone and inserts into the lateral borders of the tongue. Because of its fixed styloid attachment, contraction of the muscle causes the rear of the tongue to elevate. When the tongue is protruded, contraction of the styloglossus causes the tongue to retract.

The **hyoglossus muscle** originates at the greater cornu of the hyoid bone and inserts into the lateral aspects of the posterior tongue. When the hyoid is fixed, contraction of this muscle causes the tongue to depress and retract.

The **genioglossus muscle** is complicated in its orientation. It originates at the lingual surface of the mandible (inside the chin) and inserts into the intrinsic tongue muscles along the entire length of the inferior portion of the tongue dorsum. Thus, the anterior fibers of the genioglossus muscle are quite short because their trip is merely to the tongue tip. The inferior fibers, on the other hand, travel from the mandible to the body of the hyoid bone. In between are midlength fibers that insert into the dorsum of the tongue. To make matters more complicated (and to give the tongue more finesse!) contraction of the genioglossus can be quite discrete. When the anterior fibers contract, the tip of the tongue is pulled into the mouth and depressed. If the anterior fibers contract unilaterally, the tongue tip is pushed, or deviates, to the side that is not contracting. When the anterior and middle portions co-contract, a depression or channel along the superior surface of the tongue is formed. This tongue configuration is common and important in sucking, or the generation of negative intraoral pressure. When the middle fibers of genioglossus act alone, the posterior portion of the tongue is drawn forward, which forces the tongue tip to protrude anteriorly. The inferior fibers of the genioglossus are critical in the oral transport and pharyngeal stages of swallowing because they serve to pull the hyoid bone up and forward. Finally, the genioglossus and styloglossus have an antagonistic relationship. Their relative contractions permit positioning of the tongue within the oral cavity.

Like the intrinsic tongue muscles, all three of these extrinsic muscle pairs are innervated by the hypoglossal nerve (CN XII). However, the fourth pair of extrinsic tongue muscles, the palatoglossus, is innervated by the glossopharyngeal and vagus nerves (CN IX and X). It also is different from the other extrinsic muscles because its primary role is to lower the velum when the tongue is held still. However, when the velum is held steady in an elevated position by velar levator muscles, the contraction of the palatoglossus serves to raise the posterior tongue. This makes sense when you consider that this muscle arises from the lateral aspects of the posterior tongue and courses upward to insert laterally into the velum. This movement is critical in the initial stages of bolus transport.

Despite the seemingly infinite number of tongue configurations that can be accomplished by selective contraction of the various intrinsic and extrinsic lingual muscles, studies have shown that general tongue movement patterns for bolus transport is quite stereotypical (Hamlet, 1989; Martin, 1991; Stone & Shawker, 1986), even in the context of significant inter- and intrasubject variability (Söder & Miller, 2002; Tasko, Kent, & Westbury, 2002). Chi-Fishman and Stone (1996), using electropalatography, found that the tongue pressed against the hard palate segmentally and sequentially in two directions—from front to back and from lateral to midline—as the bolus was propelled to the oropharynx. Although the timing of the individual movement components varied with different bolus properties, the movement pattern did not vary. Adding ultrasound to electropalatography, Chi-Fishman, Stone, and McCall (1998) replicated the results of the earlier study and reported some new findings. First, the timing of lingual movements for continuous swallowing (as in drinking continuously from a cup) differed substantially from the movement timing in discrete swallows (one sip at a time). Although the fundamental components of movement in the discrete swallow were apparent in continuous swallowing (tongue tip lowering, tongue body elevation, tongue tip elevation, tongue body lowering), they occurred closely in time and even overlapped. Second, full contact of the tongue with the palate was not seen in all continuous swallows. This led to the conclusion that the motor control for the deglutive action of the tongue is largely fixed, but that task demands influence timing (and thus the appearance) of the motor pattern.

Muscles of Mandibular Movement

In the earlier section on the skeletal framework, we described how the mandible moves relative to the maxillae at the TMJ. The mandible may move up or down (elevation/depression), forward or backward (protrusion/retraction), and side to side (lateralization). Although these movements may occur in relative isolation—for example, lowering the jaw to allow food to be admitted into the oral cavity—it is more common for these movements to co-occur in varied combinations when we bite, chew, and grind. These movements are accomplished by contractions of the muscles of mastication. The muscles of mastication consist of four pairs that arise from the cranium and insert into the mandible. They are innervated by the mandibular branch of the trigeminal nerve (CN V). Three of these muscles produce mandibular elevation, or jaw closure. The other pair is involved in mandibular depression, or jaw opening.

Mandibular Closing
The muscles responsible for jaw elevation include the temporalis, masseter, and medial pterygoid muscles. Two of these muscles can be palpated easily on the external surface of the face when the teeth are alternately clenched and released. The fanlike origin of the temporalis muscle can be felt at the region of the temples. The temporalis muscle arises broadly from the temporal fossa where the fibers run just below the skin of the external face (Figure 1-24a). The muscle fibers then converge as they attach, via temporalis tendon, to the coronoid process and anterior ramus of the mandible. Because the temporalis is a flat, thin, broad muscle, it is at a mechanical advantage for producing quick elevation and retraction of the mandible, such as for biting and tearing food. Its posterior portions also contribute to lateral movements of the jaw.

The second mandibular elevator that can be palpated on the external face is the masseter (Figure 1-24b). The bulk of the masseter can be felt over the angle and ramus of the mandible when the teeth are clenched and released. This thick, powerful muscle consists of three overlapping layers, all of which arise from the zygomatic bone and arch and fuse before inserting onto the lateral surface of the angle, ramus, and coronoid process of the mandible.

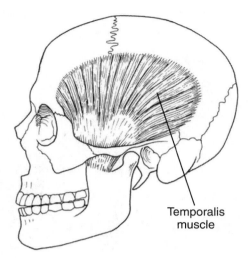

Figure 1-24a. Temporalis muscle on lateral view of skull.

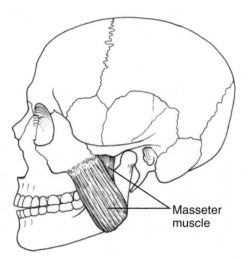

Figure 1-24b. Masseter muscle on lateral view of skull.

Though powerful alone, the masseter is functionally linked to the medial pterygoid (the third mandibular elevator) (Figure 1-24c). These two muscles can be thought of as creating a sling under each side of the mandible (**mandibular sling**). The masseter forms the external portion of the sling and the medial pterygoid forms the internal portion. The medial pterygoid muscle originates primarily from the medial surface of the lateral pterygoid plate of the sphenoid bone and inserts into the medial surface of the angle and ramus of the mandible. When the

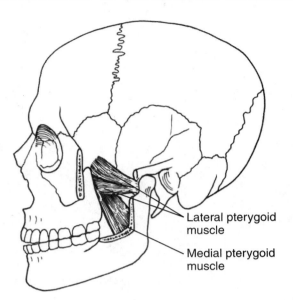

Figure 1-24c. Pterygoid muscles on lateral view of skull.

masseter and medial pterygoid muscles co-contract, they produce a powerful elevation of the mandible. The medial pterygoid, in conjunction with the lateral pterygoid muscle that we will discuss in the next section, contributes to jaw protrusion.

Mandibular Opening

The only muscle of mastication associated with active mandibular depression and protrusion is the **lateral pterygoid muscle** (Figure 1-24c). This muscle originates from the lateral portion of the greater wing of the sphenoid bone and from the lateral surface of the surface of the lateral pterygoid plate of the sphenoid bone (contrast this origin to that of the medial pterygoid muscle). It then courses horizontally and inserts into the anterior neck of the condyle of the mandible. Because of this orientation, the lateral pterygoid also participates in mandibular protrusion and lateralization. Unilateral activation is particularly important in the grinding action associated with chewing a portion of food that is positioned between the occlusal surfaces on one side of the mouth.

Three other muscles that are associated with mandibular depression and retraction are not among the *muscles of mastication*. The **digastric** (anterior belly), **geniohyoid**, and **mylohyoid muscles** attach to the mandible and to the hyoid bone, such that they depress and retract the mandible when the hyoid is fixed (Figure 1-25). The **anterior belly of the digastric** and mylohyoid muscles are innervated by the mandibular branch of the trigeminal nerve (CN V), but the geniohyoid

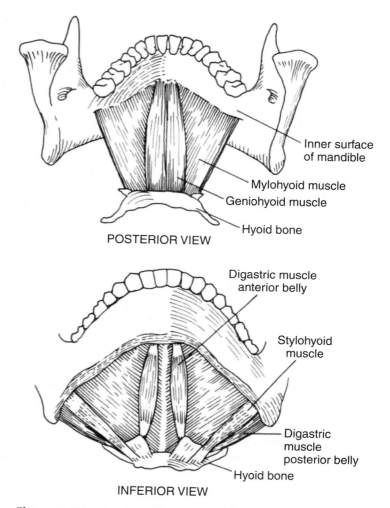

Inner surface
of mandible

Mylohyoid muscle
Geniohyoid muscle
Hyoid bone

POSTERIOR VIEW

Digastric muscle
anterior belly

Stylohyoid
muscle

Digastric
muscle
posterior belly
Hyoid bone

INFERIOR VIEW

Figure 1-25. Muscles of mandibular depression and retraction.

receives its motor supply from the hypoglossal nerve (CN XII) and branches from the **ansa cervicalis**. The **ansa cervicalis** is a complex grouping of nerve fibers from the first three cervical nerves at the level of the cervical spine C-1 to C-3. *Ansa* means loop or arc and describes two loops in the cervical plexus between C-1 and C-2 and C-2 and C-3. When the fibers from the two loops rejoin as the ansa cervicalis, they give rise to innervating branches for infrahyoid muscles.

Chewing

As mentioned earlier in this chapter, movement in the TMJ can be quite complex. Jaw movement for chewing has been found to be a highly stereotyped behavior—much less variable than for speech production—and likely under the jurisdiction of a **central pattern generator (CPG)** in the brainstem (Ostry, Vatikiotis-Bateson, & Gribble, 1997; Moore, Smith, & Ringel, 1988). You can gain an appreciation for this stereotypy simply by watching the regular pattern of jaw excursions of a friend as she mindlessly chews gum. However, stereotypy does not mean simplicity of movement around the TMJ (see Komiyama, et al., 2003). The movements associated with chewing can be categorized as those that involve **translation**, **rotation**, and a **combination** of the two (refer to Figure 1-9). Translational movements occur when the jaw is displaced in a gliding action in a single direction around the TMJ, as in mandibular protrusion, retraction, and lateralization. Rotation refers to the swinging action around the TMJ, as would be evident on mandibular elevation and depression. During chewing, the combined actions of translation and rotation characterize mandibular movement. As the jaw opens and closes, there is a concomitant protraction, retraction, and lateralization about the TMJ. This occurs in complementary function with the tongue such that the bolus is manipulated and positioned for grinding and reducing between the occlusal surfaces of the teeth.

Based on our previous coverage of the muscles of mastication, translational movements are accomplished primarily by the medial and lateral pterygoid muscles, the posterior portion of the temporalis, and the geniohyoid, mylohyoid, and anterior belly of the digastric. Rotational movements are accomplished by the masseter, temporalis, and medial pterygoid for jaw elevation, and by the lateral pterygoid, anterior belly of the digastric, geniohyoid, and mylohyoid for jaw depression. The overlap in muscles and functions suggests that many combinations of muscle activation are likely used during any episode of chewing. In fact, this has been shown to be the case. Studies using electromyographic recordings have found that of the muscles of mastication, it is only the masseter muscle that enjoys a fairly regular pattern of activity. The masseter produces maximal contraction when the mouth is most open during the chewing cycle, and then ceases its activity when the mouth is nearly closed (Palmer, et al., 1992). The activity of other muscles associated with jaw and tongue movement in chewing have been shown to be more variable, yet perhaps still under the control of a central pattern generator.

Muscles of the Soft Palate (Velum)

Just like the tongue, lips, face, and jaw, the velum is a critical structure in the oral stage of swallowing. Unlike these other structures, however, it is the velum's lack of action that makes it critical in the early stages of deglutition. The velum rests low in the oropharynx such that contact or near-contact is made with the posterior tongue. This configuration discourages food or liquid from entering the pharynx prematurely and permits normal nasal breathing. Gravity alone is all that is needed to maintain this configuration in the upright swallower. However, once the bolus begins its journey into the oropharynx, the velum and its associated structures move quickly into action to close off the **velopharyngeal port**. Velar elevation is traditionally associated with the onset of the pharyngeal stage of swallowing and will, therefore, be discussed in the next chapter.

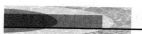

SENSORY RECEPTORS

You might be surprised to learn that the role of sensation in swallowing has been the subject of controversy over the years. Intuitively, perhaps from our experiences with dental anesthetic, we know that decreases in oral sensation interfere with the oral stage of deglutition. We also know that salivary flow and other autonomic events depend on the stimulation of sensory receptors. What remains unclear, however, is the extent to which sensation triggers motor events of swallowing. This question is most relevant to the transition between the oral and pharyngeal stage of deglutition. However, it also is relevant to the specifics of the oral stage. We automatically adjust our oral movements to accommodate the characteristics of the bolus, therefore sensory information is critical to the modulation of patterned motor behavior (Capra, 1995). This will be discussed in greater detail in Chapter 4. The characteristics of the bolus are made known to us by sensory receptors located in the oral mucosa, around the teeth, in the muscles, and in the TMJ.

For the sake of clarity, the discussion of sensory receptors has been organized by virtue of their location and function. We begin with the oral mucosa, which contains receptors that mediate touch and movement (mechanoreceptors), temperature (thermoreceptors), pain associated with tissue damage (nociceptors), and taste (chemoreceptors). In general, the anterior regions of the oral cavity are much more richly populated with these receptors than are posterior regions. Consequently, the tongue tip and lips are more sensitive than structures such as the hard palate and velum.

Mechanoreceptors fire when they are mechanically deformed. With regard to swallowing, this may result from mucosal contact with the bolus or by its contact with other oral structures during mastication. Some of these mechanoreceptors respond to light touch and adapt quickly (Meissner's corpuscles and free nerve endings). Others respond to deeper pressure or longer stimulation (Ruffini's end organs and Merkels's discs).

A specialized type of mechanoreceptors, known as **proprioceptors**, allows us to know the position of our articulators in space and relative to one another. Proprioceptors are located in muscle fibers (**neuromuscular**

spindles) and in tendons (**Golgi tendon organs**). These receptors are critical in maintaining muscle tone and facilitating controlled movement. Neuromuscular spindles are special receptors embedded in muscle tissue that fire when the length of the parent muscle is increased due to stretch. This firing, which causes the parent muscle to contract, is known as a **stretch reflex**. Neuromuscular spindles are found to varying degrees in the muscles of the tongue, jaw, and velum. Golgi tendon organs, found generously in the region of the TMJ, respond to changes in tendon tension associated with muscle contraction. When these receptors fire, they serve to relax the parent muscle to reduce tension on the tendon by mediating reflex loops on a subconscious level and in preventing injury to muscles and joints.

Thermoreceptors respond to changes in temperature and are fairly abundant in the oral mucosa. Some, such as the end bulbs of Krause, respond specifically to lowered temperature, thereby mediating the sensation of cold. Ruffini-type receptors and free nerve endings—in addition to being mechanoreceptors—are responsible for the sensation of temperature change. Free nerve endings have an additional function—they are **nociceptors** that mediate the sensation of pain in response to tissue damage.

Taste, a form of **chemoreception**, is mediated through the thousands of taste buds located throughout the oral cavity and even in the pharynx. The distribution is most heavy, however, on the tongue. The mechanism that allows us to distinguish tastes and flavors is rather complicated in that there is not a one-to-one correspondence between taste and receptor type. The primary categories of taste (salty, sweet, sour, and bitter) arise from how the food substance depolarizes given receptor cells. This information is then relayed via the facial and glossopharyngeal nerves (CN VII and IX) through the brainstem and thalamus to the mouth region of the somatosensory cortex. Here, it is influenced by collateral activation of the hypothalamus, olfactory cortex, and other brainstem regions to culminate in the subjective experience of taste. The chemical characteristics of food also stimulate the autonomic nervous system, modifying salivary flow that is a critical component in the bolus preparation.

SUMMARY

The anatomy and physiology of oral structures during a normal swallow can be explored by considering a bite of a solid bolus. The bolus is reduced and moistened during the oral preparatory phase through a combination of chewing and lingual repositioning. Cohesive or semicohesive portions are then partitioned and channeled into compartments between the tongue and hard palate. This requires:

1. Adequate lip and buccal flexibility and tension to keep the bolus in the desired intraoral locations as it was reduced and moistened

2. Proper sensory feedback about bolus properties from the sensory receptors in the oral mucosa, the taste buds, the dental receptors, and the muscles and joints; this mediates the production of the appropriate amount and consistency of saliva and the generation of appropriate chewing forces and trajectories

3. The rhythmic and patterned activation of the masseter and masticatory muscles for efficiently chewing the bolus

4. The synergistic contractions of the intrinsic and extrinsic tongue muscles to position the bolus between the occlusal surfaces of the teeth, or to temporarily store portions of the bolus in channels on the tongue or in the lateral sulci

5. Compression of the bolus against the hard palate by the tongue in anticipation of the next phase of the swallow.

STUDY QUESTIONS

1. On the skull there is only one true joint. What is it? What is its function related to oral alimentation?

2. Bolus formation is crucial to the act of deglutition. How would the absence of teeth (an edentulous state) affect this parameter of swallow?

3. What are the muscles involved in the following activities and which cranial nerves innervate these muscles?
   a. keeping the lips closed
   b. providing buccal tone
   c. creating a central lingual depression important in sucking
   d. chewing motion of jaw

4. What is the role of the velum in the first two stages of deglutition?

5. Describe the location, output, and innervation of the three major sets of salivary glands in the oral cavity.

6. What is the role of sensation in the first two stages of deglutition?

REFERENCES

Capra, N. F. (1995). Mechanisms of oral sensation. *Dysphagia, 10*(4), 235–247.

Casas, M. J., Kenny, D. J., & Macmillan, R. E. (2003). Buccal and lingual activity during mastication and swallowing in typical adults. *Journal of Oral Rehabilitation, 30*(1), 9–16.

Chi-Fishman, G., & Stone, M. (1996). A new application for electropalatography: Swallowing. *Dysphagia, 11*(4), 239–247.

Chi-Fishman, G., Stone, M., & McCall, G. N. (1998). Lingual action in normal sequential swallowing. *Journal of Speech, Language, and Hearing Research, 41*(4), 771–785.

Hamlet, S. (1989). Dynamic aspects of lingual propulsive activity in swallowing. *Dysphagia, 4*(3), 136–145.

Komiyama, O., Asano, T., Suzuki, H., Kawara, M., Wada, M., Kobayashi, K., & Ohtake, S. (2003). Mandibular condyle movement during mastication of foods. *Journal of Oral Rehabilitation, 30*(6), 592–600.

Laitman, J. T., & Reidenberg, J. S. (1993). Specializations of the human upper respiratory and upper digestive systems as seen through comparative and developmental anatomy. *Dysphagia, 8*(4), 318–325.

Martin, R. (1991). A comparison of lingual movement in swallowing and speech production. Unpublished doctoral dissertation, University of Wisconsin-Madison.

Moore, C. A., Smith, A., & Ringel, R. (1988). Task-specific organization of activity in human jaw muscles. *Journal of Speech and Hearing Research, 31*(4), 670–680.

Murray, K. A., Larson, C. R., & Logemann, J. A. (1998). Electromyographic response of the labial muscles during normal liquid swallows using a spoon, a straw, and a cup. *Dysphagia, 13*(3), 160–166.

Ostry, D. J., Vatikiotis-Bateson, E., & Gribble, P. L. (1997). An examination of the degrees of freedom of human jaw motion in speech and mastication. *Journal of Speech, Language, & Hearing Research, 40*(6), 1341–1351.

Palmer, J. B., Rudin, N. J., Lara, G., & Crompton, A. W. (1992). Coordination of mastication and swallowing, *Dysphagia, 7*(4), 187–200.

Rudney, J. D., Ji, Z., & Larson, C. J. (1995). The prediction of saliva swallowing frequency in humans from estimates of salivary flow rate and the volume of saliva swallowed. *Archives of Oral Biology, 40*(6), 507–512.

Söder, N., & Miller, N. (2002). Using ultrasound to investigate intrapersonal variability in durational aspects of tongue movement during swallowing. *Dysphagia, 17*(4), 288–297.

Stone, M., & Shawker, T. H. (1986). An ultrasound examination of tongue movement during swallowing. *Dysphagia, 1*(2), 78–83.

Tasko, S. M., Kent, R. D., & Westury, J. R. (2002). Variability in tongue movement kinematics during normal liquid swallowing. *Dysphagia, 17*(2), 126–138.

Thexton, A. (1992). Mastication and swallowing: An overview. *British Dental Journal, 173*(6), 197–206.

Veyrune, J. L., & Mioche, L. (2000). Complete denture wearers: Electromyography of mastication and texture perception whilst eating meat. *European Journal of Oral Science, 108*(2), 83–92.

CHAPTER 2

Examination of the Pharyngeal Swallow Component

LEARNING OBJECTIVES

After completing the chapter and reviewing the study questions, you should be able to:

- Understand the overlaid functions of the pharyngeal portion of the aerodigestive tract

- Understand the anatomy and physiology relevant to the pharyngeal phase of deglutition

- Describe the primary muscles used in the pharyngeal phase of deglutition

- Appreciate the mechanical linkage between the base of the tongue, the hyoid bone, and the larynx

- Appreciate the variability in sequential activation patterns of the involved musculature.

INTRODUCTION

Unlike the oral preparatory and oral transport phases of deglutition, the pharyngeal phase is largely outside voluntary control. Once the swallow response has been triggered, the bolus proceeds past the elevated velum, past the epiglottis and protected laryngotracheal region, and through the upper esophageal sphincter. This chapter focuses on the structures and functions that permit the safe journey of the bolus to the level of the esophagus.

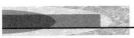

A DESCRIPTION OF THE PHARYNGEAL PHASE

The pharyngeal phase is easy to conceptualize if we continue to follow the normal swallow of a single, discrete bolus. At the end of the last chapter, the masticated bolus was beginning its journey into the oropharynx. The tongue was pressing the bolus, segmentally and sequentially, backward against the hard palate. At the same time, mastication stopped, the anterior tongue depressed and retracted, the lips pressed tightly together, and the cheeks tensed. Then, at just the right moment, the tongue dorsum rapidly depressed and retracted to create a ramp, sending the bolus back through the anterior faucial arches and into the oropharynx. By most accounts, it is the transport of the bolus—particularly past the sensory receptors of the anterior faucial arches and the base of the tongue—that triggers the pharyngeal phase of the swallow.

The pharyngeal phase consists of velopharyngeal closure, inversion of the epiglottis over the laryngeal entryway, anterior and superior displacement of the hyolaryngeal complex, closure of the false and **true vocal folds**, progressive pharyngeal contraction, and opening of the upper esophageal sphincter (UES). Thus, the pharyngeal phase is characterized by a series of involuntary airway-protective and bolus-propulsive events.

There are several important points to note before we continue with coverage of the relevant anatomy. First, as mentioned earlier, the pharyngeal phase is largely involuntary. There is little we can do to exert control over a swallow once it has been initiated. Second, for the discrete swallow, the pharyngeal phase proceeds in a relatively fixed sequence of events regardless of bolus properties or peripheral sensory inputs (although see Kendall, Leonard, & McKenzie, 2003, for a discussion of variability). Third, the swallow response does not have a single trigger point along the aerodigestive tract. The areas where stimulation most easily results in a swallow response include the anterior faucial arches, the tongue base at the level of the lower edge of the mandible, the valleculae, the pyriform sinuses, and even the larynx itself (Dua, Ren, Bardan, Xie, & Shaker, 1997; Logemann, 1998). Fourth, if the swallow response is not triggered, the airway-protective and bolus-propulsive events associated with it simply will not occur. Finally, the bolus is propelled from the oral cavity to the esophagus by both mechanical and pressure forces.

This last observation about bolus propulsion deserves some additional attention here. Were we only to consider the mechanical contributions of the anatomy, it would be tempting to conclude that the bolus is propelled back into the oropharynx by the piston-like action of the tongue, moved through the pharynx by the segmental *squeezing* action of the pharyngeal constrictors and gravity, and then channeled into the dilated upper esophageal sphincter. However, this is not the whole story. The bolus also moves because of pressure differentials that result from changes in diameter along the aerodigestive tract and the opening and closing of various valves.

The notion of pressure differentials is not as complicated as it may appear at first glance. It simply refers to the local *vacuums* that are created when one part of the aerodigestive tract decreases in size (and therefore increases in pressure) relative to adjacent portions. The aerodigestive tract from the lips to the esophagus is essentially a flexible tube that is potentially closed at both ends. Squeezing or compressing one part of the tube causes the volume (or area) of that region to decrease and the pressure in that region to increase; this is Boyle's Law. When the pressure in the adjacent region happens to be lower, a vacuum is created, causing the contents of the high-pressure region to be sucked over to the region of lower pressure.

How does this apply to the propulsion of the bolus? Simply put, the region behind the bolus decreases in size causing a build-up of pressure relative to the region in front of the bolus (Figure 2-1). This wave of pressure differential is accomplished by the contraction of muscles and the

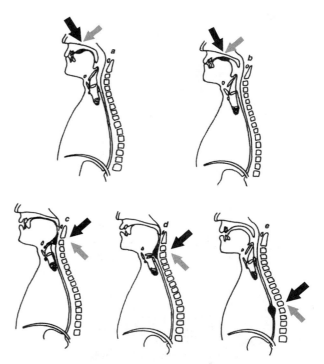

Figure 2-1. Lateral view of pressure differentials along gastrointestinal tract, with high pressure behind the bolus and low pressure in front of it.

Table 2–1. Standard definitions of swallow event terms commonly obtained in videofluorographic examinations (adapted from Logemann, 1988).

TERM	DEFINITION
Oral transit time (OTT)	Interval between posterior propulsion of the bolus and the time the bolus head passes the ramus of the mandible
Pharyngeal transit time (PTT)	Interval from offset of OTT until the tail of the bolus passes through the UES
Pharyngeal delay time (PDT)	Interval from offset of OTT until the onset of laryngeal elevation
Pharyngeal response time (PRT)	Interval from offset of PDT until the bolus tail passes through the UES
Duration of velopharyngeal closure	Interval from first to last contact of the velum with the posterior pharyngeal wall
Duration of laryngeal closure	Interval of closure of the laryngeal vestibule
Duration of UES opening	Interval of opening of the UES during swallow
Duration of hyoid movement	Interval from start of elevation to completion of descent of the hyoid
Duration of laryngeal elevation	Interval from start of elevation to completion of descent of the larynx

constriction of structures behind the bolus (to create high pressure) and the relaxation of muscles and widening of lumen in front of the bolus (to create low pressure). Although the precise relationship between levels of muscle activity and pressure generation is not well understood, passage of the bolus through the pharynx is accomplished by segmental constriction of the pharynx (to decrease volume and increase pressure behind the bolus) and the opening of the UES (to decrease pressure in front of the bolus) (McConnel, Cerenko, & Mendelsohn, 1988; Olsson, Kjellin, & Ekberg, 1996; Rademaker, Pauloski, Colangelo, & Logemann, 1998).

Now that the general framework for the pharyngeal stage has been established, let us consider the structures and functions associated with the specific events. The standard definitions of various swallow events are provided in Table 2-1, for your reference.

PHARYNGEAL ANATOMY

The pharynx is a tube-like structure that extends from the base of the skull behind the nasal cavity to the upper esophageal sphincter. It is important to point out that the pharynx is not a complete tube. It is essentially a semicircle, closed at the back. The anterior aspects of the pharynx are really just adjacent structures and cavities. The pharynx is divided into three sections: the **nasopharynx**, the **oropharynx**, and the **laryngopharynx** (Figure 2-2). The nasopharynx lies immediately behind the nasal cavity and it is potentially separated from the oropharynx by the velum. The oropharynx lies immediately behind the anterior faucial arches of the oral cavity and extends to the level of the hyoid bone. The laryngopharynx refers to the region posterior to the larynx that extends from the hyoid to the esophagus at the level of the sixth cervical vertebra.

The pharynx consists of three sets of rather semicircular muscles that are suspended from the base of the skull by a strong layer of pharyngeal aponeurosis. These muscles are called the **superior**, **middle**, and **inferior pharyngeal constrictors** (Figure 2-3a). The inferior pharyngeal constrictor is the strongest of the pharyngeal muscles and has two main components, the **thyropharyngeus** and **cricopharyngeus muscles**. The thyropharyngeus originates from the thyroid lamina while the cricopharyngeus arises from the cricoid cartilage. The muscles extend posteriorly from anterior attachments to blend at midline along the posterior pharynx to create the **posterior pharyngeal raphe** (Figure 2-3b). Thus, when these muscles contract, they primarily serve to constrict or reduce the

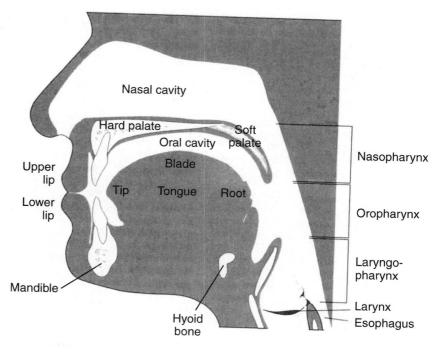

Figure 2-2. Lateral view of pharyngeal cavity divisions.

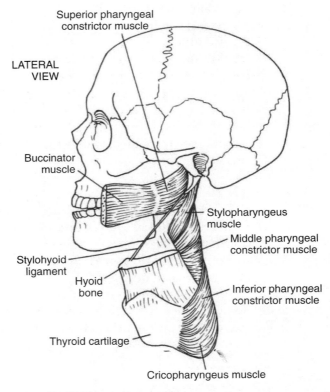

Figure 2-3a. Lateral view of pharyngeal constrictor muscles.

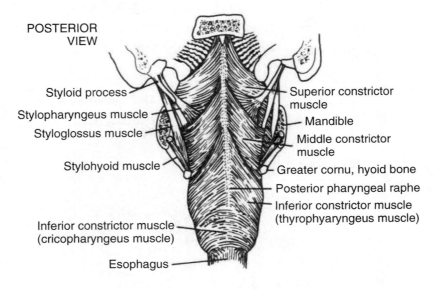

Figure 2-3b. Posterior view of pharyngeal constrictor muscles.

diameter of the pharynx. The pharynx is covered with a mucosal membrane that is continuous with the adjacent structures of the oral and nasal cavities, the larynx, and the esophagus.

The posterior wall of the pharynx lies against the anterior face of the cervical vertebrae, however, the pharynx and vertebral column are completely separated by layers of fascial sheath. Because the pharynx is not attached to the vertebral column and it is configured with special **fasciae** and **areolar** tissue, it is free to be shortened and lengthened in the vertical dimension. It can literally slide along the vertebral column. At least three sets of muscles, the **stylopharyngeus**, **salpingopharyngeus**, and **palatopharyngeus**, produce elevation of portions of the pharynx when they contract (Figure 2-3b). Because all three pharyngeal constrictor muscles converge in an upward direction on to the posterior pharyngeal raphe, they also can elevate the pharynx. All of these muscles, except for stylopharyngeus, are supplied by the **pharyngeal plexus**. This bundle of nerves consists of fibers from the glossopharyngeal, vagus, and spinal accessory nerves (CN IX, X, and XI). The stylopharyngeus is supplied by the motor branch of the glossopharyngeal nerve (CN IX).

The tube created by the pharynx and anterior structures is not smooth and uniform. There are two sets of pharyngeal recesses through which the bolus passes on its journey through the pharynx. These recesses are most clearly visible on videofluoroscopic displays of liquid swallows. The bolus first fills then outlines the L-shaped recesses of the **valleculae**, and then passes through the inferior recesses which are known as the **pyriform sinuses** (Figure 2-4). The bolus moves through lateral channels in the larygopharynx. This can be observed on videofluoroscopy in an anterior-posterior view.

The valleculae are located between the base of the tongue and the epiglottis. The epiglottis is a leaf-shaped cartilage whose stem attaches inferiorly to the thyroid angle of the larynx by way of the **thyroepiglottic ligament**. The broad leaf-like portion of the epiglottis attaches to the hyoid bone via the **hyoepiglottic ligament** where it rests against the base of the tongue. The valleculae then, are the spaces created on either side of the hyoepiglottic ligament, between the tongue base and the epiglottis. They can be easily visualized on a videofluoroscopic exam in either the A-P or lateral view. These spaces are nearly obliterated during the pharyngeal swallow when the epiglottis tilts down and back over the laryngeal entryway.

The second set of recesses in the pharynx is the pyriform sinuses. These spaces lie on either side of the thyroid cartilage, at the very bottom of the pharynx, just above the UES. They are created as the fibers of the inferior constrictor muscle wrap around to attach to the anterior thyroid cartilage. Like the valleculae, the pyriform sinuses are visible on

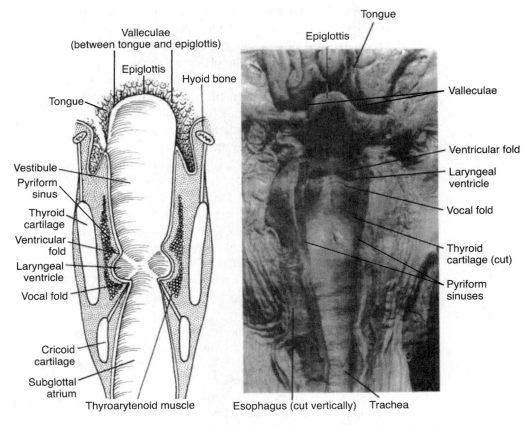

Figure 2-4. Posterior view of pharyngeal recesses in a coronal section.

videofluoroscopic exam. However, they are frequently difficult to visualize without the benefit of barium residue.

Before the pharyngeal swallow response is initiated, the pharynx is also open to the airway. The entry to the airway has several names describing slightly different locations in the entryway. The **laryngeal aditus** is the uppermost portion of the entryway and the **laryngeal vestibule** is the supraglottic space between the aditus and the ventricular or false vocal folds. The pharyngeal swallow response evokes the response of a number of structures to close off this opening during swallowing.

TRIGGERING THE PHARYNGEAL SWALLOW RESPONSE

Take a moment now and try an experiment. Without taking in any liquid or food, see how many times you can swallow in rapid succession.

You probably can do it only a couple of times after your saliva is depleted (Kennedy & Kent, 1988). Even though we can voluntarily initiate swallows, we cannot repetitively swallow without some sort of sensory input. And it is the bolus that provides this sensory input as it moves through the oral and pharyngeal cavities. The bolus stimulates superficial and deep sensory receptors, many of which project—via the glossopharyngeal, vagus, and spinal accessory nerves (CN IX, X, and XI)—to a region of the medullary **reticular formation** called the **nucleus tractus solitarius (NTS)**. This brainstem region is commonly known as the *swallowing center* and likely incorporates sensory input from trigeminal, facial, and hypoglossal nuclei (CN V, VII, and XII) as well. (Note that standard neuroanatomy references vary in their descriptions of the nerves that project to NTS.) When the sensory input to this region is of the appropriate pattern and intensity, the NTS signals motor nuclei, particularly the **nucleus ambiguus,** where the cell bodies for cranial nerves IX, X, and XI are located vertically in the brainstem, to fire. The nucleus ambiguus innervates muscles of the velum, pharynx, larynx, and upper esophagus primarily through the glossopharyngeal, vagus, and spinal accessory nerves (CN IX, X, and XI). The resulting stereotyped motor output is known as the *pharyngeal swallow response.*

There are many regions across the aerodigestive tract that, when provided with the appropriate type, intensity, and duration of stimulation, can trigger the pharyngeal swallow response. However, there are certain regions within the oropharynx that are especially efficient trigger points. It is probably the case that these regions have the strongest ties to the NTS. These include the anterior faucial arches, the posterior tongue at the level of the lower edge of the mandible, the valleculae, the pyriform sinuses, and the laryngeal aditus (Dua, et al., 1997; Robbins, et al., 1992).

Of these sites, the anterior faucial arches deserve some special attention in this chapter. They have been the topic of countless clinical and research endeavors in swallowing. We may ask ourselves why this might be the case. After all, the morphology of the sensory receptors located in the mucosa and muscles of this region is not different from that of other receptors in the oral cavity (see Kuehn, Templeton, & Maynard, 1990; Liss, 1990). What does make this region special, however, is the apparently strong connection between these sensory receptors and the NTS via afferent fibers of the glossopharyngeal nerve (CN IX). Mechanical stimulation to the anterior faucial arches is particularly efficient in triggering the pharyngeal swallow response. In fact, the first edition of Logemann's classic text on dysphagia names the anterior faucial arches as *the* trigger point for the pharyngeal swallow stage (Logemann, 1983). Since that time, additional studies have demonstrated that the anterior faucial arches are a common trigger point for many younger adults, but not necessarily for older adults who may trigger much lower in the oropharynx (Robbins, Hamilton, Lof, & Kempster, 1992). Lower regions of the pharynx also have been shown to be trigger points during normal eating (Dua, et al., 1997). Nonetheless, the anterior faucial arches are targeted for special treatment in remediating slow swallow responses in dysphagic persons. The clinical procedure of **thermal tactile application (TTA)** involves stroking the arches with a cooled metal dental mirror to increase the speed at which the pharyngeal response is triggered. Although some studies have shown immediate effects, sustained improvements in swallowing have not been demonstrated definitively (Ali, Laundl, Wallace, deCarle, & Cook, 1996; Chi-Fishmann, Capra, & McCall, 1994; Fujiu, Toleikis, Logemann, & Larson, 1994; Kaatzke-McDonald, Post, & Davis, 1996; Knauer, Castell, Dalton, Nowak, & Castell, 1990; Lazzara, Lararus, & Logemann, 1986; Rosenbek, Robbins, Fishback, & Levine, 1991; Rosenbek, Robbins, Willford, Kirk, Schiltz, Sowell, Deutsch, Milanti, & Ashford, et al., 1998; Rosenbek, Roecker, Wood, & Robbins, 1996).

CLINICAL NOTE 2-1

Sensory Stimulation Techniques

It has become common practice in many settings to include sensory stimulation techniques in the dysphagia therapy armamentarium. Thermal tactile application, **thermal gustatory treatment,** and **deep pharyngeal neuromuscular stimulation (DPNS** or **DPNMS)** are among these techniques. At the heart of these therapies is the assumption that stimulating the oral and/or pharyngeal mucosa serves to promote improved neuromuscular function for swallowing by facilitating proper tone and reflex response. However, to date, there are no published data that demonstrate the efficacy of any stimulation technique for the sustained improvement of swallow function in dysphagia. Because sensory stimulation techniques are, by their nature, invasive, clinicians must be circumspect in their use of these techniques.

In summary, when the NTS receives the appropriate intensity of patterned sensory input from peripheral receptors, a stereotyped efferent response is triggered at the nucleus ambiguus. Although the input can arise from many discrete points along the aerodigestive tract, it is probably the overall pattern of stimulation that elicits the pharyngeal swallow response. In most cases, a swallow response is triggered by the time the bolus reaches the base of the tongue at the level of the lower edge of the mandible. The next several sections describe, in detail, the anatomy and physiology associated with the pharyngeal swallow response. Keep in mind that unless the swallow response is triggered these actions will not occur.

Velopharyngeal Closure

You have learned in your previous coursework that velopharyngeal closure for speech production is not an all-or-none proposition. Even though phoneme manner is designated as nasal or non-nasal, the velum is a rather slow and sluggish articulator. As a result, our perceptual systems tolerate the effects of nasal coarticulation, particularly the nasalization of vowels that are embedded in nasal contexts (like the /ae/ in *man*). However, the swallowing mechanism is not so forgiving. It requires that velopharyngeal closure be rapid, be high in the pharynx, and form a complete seal with the posterior pharyngeal wall. Fortunately, the motor commands associated with the swallow response specify these movement requirements.

Interestingly, velar elevation for swallowing has been shown to be more complex than the simple vertical displacement of the velum for speech (Hamlet & Momiyama, 1992). Frequently, there is a high velocity anterior movement of the velum that precedes its rapid posterior displacement toward the pharyngeal wall. Nonetheless, the muscles responsible for the rapid, high, and complete closure of the velopharyngeal port are the very same ones responsible for closure in speech production. Together, they produce three distinct movements: 1) velar elevation first anteriorly, then rapidly back toward the posterior wall of the pharynx at the oro-nasopharyngeal junction, 2) medial movement of the lateral pharyngeal walls, and 3) forward displacement of the posterior pharyngeal wall. This closure is maintained for one-half to one second in duration (Smith, Hamlet, & Jones, 1990). The muscles that accomplish these movements are innervated by the pharyngeal plexus, with the pharyngeal branch of the vagus nerve (CN X) playing a prominent role.

Let us begin with the muscles responsible for velar elevation (Figure 2-5). The **levator veli palatini** comprises the bulk of the velum. Each superior end of this muscle extends down from its attachment at the base of the skull near the **torus tubarius** to blend with its mate at the midline of the velum. Its anterior fibers insert into the palatal aponeurosis. Its contraction forcefully and rapidly elevates the velum toward the posterior pharyngeal wall. Simultaneous contraction of the small **musculus uvulae** gives added lift to the posterior quadrant of the velum for even tighter velopharyngeal contact. This muscle extends from the posterior nasal spine to the body of the uvula. You may have learned that the **tensor veli palatini muscle** does little to tense or elevate the velum during speech production, and this is the case. However, the muscle which extends from the hamulus of the medial pterygoid plate of the sphenoid bone and torus tubarius to the palatal aponeurosis is active during velar elevation for swallowing (Hamlet & Momiyama, 1992). It contracts in

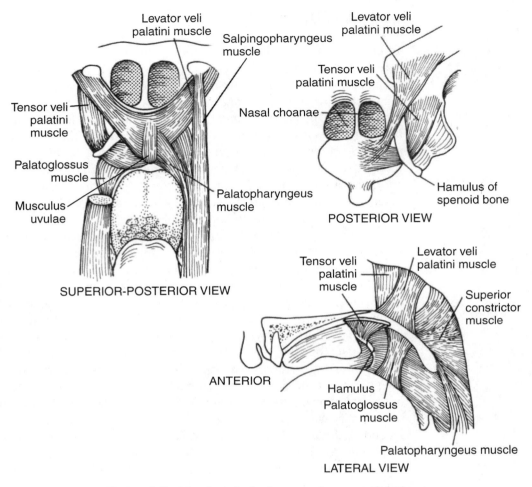

Figure 2-5. Muscles of velopharyngeal port modulation.

tandem with levator veli palatini and likely serves to tense the anterior velum during elevation for swallowing. It also opens the **auditory tube**, which explains why our ears often *pop* when we swallow. Unlike the other muscles of the velum, tensor veli palatini receives its motor innervation from the trigeminal nerve (CN V).

It is not clear which muscles are responsible for the initial high-velocity anterior displacement of the velum that precedes its rapid excursion toward the posterior pharyngeal wall. Hamlet and Momiyama (1992) reported that this movement was temporally linked to tensor and levator activity, but these muscles are not in an optimal position to displace the velum anteriorly. They postulated that the velar depressor, palatoglossu, might be responsible. Furthermore, this action may be part of an initial *set up* for the swallow response, getting the velum in motion and ready to make its critical journey to the posterior pharyngeal wall.

The next component of velopharyngeal closure, the lateral displacement of the pharyngeal walls, is accomplished largely by contraction of the horizontal fibers of the palatopharyngeus muscle. You may recall that the bulk of the palatopharyngeus is regarded as a velar depressor so it is not active during closure of the velopharyngeal port. However, some bands of fibers from this muscle course horizontally at the level of the velum to insert into the pharyngeal walls. When these fibers contract, they serve to pull the lateral pharyngeal walls toward midline, thus hugging the sides of the elevated velum.

The last component of velopharyngeal closure is accomplished by the **superior constrictor** muscle of the pharynx. This muscle arises from the pterygomandibular ligament which extends vertically from the hamulus of the medial pterygoid plate of the sphenoid bone at the base of the skull. This ligament is also the posterior attachment for the buccinator muscle as we learned in the last chapter. As the fibers from these two muscles blend together in their attachment to the ligament, they form the pterygomandibular raphe. The fibers of the superior constrictor then course posteriorly to blend with their mate at midline creating the posterior pharyngeal raphe of the pharynx. When this muscle contracts, it pulls the posterior pharyngeal wall forward. In some people, simultaneous contraction of the horizontal fibers of the palatopharyngeus and the superior constrictor creates a bulge on the posterior pharyngeal wall. This is known as **Passavant's pad**. This term is covered in the speech-language pathology curriculum when learning about velopharyngeal closure for speech production.

Hyolaryngeal Elevation

Just about the same time as velopharyngeal closure commences, so too does the upward and anterior movement of the hyoid bone and the column of laryngeal cartilages that are suspended from it (the **hyolaryngeal complex**). It takes roughly one-half second for maximal elevation and anterior displacement of the hyolaryngeal complex to occur, and it stays elevated for about another quarter second longer (Logemann, 1983). Keep in mind the mechanical linkage between the base of the tongue, the hyoid bone, and the larynx. Although these structures can move independently to some degree, they are inextricably linked by muscles and tendons. Thus, it makes sense that as the tongue muscles that comprise the mouth floor contract, the hyoid bone is pulled up, which, in turn, tends to elevate the larynx. Several muscles that extend from the floor of the mouth to the hyoid bone instigate this movement (Figure 2-6). They include the anterior belly of the digastric, the mylohyoid, and the geniohyoid. Laryngeal elevation relative to the hyoid bone is assisted by the **thyrohyoid muscle**. Contraction of this muscle also contributes to the dilation of the upper esophageal sphincter, a phenomenon that will be discussed in greater detail in the next chapter.

In the previous chapter, the anterior belly of the digastric, and its role as a mandibular depressor in the oral stage of deglutition, was discussed. The digastric muscle has a second function, and another portion called the **posterior belly of the digastric**. The anterior and posterior bellies of the digastric muscle meet up at the hyoid bone by way of a tendonous loop. While the anterior portion arises from the

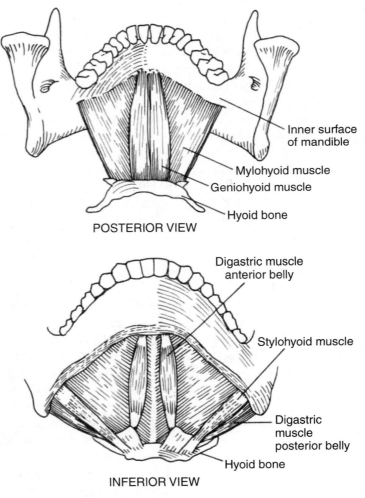

Inner surface of mandible

Mylohyoid muscle
Geniohyoid muscle

Hyoid bone

POSTERIOR VIEW

Digastric muscle anterior belly

Stylohyoid muscle

Digastric muscle posterior belly

Hyoid bone

INFERIOR VIEW

Figure 2-6. Hyolaryngeal muscles.

mandible, the posterior portion arises from the mastoid process of the temporal bone. When the mandible is fixed and these muscles contract simultaneously, the hyoid bone is raised. Because the movement of the hyoid at the initiation of the pharyngeal swallow response is in the superior and anterior direction, the anterior belly of the digastric is at a mechanical advantage to assist in hyolaryngeal elevation.

The fibers of the mylohyoid muscle form the floor of the mouth. They extend from the inner border of the mandible and course inferiorly and medially to blend with their mates at the **midline raphe**. The posterior fibers of this muscle attach to the body of the hyoid bone. Thus, when they contract they draw the hyoid up and forward.

The geniohyoid muscle also draws the hyoid up and forward. It originates at the mental symphysis and courses posteriorly and inferiorly to attach to the front of the hyoid bone. Unlike the anterior belly of the digastric and the mylohyoid muscles, which are innervated by the trigeminal nerve (CN V) and facial nerve (CN VII), respectively, the geniohyoid is innervated by hypoglossal nerve (CN XII).

The thyrohyoid is a deep muscle that extends from the lateral thyroid lamina to the lower border of the greater horn of the hyoid bone. When the hyoid is fixed (or is being pulled upward), contraction of the thyrohyoid elevates the thyroid cartilage. This muscle, like other infrahyoid muscles, is innervated by the hypoglossal nerve (CN XII) and fibers from upper cervical nerves.

Several studies have attempted to characterize the activation pattern of muscles involved in the elevation of the hyolaryngeal complex in swallowing. The conclusion, not surprisingly, is that there is a great deal of temporal overlap between tongue movements associated with bolus transport and the activation of the suprahyoid muscles. It may be best to think of hyolaryngeal elevation as a critical component of the pharyngeal swallow stage that is highly plastic and adjustable to meet the requirements of the swallowing conditions (Gay, Rendell, & Spiro, 1994; Spiro, Rendell, & Gay, 1994).

Despite the variability in activation patterns among muscles of hyolaryngeal elevation, recent investigations have challenged commonly held beliefs about hyoid kinematics. Ishida, Palmer, and Hiiemae (2002) measured the upward and forward movements of the hyoid during liquid and solid swallows, and discovered that the upward movements frequently were extremely small. However, the forward displacement of the hyoid was more similar and robust across swallows. Their finding supports the observations of others that hyoid movement is indeed variable, but that the mechanical linkage between the hyolaryngeal complex and UES results in fewer degrees of freedom for the forward movement leg of hyoid elevation. Chi-Fishman and Sonies (2002) also investigated hyoid kinematics using ultrasonography. They discovered, among other things, a great deal of task-dependent patterning of hyoid movement based on bolus size and viscosity.

Laryngeal Protection

Perhaps the most critical result of the swallow response is the three-tiered protection of the airway that is set into motion. These tiers include inversion of the epiglottis over the laryngeal aditus and closure of the true and false vocal folds. It was previously believed that these events occurred in a relatively fixed sequence, with the true vocal folds closing first, followed by the false folds, and then epiglottic inversion. However, discovering the actual sequence has been difficult to ascertain because of limitations in technology. Visualization techniques, such as endoscopy, do not permit the viewing of the vocal folds throughout the entire swallow sequence. The view is obscured at the most critical moments—when the epiglottis inverts and the bolus traverses the pharynx. Vocal fold movement also is difficult to view on videofluorographic images because of the tissue density and lack of visual contrast in that region. Electromyography and electroglottography offer indirect evidence of vocal fold closure, but these methods suffer from lack of specificity. Recent studies, using multiple and more sophisticated imaging technologies, have caused us to question the stability of the *bottom-up* sequence (Dua, Ren, Barden, Xie, & Shaker, 1997; Flaherty, Seltzer, Campell, Weisskoff, & Gilbert, 1995; Kendall, Leonard, & McKenzie, 2003; Ohmae, Logemann, Kaiser, Hanson, & Kahrilas, 1995). Regardless of the order of closure, the events serve to move out any swallowed material that has entered the laryngeal vestibule and to prevent other material from entering the area.

Closure of the **true vocal folds** is believed to occur closely around the time of elevation of the hyolaryngeal complex (Flaherty, et al., 1995). Vocal fold adduction for swallowing is accomplished by contraction of the following muscles: **lateral cricoarytenoid**, **interarytenoids**, **vocalis (thyroarytenoid** or **thyrovocalis)**, and **thyromuscularis** (Figure 2-7a). These intrinsic muscles, all innervated by the recurrent laryngeal branch of the vagus nerve (CN X), are the same muscles that serve to adduct the vocal folds for the purpose of phonation; however, the vocal fold closure pressure during volitional swallowing has been found to exceed the pressure for phonation (Shaker, Dua, Ren, Xie, Funahashi, & Schapira, 2002). The only intrinsic laryngeal muscle not directly implicated in swallowing is the **cricothyroid** which is innervated by the superior laryngeal nerve of the vagus (CN X).

The lateral cricoarytenoid extends from the cricoid lamina to the muscular process of the arytenoid cartilage. Contraction of this muscle causes the vocal processes of the arytenoids to displace medially, thereby

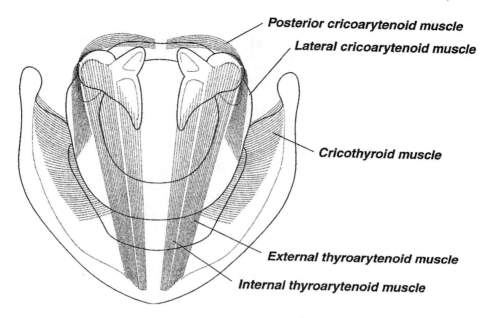

Posterior cricoarytenoid muscle

Lateral cricoarytenoid muscle

Cricothyroid muscle

External thyroarytenoid muscle

Internal thyroarytenoid muscle

Figure 2-7a. Instrinsic laryngeal muscles.

creating adduction of the vocal folds. The two interarytenoid muscles assist in this adduction by pulling the arytenoids closer together (Figure 2-7b). The **oblique interarytenoid muscle** extends from the apex of one cartilage to the muscular process of the other. The transverse portions extend laterally between the posterior aspects of the cartilages. Thus, their contraction aids in medial compression of the posterior portion of the vocal folds. Finally, the thyroarytenoid muscle extends from the muscular processes of the arytenoids to the thyroid angle. Its contraction assists in shortening and relaxing the vocal folds by decreasing the distance between the arytenoids and the thyroid cartilage.

The **ventricular folds**, also known as the **false vocal folds**, are not muscular structures (though fibers from the thyromuscularis may extend into the ventricular folds). Rather, they are outcroppings of mucosal tissue that lie immediately superior to the true muscular vocal folds and attach anterolaterally to the arytenoid cartilages. Because of this lack of muscular constitution, they only can be adducted when the arytenoid cartilages are displaced medially and anteriorly. Two muscles have been credited with this displacement: the oblique interarytenoids and the **aryepiglottic** muscle (Figure 2-7c). The aryepiglottic muscle, when present, is notoriously poorly developed. It arises from the apex of the arytenoids and often appears to blend with the oblique interarytenoid fibers. It sometimes extends to the superior edge of the epiglottis. Because the muscle fibers tend to be scarce and thin, this muscle may or may not play a role in

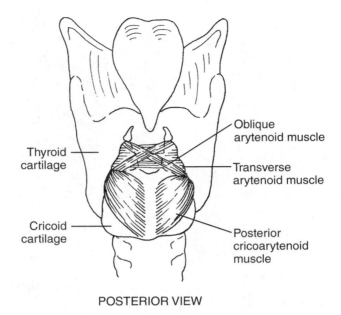

POSTERIOR VIEW

Figure 2-7b. Posterior view of intrinsic laryngeal muscles.

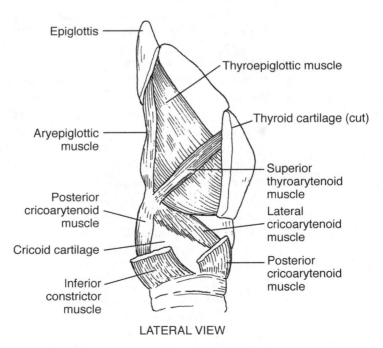

LATERAL VIEW

Figure 2-7c. Lateral view of laryngeal muscles.

moving the arytenoids, and hence the false vocal folds. The oblique inter-arytenoids are at a mechanical advantage to displace the false vocal folds, however, so their contribution to this movement is more certain.

As mentioned earlier, the epiglottis is tethered to the thyroid angle of the larynx and to the hyoid bone by ligaments. Thus, as hyolaryngeal elevation occurs, muscular and nonmuscular forces contribute to two distinct movements of the epiglottis as it covers the airway (VanDaele, Perlman, & Casell, 1995). The first movement is from its vertical resting position to a horizontal position. This occurs at the level of the thyroepiglottic attachment and results most likely from the initial anterior-superior displacement of the hyoid bone. Then, as the larynx rises further due to thyrohyoid contraction, the upper third of the epiglottis bends into the pharynx at the level of the hyoepiglottic ligament. Together, these movements serve to cover the laryngeal aditus and split the bolus and channel it down the lateral aspects of the pharynx. Or, if the bolus does not split, the movement will serve to channel it down one side of the pharynx, or safely over the midline of the covered laryngeal aditus (Dua, et al., 1997).

Proper channeling of the bolus to the esophagus characterizes the majority of normal swallows. However, the mechanical barriers that protect our larynx are not foolproof. All of us have experienced an occasional case of *it went down the wrong pipe*. We cough and sputter, our eyes tear, and we recover within a few seconds or minutes. This occurs because of a reflexive second line of defense. The larynx and trachea contain highly sensitive receptors that convey information, via superior laryngeal and recurrent branches of the vagus nerve (CN X), about the entry of foreign material into the larynx and airway. The mucosal surface of the larynx above the vocal folds is subserved by the internal branch of the superior laryngeal nerve (Sasaki & Weaver, 1997). The inferior surface of the vocal folds and the trachea are subserved by the recurrent laryngeal nerve branch. Stimulation of receptors in this region instigates a reflexive cough until the intruding material is forcefully expelled.

CLINICAL NOTE

2-2

Laryngeal Cough Reflex

The last line of defense for the larynx is forcefully coughing out any material that manages to slip into the region of the vocal folds or below. At least one study has suggested that an absent or weakened laryngeal cough reflex is associated with the risk of developing aspiration pneumonia in stroke patients (Addington, Stephens, Gilliland, & Rodriguez, 1999; see also Aviv, Sacco, Mohr, Thompson, Levin, Sunshine, Thomson, & Close, 1997; Smith-Hammond, Goldstein, Zajac, Gray, Davenport, & Bolser, 2001). Although the validity of this premise remains to be established, research protocols have been developed to test the integrity of the laryngeal cough reflex in patients with dysphagia.

Progressive Pharyngeal Contraction

The modification of terminology is common during the development of any field, and the study of swallowing is no exception. Until quite recently, the term **pharyngeal peristalsis** was used to characterize the segmental and sequential contraction of the pharyngeal wall that is triggered by the pharyngeal swallow response. Peristalsis is the same term that is applied to the movement of esophagus and the gastrointestinal tract as they move the bolus through the system. There are two reasons, however, that peristalsis is not the appropriate term for pharyngeal movement. First, peristalsis refers to movement of a muscular tube, and you will recall that the pharynx is really more of a muscular semicircle. Second, peristalsis is more formally associated with the sequential and segmental action of involuntary muscle. Even though we cannot voluntarily alter the pattern of contraction of the pharyngeal constrictors during a swallow, all of the pharyngeal constrictor muscles are striated and voluntary. Therefore, many authors have chosen to abandon the term peristalsis, altogether, in favor of other terms such as **progressive contraction**.

The muscles responsible for this segmental contraction were mentioned earlier in this chapter. Recall that the superior, middle, and inferior constrictor muscles are three semicircular bands of muscle that are suspended from the skull and comprise the lateral and posterior walls of the pharynx. Their primary function is to constrict the lumen of the pharynx and to elevate it. All three of these muscles terminate at midline on the posterior pharyngeal wall creating a seam called the posterior pharyngeal raphe. The superior constrictor extends back from the pterygomandibular raphe to the posterior pharyngeal raphe. Recall that the pterygomandibular raphe is created as the fibers from the superior constrictor blend with those of the buccinator at the pterygomandibular ligament. The middle constrictor originates in a narrow band on the greater horn of the hyoid bone and courses back to the posterior pharyngeal raphe just below the superior constrictor. The inferior constrictor has a broad origin along the thyroid and cricoid cartilages (thyropharyngeus arising from the thyroid cartilage; cricopharyngeus from the cricoid cartilage) and extends to the posterior pharyngeal raphe below the middle constrictor. These muscles are innervated by the pharyngeal plexus.

The pharyngeal contraction, set into motion by the swallow response, is critical in generating the forces and pressures necessary for guiding the bolus efficiently to the UES—all in about the space of one second. The wave begins as the tongue base makes firm contact with the posterior pharyngeal wall. This occurs as the tail-end of the bolus is delivered to the oropharynx. The mechanical force of the tongue and the pressure increase created by the decrease in supra-bolus space serve to propel the bolus downward. The segmental and sequential contractions of the pharyngeal constrictors follow along the tail-end of the bolus, acting at once to guide and clear residue that remains in the pharynx at a rate of about 13 cm/sec (McConnell, et al., 1988; Olsson, Kjellin, & Ekberg, 1996).

The pressures generated along the pharynx, by the constriction of the muscles, are not uniform. Peak pressures in the region of the tongue base and superior constrictor are less than those in the region of the inferior constrictor. Olsson and his colleagues (1996) speculated this is likely due to both mechanical and neurological factors. First, recall that the pharynx is not uniform along its length: the diameter of the upper segments is greater than that of the lower segments. This means—remembering the pressure-volume relationship discussed earlier—that, for a given level of contraction, it would be easier to generate high pressure levels when the volume is already small. It makes sense that, for the same amount of muscle contraction and pharyngeal constriction, pressure in smaller areas of the pharynx will be higher than pressure in larger areas. Second, the mobility of the anterior origins of the three constrictor muscles varies—this determines how much the lumen can be reduced by pulling the anterior structures backward. Finally, it is possible that the three muscles derive innervation from different motor neuron pools within the brainstem. This would allow for the swallow center to organize the sequential contraction of these muscles. Palmer, Tanaka, and Ensrud (2000) found additional evidence to support the notion of a distinct innervation pattern. They discovered that pharyngeal shortening during a swallow is achieved by greater elevation of the hypopharynx than for the oropharynx. Additionally, laryngeal elevation is less extreme than pharyngeal elevation, such that simple biomechanical linkage cannot account for both movements. Distinct neural activation sources must be operative.

In any case, the sequence of muscle activation appears to be fixed and relatively unaffected by bolus characteristics—even though the duration and intensity of muscle activation is affected by bolus characteristics. It should be noted that body position does have an effect on tongue force and pharyngeal pressure relationships. When supine or upside down, the tongue driving force increases and the hypopharyngeal pressure dyamics change (Dejaeger, Pelemans, Ponette, & Vantrappen, 1994).

Opening of the Upper Esophageal Sphincter

The final component of the pharyngeal swallow response is the opening of the UES. This sphincter, which will be covered in great detail in the next chapter, is created by the thyropharyngeus and cricopharyngeus muscles that comprise the inferior pharyngeal constrictor muscle, and **upper cervical esophagus** muscle fibers. The UES is the boundary between the pharynx and the esophagus and it is tonically closed. When the pharyngeal swallow response is triggered, however, the fibers of the cricopharyngeus relax and the UES begins to dilate. This corresponds with elevation of the hyolaryngeal complex that mechanically *stretches* the opening further by pulling the cricoid cartilage away from the pharyngeal wall. This opening is important long before the bolus reaches the UES. Recall that UES dilation is thought to be responsible for the pressure differential that is created along the pharynx—with high pressure behind the bolus due to pharyngeal elevation and constriction, and low pressure in front of the bolus due to UES dilation. This corresponds favorably with the finding of Kendall, Leonard, and McKenzie (2003) that the maximal pharyngeal constriction always occurred after the UES was maximally opened. This helps pull and push the bolus along.

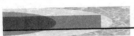

SWALLOWING AND RESPIRATION

In the very beginning of this book we emphasized that speech, swallowing, and respiration are overlaid functions of the aerodigestive tract. In this chapter, the great care taken by structures of the upper tract to protect the airway from the bolus has been discussed. Because of the organization of neural control for swallowing and breathing, it is virtually impossible to breathe and swallow at the same time. Numerous investigations have examined the coordination of respiration and swallowing and have reached similar conclusions (Edgar, 1994; Hiss, Treole, & Stuart, 2001; Klahn & Perlman, 1999; Nilson, Ekberg, Olsson, Kjellin, & Hindfelt, 1996; Preiksaitis, Mayrand, Robins, & Diamant, 1992; Selley, Ellis, Flack, Bayliss, & Pearce, 1994; Smith, Wolkove, Calacone, & Kreisman, 1989). First, swallows typically occur during the expiratory cycle of breathing. That is to say, in preparation for swallowing, we stop breathing after we have exhaled a bit. We then swallow, while holding our breath (**apneic period**) for less than a second as the bolus travels safely to the esophagus, then we complete our exhalation. This EXHALE-SWALLOW-EXHALE pattern appears to account for the vast majority of normal swallows, with INHALE-SWALLOW-EXHALE trailing a distant second. In either case, exhalation following a swallow makes perfect sense for airway protection. Inhaling immediately after a swallow does occur on a small percentage of normal swallows. However, this pattern may be regarded as less safe. It may encourage any pooled residue in the pharynx to be sucked into the laryngeal vestibule and trachea. Studies of populations with respiratory deficits have shown that the need for oxygenation may interfere with safe breathing-swallowing patterns, putting patients at risk for aspiration (Edgar, 1994). All of the research to date suggests that maximal airway protection comes when:

- Expiration occurs before and after the swallow
- The larynx is maximally isolated from the pharynx during the swallow
- The laryngeal cough reflex is intact.

Any problem that interferes with these protective components will increase the risk of choking and aspiration.

SUMMARY

The pharyngeal stage begins as the bolus is propelled back into the oropharynx. The proper pattern and intensity of sensory stimulation to the NTS triggers a patterned sequence of motor events at the nucleus ambiguus. This sequence includes both airway-protective and bolus-propulsive events that are not under the jurisdiction of voluntary control. These include:

1. Velopharyngeal closure, characterized by a brief anterior displacement of the velum followed by rapid elevation and solid contact with the lateral and posterior pharyngeal walls
2. Elevation and anterior displacement of the hyolaryngeal complex
3. Closure of the true and false vocal folds and the cessation of breathing
4. Inversion of the epiglottis over the laryngeal aditus
5. Progressive pharyngeal contraction following the tail end of the bolus
6. Opening of the upper esophageal sphincter.

The bolus is propelled through the pharynx by mechanical as well as pressure-dynamic forces. Pressure differentials are generated by constriction of the pharynx above the bolus and the opening of the UES below the bolus. In breathing, exhalation usually follows the pharyngeal stage of the swallow.

STUDY QUESTIONS

1. What structural events are associated with the pharyngeal swallow response?
2. Which areas along the aerodigestive tract have been shown to be efficient triggers for the pharyngeal swallow response?

3. How do *pressure differentials* contribute to bolus transport and what structures and events are responsible for their generation?

4. Which peripheral sensory structures and brain regions are associated with mediation of the pharyngeal swallow response?

5. Describe the typical coordination of breathing and swallowing. How might this be affected in certain disease states?

REFERENCES

Addington, W. R., Stephens, R. E., Gilliland, K., & Rodriguez, M. (1999). Assessing the laryngeal cough reflex and the risk of developing pneumonia after stroke. *Archives of Physical Medicine and Rehabilitation, 80*(2), 150–154.

Ali, G. N., Laundl, T. M., Wallace, K. L., deCarle, D. J., & Cook, I. J. S. (1996). Influence of cold stimulation on the normal pharyngeal swallow response. *Dysphagia, 11*(1), 2–8.

Aviv, J. E., Sacco, R. L., Mohr, J. P., Thompson, J. L. P., Levin, B., Sunshine, S., Thomson, J., & Close, L. G. (1997). Laryngopharyngeal sensory testing with modified barium swallow as predictors of aspiration pneumonia after stroke. *The Laryngoscope, 107*(9), 1254–1260.

Bosma, J. F., & Barner, H. (1993). Ligaments of the larynx and the adjacent pharynx and esophagus. *Dysphagia, 8*(1), 23–28.

Chi-Fishman, G., Capra, N. F., & McCall, G. N. (1994). Thermomechanical facilitation of swallowing evoked by electrical nerve stimulation in cats. *Dysphagia, 9*(3), 149–155.

Chi-Fishman, G., & Sonies, B. C. (2002). Effects of systematic bolus viscosity and volume changes on hyoid movement kinematics. *Dysphagia, 17*(4), 278–287.

Dejaeger, E., Pelemans, W., Ponette, E., & Vantrappen, G. (1994). Effect of body position on deglutition. *Digestive Diseases and Sciences, 39*(4), 762–765.

Dua, K. S., Ren, J., Bardan, E., Xie, P., & Shaker, R. (1997). Coordination of deglutitive glottal function and pharyngeal bolus transit during normal eating. *Gastroenterology, 112*(11), 73–83.

Edgar, J. (1994). Meal-related patterns of respiration and deglutition in patients with chronic obstructive pulmonary disease. Unpublished dissertation, University of Minnesota.

Flaherty, R. F., Seltzer, S., Campbell, T., Weisskoff, R. M., & Gilbert, R. J. (1995). Dynamic magnetic resonance imaging of vocal cord closure during deglutition. *Gastroenterology, 109*(3), 843–849.

Fujiu, M., Toleikis, J. R., Logemann, J. A., & Larson, C. R. (1994). Glossopharyngeal evoked potential in normal subjects following mechanical stimulation of the anterior faucial pillar. *Electroencephalography and Clinical Neurophysiology, 92*(3), 183–195.

Gay, T., Rendell, J. K., & Spiro, J. (1994). Oral and laryngeal muscle coordination during swallowing. *Laryngoscope, 104*(3 Pt 1), 341–349.

Hamlet, S. L., & Momiyama, Y. (1992). Velar activity and timing of eustachian tube function in swallowing. *Dysphagia*, 7(4), 226–233.

Hiss, S. G, Treole, K., & Stuart, A. (2001). Effects of age, gender, bolus volume, and trial on swallowing apnea duration and swallow/respiratory phase relationships of normal adults. *Dysphagia*, 16(2), 128–135.

Ishida, R., Palmer, J. B., & Hiiemae, K. M. (2002). Hyoid motion during swallowing: Factors affecting forward and upward displacement. *Dysphagia*, 17(4), 262–272.

Kaatzke-McDonald, M. N., Post, E., & Davis, P. J. (1996). The effects of cold, touch, and chemical stimulation of the anterior faucial pillar on human swallowing. *Dysphagia*, 11(3), 198–206.

Kendall, K. A., Leonard, R. J., & McKenzie, S. W. (2003). Sequence variability during hypopharyngeal bolus transit. *Dysphagia*, 18(2), 85–91.

Kennedy, J., & Kent, R. D. (1988). Physiological substrates of normal deglutition. *Dysphagia*, 3(1), 27–34.

Kent, R. D. (1997). *The speech sciences*. Clifton Park, NY: Thomson Delmar Learning.

Klahn, M. S., & Perlman, A. L. (1999). Temporal and durational patterns associating respiration and swallowing. *Dysphagia*, 14(3), 131–138.

Kuehn, D. P., Templeton, P. J., & Maynard, J. A. (1990). Muscle spindles in the velopharyngeal musculature of humans. *Journal of Speech and Hearing Research*, 33(3), 488–493.

Lazzara, G., Lararus, C., & Logemann, J. A. (1986). Impact of thermal stimulation on the triggering of the swallowing reflex. *Dysphagia*, 1(2), 73–77.

Liss, J. M. (1990). Muscle spindles in the human levator veli palatini and palatoglossus muscles. *Journal of Speech and Hearing Research*, 33(4), 736–746.

Logemann, J. A. (1983). *Evaluation and treatment of swallowing disorders*. San Diego, CA: College-Hill Press.

Logemann, J. A. (1998). *Evaluation and treatment of swallowing disorders* (2nd ed.). Austin, TX: Pro-Ed.

McConnell, F. M. S., Cerenko, D., & Mendelsohn, M. S. (1988). Manofluorographic analysis of swallowing. *Otolaryngologic Clinics of North America*, 21 (4), 625–635.

Nilsson, H., Ekberg, O., Olsson, R., Kjellin, O., & Hindfelt, B. (1996). Quantitative assessment of swallowing in healthy adults. *Dysphagia*, 11(2), 110–116.

Ohmae, Y., Logemann, J. A., Kaiser, P., Hanson, D. G., & Kahrilas, P. J. (1995, September/October). Timing of glottic closure during normal swallow. *Head & Neck*, 17(5), 394–402.

Olsson, R., Kjellin, O., & Ekberg, O. (1996). Videomanometric aspects of pharyngeal constrictor activity. *Dysphagia*, 11(2), 83–86.

Palmer, J. B., Tanaka, E., & Ensrud, E. (2000). Motions of the posterior pharyngeal wall in human swallowing: A quantitative videofluorographic study. *Archives of Physical Medicine and Rehabilitation*, 81(11), 1520–1526.

Preiksaitis, H. G., Mayrand, S., Robins, K., & Diamant, N. E. (1992). Coordination of respiration and swallowing: Effect of bolus volume in normal adults. *American Journal of Physiology*, 263 (3 Pt 2), R624–R630.

Rademaker, A. W., Pauloski, B. R., Colangelo, L. A., & Logemann, J. A. (1998). Age and volume effects on liquid swallowing function in normal women. *Journal of Speech, Language, and Hearing Research, 41*(2), 275–284.

Robbins, J., Hamilton, J. W., Loff, G. L., & Kempster, G. B. (1992). Oropharyngeal swallowing in normal adults of different ages. *Gastroenterology, 103*(3), 823–829.

Rosenbek, J. C., Robbins, J., Fishback, B., & Levine, R. (1991). Effects of thermal application on dysphagia after stroke. *Journal of Speech and Hearing Research, 34*(6), 1257–1268.

Rosenbek, J. C., Robbins, J., Willford, W. O., Kirk, G., Schiltz, A., Sowell, T. W., Deutsch, S. E., Milanti, F. J., Ashford, J., Gramigna, G. D., Fogarty, A., Dong, K., Rau, M. T., Prescott, T. E., Lloyd, A. M., Sterkel, M. T., & Hansen, J. E. (1998). Comparing treatment intensities of tactile-thermal application. *Dysphagia, 13*(1), 1–9.

Rosenbek, J. C., Roecker, E. B., Wood, J. L., & Robbins, J. (1996). Thermal application reduces the duration of stage transition in dysphagia after stroke. *Dysphagia, 11*(4), 225–233.

Sasaki, C. T., & Weaver, E. M. (1997). Physiology of the larynx. *The American Journal of Medicine, 103*(5A), 9S–18S.

Seikel, J. A., King, D. W., & Drumright, D. G. (2000). *Anatomy and physiology for speech, language, and hearing* (2nd ed.). Clifton Park, NY: Thomson Delmar Learning.

Selley, W. G, Ellis, R. E., Flack, F. C., Bayliss, C. R., & Pearce, V. R. (1994). The synchronization of respiration and swallow sounds with videofluoroscopy during swallowing. *Dysphagia, 9*(3), 162–167.

Shaker, R., Dua, K. S., Ren, J., Xie, P., Funahashi, A., & Schapira, R. M. (2002). Vocal cord closure pressure during volitional swallow and other voluntary tasks. *Dysphagia, 17*(1), 13–18.

Smith, D., Hamlet, S., & Jones, L. (1990). Acoustic technique for determining timing of velopharyngeal closure in swallowing. *Dysphagia, 5*(3), 142–146.

Smith, J., Wolkove, N., Colacone, A., & Kreisman, H. (1989). Coordination of eating, drinking, and breathing in adults. *Chest, 96*(3), 578–582.

Smith-Hammond, C. A., Goldstein, L. B., Zajac, D. J., Gray, L., Davenport, P. W., & Bolser, D. C. (2001). Assessment of aspiration risk in stroke patients with quantification of voluntary cough. *Neurology, 56*(4), 502–506.

Spiro, J., Rendell, J. K., & Gay, T. (1994). Activation and coordination patterns of the suprahyoid muscles during swallowing. *Laryngoscope, 104* (11 Pt 1), 1376–1382.

VanDaele, D. J., Perlman, A. L., & Cassell, M. D. (1995). Intrinsic fibre architecture attachments of the human epiglottis and their contributions to the mechanism of deglutition. *Journal of Anatomy, 186* (Pt. 1), 1–15.

CHAPTER 3

Examination of the Esophageal Swallow Component

LEARNING OBJECTIVES

After completing the chapter and reviewing the study questions, you should be able to:

- Describe esophageal anatomy and physiology during deglutition

- Explain neural regulation and blood supply of the esophagus

- Discuss the coordination of structures for successful deglutition

- Describe similarities and differences between the upper esophageal sphincter (UES) and lower esophageal sphincter (LES)

- Differentiate between oropharyngeal and esophageal component disturbances during deglutition.

INTRODUCTION

It may seem odd that an entire chapter is dedicated to the structures involved in the esophageal phase of swallowing–a phase that is not under volitional control or amenable to behavioral intervention strategies used by clinicians. Understanding these structures and this phase is critical, however, to identifying problems that may present as oropharyngeal dysphagia that are related to an esophageal structural or motility disorder. Up to 25% of distal esophageal lesions present with oropharyngeal symptoms (Low & Rubesin, 1993). As well, oropharyngeal and esophageal dysphagia often co-occur (Triadafilopoulos, Hallstone, Nelson-Abbott, & Bedinger, 1992). As a member of the health care team, the speech-language pathologist needs to recognize when problems in the esophageal phase need to be further explored and be fluent in the anatomy and physiology of this important phase. They should be able to identify gross problems videofluoroscopically and request that the radiologist or primary care phsyician follow up on any irregularities observed. Perhaps most critical to the hospital-based clinician, the speech pathologist must be able to differentiate between dysphagia resulting from poor oral or pharyngeal phase dynamics from problems with upper

67

esophageal sphincter opening. A thorough understanding of the timing and coordination between structures of the oropharynx and upper esophagus is essential to accurate diagnosis and treatment planning.

Like the layers of an onion, the level of esophageal detail presented can range from very basic to extremely detailed and complex. It is an amazing organ with many functional neural, lymphatic, and circulatory interconnections with organs in the abdominal cavity and elsewhere in the body. The goal of this chapter is to provide enough detail on esophageal anatomy and physiology so that the speech-language pathologist understands the function of this important structure. The informed clinician must be able to differentiate pharyngeal and esophageal symptoms, when possible, and understand the overlapping of the pharyngeal and esophageal phases. This will allow effective communication with physicians/medical personnel, and enable the clinician to make an informed referral to a gastroenterologist, when appropriate.

ESOPHAGEAL STRUCTURE

The esophagus is a *food tube* designed to move ingested material to the stomach quickly and efficiently. In adults, the esophagus is approximately 18 to 25 cm long. At rest, the esophagus is collapsed or flattened and lies behind the pulmonary and cardiac systems and anterior to the spinal vertebrae. Figure 3-1 shows the positional relationship between the trachea and esophagus. It is wider laterally than it is thick in the anterior-posterior plane (Figure 3-2). It can stretch approximately 3 cm in the lateral plane and 2 cm in the anterior-posterior plane, accommodating a large bolus when necessary. For this reason, the interior appears wrinkled, allowing for additional stretch (Figure 3-3). Its flattened rest position is designed to prevent excess air from entering the esophagus or stomach or allowing previously ingested material from traveling in a retrograde manner (back up the way it came). The esophagus runs vertically from the bottom of the posterior pharynx at the cervical vertebral level of C5–6, pierces through the diaphragm, and enters the abdominal cavity where it connects to the stomach at the thoracic T-10 vertebral level (Boyce & Boyce, Jr., 1995).

The esophagus may be divided into three relatively distinct areas related to its position along the spinal vertebrae–the cervical esophagus, the thoracic esophagus, and the abdominal esophagus. The **cervical esophagus** extends from the upper esophageal sphincter (UES) and is composed of striated muscle fibers. It measures about four to five cm long from the junction of the pharynx and esophagus to the top of the sternum (suprasternal notch). The **thoracic esophagus** forms the bulk of the esophagus and is located in the thorax or chest cavity. It runs

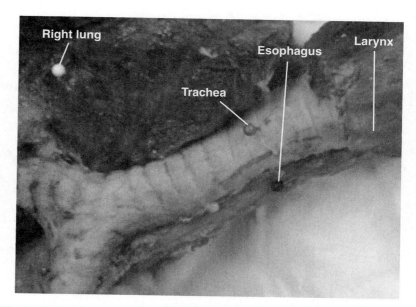

Figure 3-1. Relationship between trachea and esophagus in cervical region of the neck.

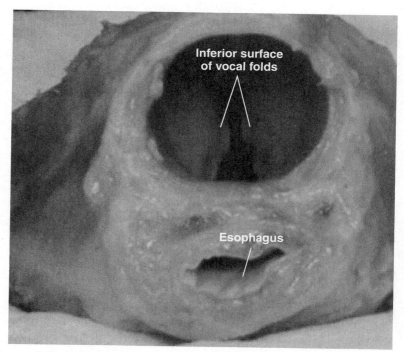

Figure 3-2. Inferior view of cross-section of trachea and esophagus just below excised larynx.

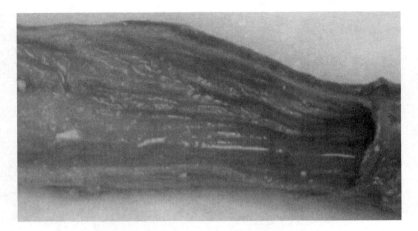

Figure 3-3. Section of interior thoracic esophagus.

behind the trachea and to the right of the aortic arch slightly off midline because of the presence of the mediastinum, the sac that houses the heart. At the level of the diaphragm (approximately thoracic vertebrae T-8) the thoracic esophagus courses anteriorly to the aorta and crosses over to the left side. The upper portion of the thoracic esophagus includes both types of esophageal muscle fibers, striated and smooth. Near the level of the tracheal bifurcation, where the right and left bronchus course to each lung, a transition zone of a few centimeters consists of mixed striated muscle fibers and smooth muscle tissue. The distal thoracic esophagus (or part farthest away from the mouth) consists of smooth muscle fibers. The **abdominal esophagus** is the short 0.5 to 2.5 cm portion that is located on the left side in the abdominal cavity after the organ has pierced the diaphragm at the T-10 level of the vertebral column. The esophagus enters the stomach, which is left of midline, at an angle. The distal abdominal esophagus terminates as the **lower esophageal sphincter** (LES) that forms the entrance into the stomach. Figure 3-4 shows examples of esophageal divisions most commonly found in the literature (Pope, 1997). The distal esophagus is the area most susceptible to motor disorders, also known as **motility disorders** (Orr, 1986).

The esophagus can be conceptualized as a valved structure. As mentioned earlier, its superiormost valve is the upper esophageal sphincter (UES), also termed the **cricopharyngeal (CP) sphincter**, or the **pharyngoesophageal (PE) segment**, that is likely composed of multiple muscle contributors (hence the various terms used across medical specialties). Generally it is agreed that the cricopharyngeus muscle, which is a major contributor to the sphincter, is a component of the inferior pharyngeal constrictor muscle. In this textbook we have chosen

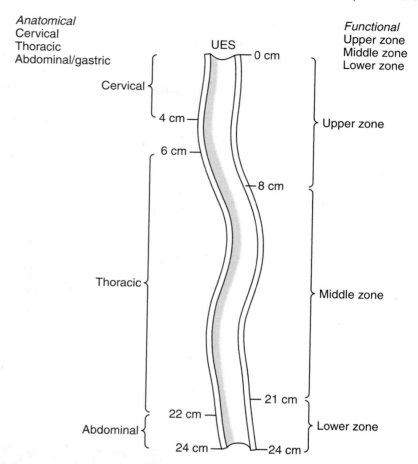

Anatomical
Cervical
Thoracic
Abdominal/gastric

Functional
Upper zone
Middle zone
Lower zone

UES

Cervical

0 cm

4 cm

6 cm

8 cm

Upper zone

Thoracic

Middle zone

21 cm

22 cm

Abdominal

Lower zone

24 cm — 24 cm

Figure 3-4. Common divisions of the esophagus (anatomical vs. functional labeled drawing).

to use the more generic term *UES* that is most often found in the medical literature. The lower esophageal sphincter (LES) acts as the valve at the top of the stomach. Both the UES and LES sphincters are tonically closed (maintenance of muscle contraction for long periods) and designed to prevent material moving in an inferior direction from refluxing into the pharynx from the esophagus or into the esophagus from the stomach. In this manner, we can think of the two sphincters as *valve-like*, though they are not true valves.

The esophagus has four tissue layers with muscle fibers arranged in different directions to facilitate bolus transport. The innermost layer (closest to the bolus traveling through the esophagus) is a thick covering of **mucosa**. This tissue is generally pinkish-gray with noticeable vascularization from the UES to the LES. At the LES, the mucosa makes an abrupt change to a deep reddish orange color without visible vascularization.

Deep to the mucosa is a **lamina propria** (similar to that found in the vocal folds) consisting of connective tissue and mucous-secreting glands, followed by **muscular mucosa** and a **submucosa** (Boyce & Boyce, Jr., 1995). In addition to mucous secretion that can aid in bolus transport, the esophageal glands also produce bicarbonate ions that can neutralize gastric acid if, and when, reflux occurs.

The depth or thickness of mucosal tissue in the esophagus has a protective function against abrasion injuries. The muscular layers deep to the mucosa have circular fibers first, with the outermost layer consisting of longitudinal fibers. On cross-section, the various layers from mucosa to muscle can be visualized (Figure 3-5).

Muscle fiber types vary in the esophagus (see Table 3-1). In the top third of the esophagus, the muscle fibers are striated (the fiber type of voluntary muscle), in the middle third the fibers are mixed (striated and smooth) and in the lower third the fibers are smooth muscle tissue similar to the remaining tissue of the digestive tract. Understanding the location of fiber-type change within the esophagus is important when examining physiological function in normal and disordered swallowing since neurologic control differs in distal and proximal parts, in part, based on the muscle fiber types. It is interesting to note that the upper striated portion differs from skeletal muscle in that it developed embryologically from the caudal branchial arches and not **somites** (as did limb musculature). It also differs histologically from other striated muscles by having different types of motor end plates, different fiber

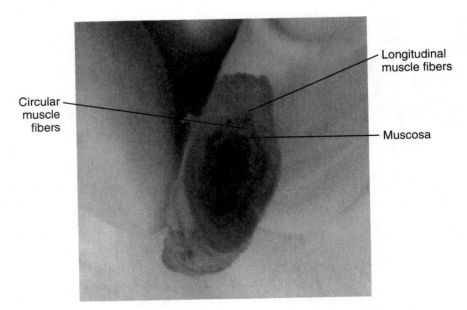

Figure 3-5. Mucosa and muscle layers of esophagus on cross-section.

Table 3-1. Human muscle fiber types.

FIBER TYPE	DEFINITION	DESCRIPTION AND LOCATION
Striated	*Striped* fiber appearance due to myofilament overlapping	Voluntary or skeletal muscle tissues, i.e., arms, legs
Smooth	Contractile fibers with spindle-shaped cells without visible striations	Involuntary muscle of internal organs, blood vessels, and hair follicles
Cardiac	Specific connecting transverse striated muscle fibers	Specialized to the heart or myocardium

diameters, and a different type of metabolic component (**myosin ATPase**). This is understandable given the very specific function of efficiently moving material through the esophagus.

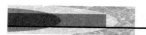# ESOPHAGEAL INNERVATION

The amazingly complex gastrointestinal tract has different control systems operating at various levels along the digestive tract to accomplish **peristalsis,** or the sequential, phasic muscle contractions that carry the food bolus from the oral cavity to the stomach. This highly coordinated movement includes the proximal contraction of muscle fibers with concurrent distal relaxation of muscle fibers that allow efficient progress of the bolus to the stomach. Peristaltic waves can be further subdivided into **primary, secondary,** and **tertiary peristaltic waves.** Primary waves are initiated by a pharyngeal swallow while secondary waves are normal peristaltic waves that are not initiated by a swallow. Secondary waves may result from the distention and localized pressure of a partial bolus within the esophagus (Biancani & Behar, 1995). Tertiary waves, most often seen in older individuals, are defined as contractions that occur in the body of the esophagus at the same time as primary or secondary waves. Tertiary waves may occur without noticeable effect on a person or they may be of a magnitude that is experienced as dysphagia or chest pain (Orr, 1986). In younger individuals tertiary waves are often considered an abnormal finding.

The different control systems in use to regulate peristalsis are related to the differences in muscle type composition along the tract. The striated muscles of the oropharynx and cervical esophagus are controlled by the peripheral nervous system at the brainstem level. The smooth muscle fibers of the thoracic and abdominal esophagus are controlled by a specific part of the peripheral nervous system called the

enteric nervous system. The enteric system is intrinsic to the digestive tract meaning that cell bodies controlling the structures are embedded into the peripheral tract tissues. This is a unique control system that is not found in other organ systems. This intrinsic neural system controls gastrointestinal motility, blood flow, water and electrolyte transport, and acid secretion. Because of the unique nature of the enteric nervous system, it is discussed separately, in detail, below.

Peripheral Nervous System Control

The esophagus receives information from many levels of the nervous system. A quick review of nervous system divisions is provided in Table 3-2. In studying speech and language production, the nervous system is typically divided into the central nervous system (CNS) consisting of the brain and spinal cord, and the peripheral nervous system (PNS) consisting of 12 pairs of cranial nerves and 31 pairs of spinal nerves. Little attention is addressed to another part of the peripheral nervous system–the autonomic nervous system (ANS). This (predominantly) motor system innervates smooth muscle, cardiac muscle, and glands. Unlike the somatic portion of the peripheral nervous system, which can innervate a structure with one neuron running from the brain or spinal cord out to the muscle (like the hypoglossal nerve to the tongue), the autonomic system requires two neurons. The cell body for the first neuron, called a **preganglionic neuron**, is located in a motor nucleus in the CNS. Its axon synapses with a second neuron's cell body located in an **autonomic ganglion** outside of the CNS. The second neuron is called a **postganglionic neuron**. The postganglioinic (or postsynaptic neuronal axon) then goes to the organ or gland it innervates. The main difference is that there are two locations for cell bodies–one in the CNS (nucleus) and one in the PNS (autonomic ganglion). A **nucleus** is an aggregate of

Table 3-2. Nervous system divisions.

CENTRAL NERVOUS SYSTEM (CNS)	PERIPHERAL NERVOUS SYSTEM (PNS)
Brain and spinal cord	Somatic function–voluntary to striated muscle
	cranial nerves
	spinal nerves
	Autonomic function–involuntary to smooth muscle, cardiac muscle, and glands
	sympathetic nerves—increase visceral activity; *fight-or-flight*
	parasympathetic nerves—decrease visceral activity; *system equilibrium*

cell bodies located together in the central nervous system. With a few exceptions, **ganglia** are clusters of nerve cell bodies located in the peripheral nervous system (outside the CNS). This detailed explanation of the ANS is important because, as we mentioned, the esophagus has proximal striated muscle and distal smooth muscle. Autonomic function is critical for normal esophageal physiology in the distal esophagus. Sensory and motor information at the central level, within the brain, does influence and modulate the swallow sequence, as described in other chapters of this book. It is the **autonomic division** of the peripheral nervous system that interacts with the enteric nervous system—specifically nerve fibers from the **parasympathetic** and **sympathetic** divisions (see ANS, Clinical Note 3-1). The cell bodies of these fibers are located in the dorsal motor nucleus of the vagus in the brainstem. Motor parasympathetic fibers are carried by the vagus nerve (CN X) and play the largest regulatory role by increasing secretory activity and motility of the gastrointestinal tract. Gastrointestinal activity is highest during times of normal bodily function, not while in a *fight-or-flight* stress situation; hence, the parasympathetic system is hard at work most often. These preganglionic parasympathetic fibers traveling to the esophagus end in ganglia within the esophageal wall.

CLINICAL NOTE 3-1

Function of ANS Divisions

The autonomic nervous system is the great regulator of internal organ systems such as the heart, smooth muscles, and glands. The digestive tract is one system that consists of smooth muscle. A general rule of thumb to remember autonomic nervous system function is that sympathetic function is usually to increase activity (*fight-or-flight* response) while parasympathetic function decreases or calms activity and brings organ systems back into equilibrium. The visceral organs that are innervated by the autonomic nervous system include salivary glands, esophagus, stomach, intestinal tract, lungs, heart, kidneys, bladder, and blood vessels.

The **vagus nerve** (CN X) plays a substantial role in nervous system influence on the esophageal phase. A few of the sensory and motor branches of this nerve, related to pharyngeal and laryngeal sensation, velopharyngeal function, and voice production, are familiar to speech-language pathologists. Recall that the sensory division of the pharyngeal branch of the vagus nerve is responsible for sensation to the mucous membrane of the soft palate, tonsils, and pharynx. The pharyngeal branch supplies motor function to the muscles of the soft palate (except for the tensor veli palatini). Motor function to the larynx is supplied by the external branch of the superior laryngeal nerve to the cricothyroid muscle and the recurrent laryngeal nerve to all intrinsic laryngeal muscles excluding the cricothyroid muscle. The recurrent laryngeal nerve is also responsible for sensation from the vocal folds and subglottic larynx. The internal branch of the superior laryngeal nerve carries sensory information from the larynx and epiglottis, however, the vagus is much larger with 13 main branches. A complete listing is provided in Table 3-3 and a detailed listing of its regulatory role is provided in Clinical Note 3–2. The vagus has a large representation in the brainstem related to its many sensory and motor functions. As you may recall from your general anatomy course, there are three main nuclei that have a large number of vagal cell bodies–the **dorsal motor nucleus**, the nucleus tractus solitarius (which receives sensory information from the facial, glossopharyngeal, and vagus nerves [CN VII, IX, and X]), and the nucleus ambiguus (which houses motor nuclei to the glossopharyngeal, vagus, and spinal accessory nerves [CN IX, X, and XI]).

Table 3-3. Vagus nerve branches.

NERVE BRANCH	SUBDIVISION
Meningeal	
Auricular	
Pharyngeal	
Superior cervical cardiac	
Carotid body	
Superior laryngeal	Internal laryngeal External laryngeal
Inferior cervical cardiac	
Recurrent laryngeal	Tracheal Esophageal Inferior laryngeal
Thoracic cardiac	Bronchial
Esophageal plexus	
Anterior vagal trunk	Gastric Hepatic
Posterior vagal trunk	Celiac Gastric

CLINICAL NOTE

3-2

Vagus Nerve (Cranial Nerve)

The vagus nerve, in its long and circuitous route, serves many types of muscles and organs. Even though speech-language pathologists concentrate on its motor function, the vagus is predominately (90%) a sensory nerve (Bhatnagar & Andy, 1995). This important nerve has fibers that can be classified into four main functional types. **General visceral afferent** (GVA) fibers carry sensory information from the muscles of the pharynx, larynx, chest cavity, and abdomen to the nucleus solitarius in the brainstem. **General visceral efferent (GVE) fibers** originate in the dorsal motor nuclei of the upper brainstem and provide motor commands to the esophagus, intestinal tract, respiratory system, and cardiac system. **Special visceral afferent (SVA) fibers** carry taste information from the pharynx and epiglottis to the nucleus solitarius in the medulla. **Special visceral efferent (SVE) fibers**, from the nucleus ambiguus in the medulla, provide motor commands to the muscles of the soft palate, pharynx, and larynx for resonation, phonation, and swallow (Bhatnagar & Andy, 1995).

The cervical esophagus is innervated by the recurrent laryngeal nerve, the same nerve that supplies motor function to the intrinsic laryngeal muscles for voice production. The fact that airway protection and control of the UES-relaxation during swallow are served by the same nerve makes sense functionally. This neural arrangement allows for a high level of coordination to prevent refluxed material from entering the airway (see the esophagoglottal closure reflex, Clinical Note 3-3). Unfortunately, damage to this single nerve, which serves multiple functions, can have the devastating results of dysphagia, dysphonia, and weakened airway protection.

CLINICAL NOTE

3-3

Esophagoglottal Closure Reflex

Distention of the proximal portion of the esophagus results in reflex closure of the vocal folds, termed the esophagoglottal closure reflex. This reflex is thought to act as an airway protection reflex from reflux material (Shaker & Lang, 1997; Shaker, et al., 1992).

The right and left branches of the vagus nerve intermingle with sympathetic fibers to form the **esophageal plexus.** Inferior to this plexus but still above the diaphragm, the main vagal nerve trunks consist of an **anterior vagal trunk** (left) and a **posterior vagal trunk** (previously the right vagus). After they pierce the diaphragm, the anterior (or left) vagal trunk divides into **anterior gastric branches** to supply the stomach and a **hepatic branch** to supply the liver. The posterior (or right) vagal trunk divides in a similar manner to become the **posterior gastric branches** and a branch to the **celiac plexus**, a very large neural plexus responsible for the abdominal viscera (Boyce & Boyce, Jr., 1995). Sympathetic fibers arising from multiple nerve groups (superior cervical ganglion, sympathetic chain, major splanchnic nerve, thoracic aortic plexus, and celiac ganglion) have an inhibitory effect and are primarily responsible for sphincter relaxation (inhibition of muscle contraction) during bolus transport.

Enteric Nervous System Regulation

The term enteric comes from the Greek word **enteron** meaning intestine or bowels. The enteric neural system, then, is the nervous system of the intestines. These nerves are located within the walls of the esophagus and intestinal tract. In the esophageal portion of the tract the nerves reside between the layers of the longitudinal and circular muscles. This coalescing of nerve fibers, or plexus, is called **Auerbach's plexus**. Another plexus, **Meissner's plexus**, is located in the submucosa of the esophagus. This arrangement allows reflexes, such as secondary peristaltic waves, to be mediated locally, independent of the central nervous system (Conklin & Christensen, 1994). This is not to say, however, that the central nervous system does not play a role in regulation of the esophagus and intestinal tract. While capable of working independently, central control or influence is often part of digestive function (Diamant, 1997). The enteric system sends information to the CNS by way of different ganglia–the **celiac ganglia** and **adrenergic ganglia** in the thoracic sympathetic chain (Furness & Bornstein, 1995).

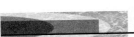

ESOPHAGEAL BLOOD SUPPLY

Blood supply to the esophagus is largely segmental–that is, with little overlap or compensatory supply from other arterial sources. The cervical esophagus is served primarily by branches of the **inferior thyroid artery**. The thoracic esophagus receives blood from branches of the **aorta, right intercostal**, and **bronchial** arteries. Branches of the **left gastric, short gastric**, and **left inferior phrenic** arteries supply the abdominal esophagus. A view of the arterial blood supply can be seen in Figure 3-6.

Venous drainage consists of numerous levels leading from the surface or mucosal level through the esophageal tissues finally reaching large veins. It is easiest visualized as steps leading down or away from the digestive organs–at first, rather fine and narrow vessels or tributaries, gradually growing larger.

Intraepithelial channels lead to a **subepithelial superficial plexus** or communicating network. This plexus leads to **deep intrinsic**

Figure 3-6. Arterial blood supply to the esophagus.

Cervical esophagus supplied by:

      ↳ Branches of inferior thyroid artery with possible assistance from:

            ↳ Common carotid, subclavian, vertebral, ascending pharyngeal arteries

Thoracic esophagus supplied by:

      ↳ Branches of the aorta, right intercostals, bronchial arteries

Abdominal esophagus supplied by:

      ↳ Branches of the left gastric, short gastric, left inferior phrenic arteries

Blood supply to the esophagus is primarily segmental with minimal overlap—few vessels serve more than one esophageal region. (Based on Boyce & Boyce, Jr. 1995.)

veins in the submucosa. From deep intrinsic veins the blood drains to **adventitial veins.** In the cervical esophagus the adventitial veins empty into the **inferior thyroid vein, deep cervical vein, vertebral vein,** and **peritracheal venous plexus.** In the thoracic esophagus the adventitial veins empty into the right **azygous vein** and the left **hemiazygous** or **intercostal veins.** Drainage is different at the **esophagogastric junction.** Superficial venous plexuses and deep intrinsic veins drain to gastric vessels. At this level of the gastroesophageal junction portal, systemic circulation handles blood return from the esophagus, diaphragm, stomach, pancreas, spleen, and retroperitoneum (area behind the stomach cavity). Figure 3-7

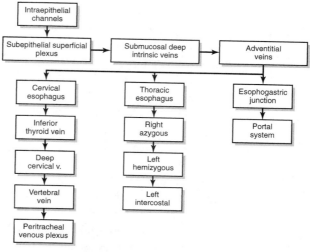

Diagram demonstrates the common shared drainage along the esophagus (Based on Boyce & Boyce, Jr. 1995).

Figure 3–7. Venous drainage of the esophagus.

provides a schematic of this branching drainage pattern. Given this intermingling of blood from many organs, it is easy to understand why **metastatic disease**, the spread of cancer to other organ sites, in this region is quite frequent with devastating results. Many types of cancer cells can easily travel from one site to another through blood vessels.

The lymphatic system is very active in the region of the esophagus and stomach in the thoracic and abdominal cavities. Its job is to carry plasma proteins that have escaped from blood capillaries back into the circulatory system. **Lymphatic drainage** for the esophageal region is similar to venous drainage in that it is not segmental. The dense network of lymph vessels in the mucosa and submucosa of the esophagus are arranged with multiple interconnections between nodal chains. The vessels lay longitudinally along the outer wall of the esophagus and pierce the muscular wall to drain into **adventitial lymph nodes**. The multiple connections between drainage sites effectively link structures of the mediastinum. As with the circulatory system, this facilitates spread of esophageal cancer to other structures in the region.

ESOPHAGEAL PHYSIOLOGY

The esophagus carries material to the stomach. It also allows for retrograde movement during vomiting and burping. The physiology of the esophagus and its two sphincters is based on maintaining appropriate pressures within the muscular structure (which differ in the esophageal body compared to the sphincters) along with carefully timed peristaltic waves to carry material to the stomach. Peristalsis is the systematic squeezing of the muscle segment behind the bolus with simultaneous relaxation of the segment preceding the bolus. The result of this is sometimes referred to as a *stripping action* within the pharynx and esophagus. It is easily visualized as the movement seen when a snake swallows a rodent. Muscle contraction behind the *meal* propels the bolus to the stomach (Biancani & Behar, 1995). This movement can also be described in terms of pressure differences behind and in front of the bolus (refer to Chapter 2 for a description of pressure differentials in the upper alimentary tract during swallowing). The superior and anterior movement of the hyolaryngeal complex at the initiation of swallow results in negative hypopharyngeal pressure while the tongue driving pressure creates a significant positive pressure behind the bolus. Any way you conceptualize it, the importance of intact, functional musculature in the oral and pharyngeal cavities is apparent. Adequate tongue driving pressure is essential to bolus propulsion. As you may expect, the opening and closing of the UES and LES sphincters must be carefully timed for an effective swallow.

Equally important, efficient bolus clearance from the pharynx into the esophagus is influenced by the initial propulsive force of the bolus by the tongue during the oral phase of deglutition to initiate the primary (or first) peristaltic wave (Biancani & Behar, 1995; Kahrilas, 1997). Once through the UES, the bolus is influenced by both gravity and peristaltic movement. The role gravity plays depends on the type of bolus and the position of the person. In the upright position, liquids require less peristaltic assistance to reach the LES while a solid bolus requires more. Liquid boluses actually reach the LES before it opens and must wait for the peristaltic wave to catch up prior to being pushed through the opening. A wet swallow (bolus of water) differs from a dry swallow (or saliva swallow) by eliciting a longer duration of UES opening and a peristaltic wave with greater amplitude (Dodds, Hogan, Reid, Stewart, & Arndorfer, 1973). A solid bolus often assists in the opening of the relaxed LES by its own pressure as it is carried forward by the peristaltic contraction. If any material is left in the esophagus, a secondary peristaltic wave initiated by the enteric system (and therefore involuntary) carries the bolus down to and through the LES in order to completely clear the esophagus. This is the same mechanism by which refluxed material is cleared from the esophagus—a secondary peristaltic wave brings it back to the stomach where it belongs. The type of receptors stimulated to initiate the secondary peristalsis likely include mechanoreceptors and possibly acid or osmotic pressure receptors (Christensen, 1997). The physiology of secondary peristalsis remains a current area of research.

Upper Esophageal Sphincter

Defining the components of the UES and its neural regulation has been an ongoing problem and a controversial topic in the field of anatomy. In part, difficulties have occurred when gross dissection has identified fewer separate structures than those that have been physiologically shown to participate in sphincteric opening. For example, while it is accepted that the 1 to 2 cm wide cricopharyngeus participates in esophageal opening, physiological studies have demonstrated increased tonic closure along a 2 to 6 cm region. Obviously, there are other muscle components to the sphincter than the single cricopharyngeus muscle (Mu & Sanders, 1996). This discrepancy between morphology and physiology has had a filter-down effect on dysphagia diagnosis and management when dysphagia is attributed to problems with timing and duration of UES opening and closing. Accurate diagnosis and clinical management of UES problems continues to be challenging in current dysphagia management (see Clinical Note 3-4).

Cricopharyngeal Myotomy Outcomes

In one of the few randomized prospective studies on cricopharyngeal myotomy outcomes in post head and neck cancer tumor resection (base of tongue or supraglottal region) results indicated no difference in swallow function 6 months post surgery between those patients who received a myotomy at the time of tumor resection versus those patients who did not have a myotomy (Jacobs, et al., 1999). Cricopharyngeal opening is a complex interaction between neural control and biomechanical movements of adjacent structures that is rarely solved with a myotomy, as measured by carefully designed clinical studies.

Upper Esophageal Sphincter Anatomy and Physiology

Currently, it is widely held that the cricopharyngeal muscle, inferior constrictor muscle fibers, and the proximal esophagus contribute to sphincteric opening and closing of the UES (Lang & Shaker, 1997; Mu & Sanders, 1996). The UES is a functional term rather than one specific anatomic structure. Different from other sphincters in the body, the UES is not a fully circular ring of muscle. Rather, the cricopharyngeal and inferior constrictor fibers form a C-shape posteriorly and insert anteriorly onto the cricoid cartilage (review schematic in Figure 2–3). Figure 3-8 shows a fluorographic image highlighting the closed UES. You can see the last bolus swallowed just below the high pressure region of the UES.

The spatial arrangement of the UES fibers has clinical implications (see Zenker's diverticulum, Clinical Note 3–5). This arrangement of the UES muscle components influences how the sphincter opens. The UES is tonically contracted as indicated by constant EMG activity measured within this 2 to 6 cm region with inhibition of activity during swallow. The UES has higher measured pressure in the anterior-posterior dimension than in the lateral dimension. Relaxation of the muscle fibers is part of the swallow sequence responsible for sphincteric opening–but only part. Current thought holds that the traction placed on the sphincter by the superior and anterior movement of the hyolaryngeal complex is the most significant component of timely UES opening allowing bolus passage.

Morphology Predisposing to Zenker's Diverticulum

The arrangement of muscle fibers at the UES consists of a horizontally-placed circular loop of muscle at the top of the esophagus. Another portion consists of muscle fibers angled obliquely, attaching to the medial raphe (which runs vertically down the back of the pharynx). This positioning creates a weak triangular region in the posterior hypopharynx known as Killian's triangle. When significant pressures generated in this region during swallowing result in the outpouching, or pushing, of mucosa through this weakened area it is termed a Zenker's diverticulum. Management is usually surgical.

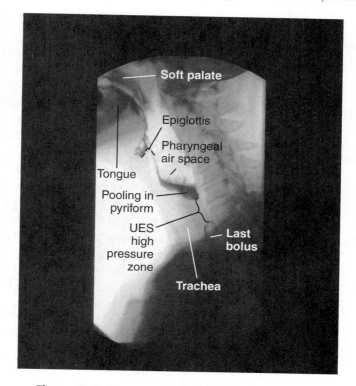

Figure 3-8. Fluoroscopic image highlighting UES.

This appreciation of the mechanical influence of the hyoid bone in pulling the UES open is critical to the speech-language pathologist. The variability of UES opening timing, amplitude, and duration, based on bolus characteristics, will be discussed in Chapter 4. Often, when bolus passage is impeded and residue is observed in the pyriform sinuses after the swallow, physicians assume that lack of adequate UES opening is a neurological concern—the primary problem that can be addressed with a cricopharyngeal myotomy. This procedure cuts the fibers of the UES and will not improve bolus transit if the actual problem is one of poor hyolaryngeal elevation. A secondary UES dysfunction, such as this, would require different management that addresses hyolaryngeal elevation. Frequently, an inappropriate myotomy results in reflux problems due to disruption of the integrity of the sphincter to prevent retrograde movement of the stomach contents toward the pharynx and the patient will be worse off than when impaired bolus clearance was the only concern.

Innervation of the Upper Esophageal Sphincter

Various nerves and nerve plexi have been attributed to the muscles that constitute the UES. As well, the pattern of nerve distribution through muscle tissue within the UES has not been defined. Recent use of newer staining techniques, which allows visualization of stained neural tissue against translucent connective and muscular tissue (Sihler's stain), has provided valuable information addressing the UES innervation pattern and specific nerve supply to the sphincteric structures.

In general, somatic nerves from the brainstem supply the striated muscles (pharyngeal and upper esophagus). Autonomic nerves supply the smooth musculature of the esophagus. Both the striated and smooth muscle of the UES are innervated by fibers of the pharyngeal plexus, primarily through somatic and autonomic branches of the vagus (CN X). The inferior pharyngeal constrictor and cricopharyngeus muscles are innervated by various components of the pharyngeal plexus. Interoperative electromyography has demonstrated that the recurrent laryngeal branch of the vagus nerve supplies these muscles in some people (Brok, et al., 1999). The esophagus receives innervation from the autonomic nervous system through branches of the vagus (CN X) and has a highly developed local circuit control system.

Lower Esophageal Sphincter

The LES opens into the stomach where the bolus is contained and digestion begins. Alternatives to oral feeding often bring nutrition directly to the stomach bypassing the esophagus and LES. See Clinical Note 3–6 for a discussion of non-oral feeding methods.

CLINICAL NOTE 3-6

The Difference Between Enteral and Parenteral Feeding

Enteral feeding methods provide nourishment directly to the gastrointestinal tract via a tube. The tube may be a nasogastric tube that travels through the nose, UES, esophagus, and LES (Figure 3–9). It may also be a tube that is placed directly into the stomach (gastrostomy) or jejunum (a part of the small intestine). The method of insertion may be surgical or, more commonly today, percutaneous (through the skin) guided by an endoscope. This procedure is called a PEG–percutaneous endoscopic gastrostomy. In Figure 3-10 the frame depicts the puncture into the stomach being viewed endoscopically; the following figure (3-11) shows the correct seating of the gastrostomy collar. The collar will be replaced approximately every six months. Subsequently, the procedure is easier when the tissue tract from the external stomach through the abdominal muscles has healed. (The procedure is similar to replacing a tracheo-esophageal voice prosthesis.)

Parenteral feedings refer to the delivery of food through some other manner than by the gastrointestinal tract–most often through intravenous (IV) injection.

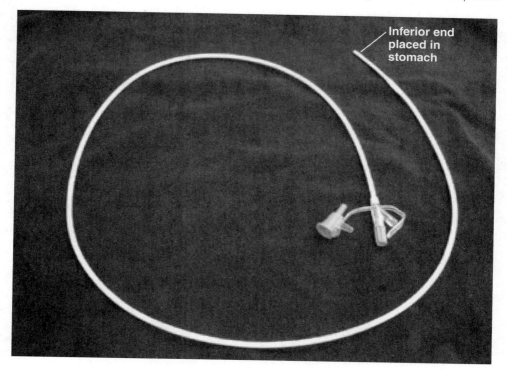

Inferior end placed in stomach

Figure 3-9. Nasogastric tube.

The LES is an important barrier to gastric contents moving in a retrograde direction with resulting damage to the mucosal lining of the esophagus. A number of comparisons between the upper and lower esophageal sphincters can be made to highlight similarities and differences between them.

Lower Esophageal Sphincter Anatomy and Physiology

First, LES morphology differs substantially from the UES. It is formed by increased thickness of the circular muscle fibers of the esophagus with a histological change in the circular muscle fibers located here. These complete rings of muscle do not insert onto cartilage as in the UES. The LES is located near or between the crural fibers of the diaphragm which may assist in closure during instances of increased pressure such as when inhaling deeply, coughing, or lifting with a closed glottis. Like the UES, it is tonically contracted in its resting state along a 3 to 5 cm high-pressure zone. Unlike the UES, this is not the result of continuous neural firing but primarily due to intrinsic characteristics of the muscle fibers (Miller, 1999). While it does not relax at the initiation

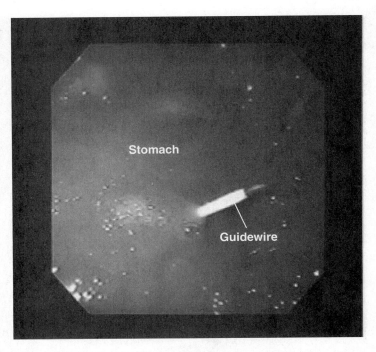

Figure 3-10. Endoscopic view of PEG insertion—guidewire. (*Courtesy of V. Duane Bohman.*)

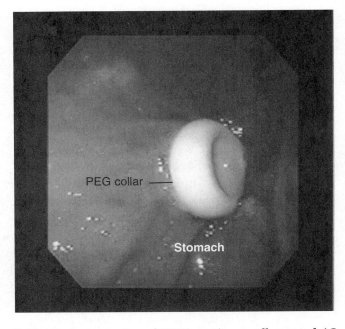

Figure 3-11. Endoscopic view of PEG insertion—collar seated. (*Courtesy of V. Duane Bohman.*)

of the swallow, it does by the time the peristaltic wave is in the mid-portion of the esophagus (in the smooth muscle region). Like the UES, the relaxed sphincter is not patent—it is closed and requires opening by an outside force. In the UES, recall that hyolaryngeal anterior and superior movement creates the opening traction. In the LES the pressure of the bolus combined with the peristaltic force opens the relaxed sphincter. It takes approximately five seconds for the LES to regain its pre-swallow pressure and is then followed by an after-contraction or rebound pressure.

The influence of bolus characteristics on the pharyngeal swallow and UES function will be addressed in the next chapter. Unlike the UES, bolus characteristics do not seem to play a significant role in regulation or modulation of LES contraction and relaxation. However, chemical composition of the bolus may influence LES function. Specific types of foods, such as fatty fried foods, have been shown to reduce LES resting pressure, predisposing an individual to gastroesophageal reflux. LES resting pressure varies depending on an individual's posture. LES pressure is higher when supine and lower when upright (Sears, Castell, & Castell, 1990). This is intuitive since the barrier between esophagus and stomach needs to be tighter when gravity is not assisting in keeping the food in the stomach, as when lying down.

 ## ESOPHAGEAL PRESSURE MEASUREMENT USING MANOMETRY

The extent to which a sphincter relaxes and contracts, and the strength of peristaltic waves, can best be described with pressure measurements. This allows for gradients of opened or closed, or amplitude of waves, to be measured and discussed. The process of measuring esophageal pressures (including at the UES and LES) is called **esophageal manometry**. Manometry is usually performed by a gastroenterologist in the clinical or hospital setting. A flexible tube with multiple pressure sensors is passed through the nose and swallowed through the UES, down the esophagus, and through the LES into the stomach. As the swallow progresses in a caudal direction, the sensors can measure the muscular forces exerted on the transducers. The amount of force at each sensor site, measured in millimeters of mercury (mm Hg) across time, is mapped for a normal swallow. More specifics about the use of this test are provided in Chapter 5, which deals with direct and indirect measures of the oropharyngeal and esophageal function.

At the UES, tonic pressure generated is higher in the anterior-posterior plane than in the lateral plane. In other words, the UES has a tighter squeeze from front to back rather than side-to-side. A number of things, including whether a person is awake or in a deep sleep, can influence the actual pressure generated at the UES. During deep sleep the UES pressure decreases. Reflux in the distal esophagus has been noted to raise the resting UES pressure. The UES has a resting pressure of approximately 50 to 60 mm Hg (Orr, 1986).

Typically, in a clinical setting, manometric measures are made with an individual in a supine (laying down) position. Normative pressure values for water swallows in this body position have been generated and are used by the gastroenterologist when evaluating and diagnosing motility disorders of the esophagus. But these norms are not appropriate comparison points for swallow function in an upright position during meal times. Currently, little is known about the effect of upright liquid and solid bolus swallows on the UES, LES, or peristalsis. Early findings indicate that in the upright posture there is a high incidence of abnormal nonperistaltic waveforms in normal individuals without reported swallowing difficulties (Sears, Castell, & Castell, 1990). Timing and duration of UES opening, based on bolus size and type, is discussed in the next chapter. Bolus characteristics also influence the amount of pressure generated at the UES (Kahrilas, Dodds, Dent, Logemann, & Shaker, 1988).

Age and Sex Effects on Esophageal Pressures

Understanding normal variation in the intraluminal esophageal pressures measured by manometry is extremely important when diagnosing disease states. We need to know what is "normal" for a given individual or a given group of individuals in order to make appropriate judgments. Two main characteristics that may significantly affect manometric values are age and sex. To date, few large-scale studies without technical limitations (due to type of transducers used, limited age range of subjects, small sample sizes) have investigated the effect of age and sex on esophageal pressures generated during motility. Preliminary evidence suggests both age and sex have a significant effect on manometric pressures of the pharynx and UES (van Herwaarden, Katz, Gideon, Barrett, Castell, Achem, & Castell, 2003). Pharyngeal contraction amplitude (measured in mmHg) was greater, and the time to reach peak pharyngeal contraction and the duration of contraction was longer in individuals over 60 years of age when compared to adults younger than 60. Resting UES pressure was found to decrease with age. The rate of UES relaxation rate in normal elderly individuals was delayed compared to young adults. When sex effects were examined, normal females had higher resting UES pressures than their male counterparts. Replication of these findings in large groups of normal individuals is necessary before interpretation is more than working hypotheses. The "take-home" message is that both age and sex may differentially affect the physiology of swallow mechanics.

SUMMARY

In this chapter we have discussed the esophageal phase of swallow in terms of the structures involved:

- UES, which mainly consists of the cricopharyngeus muscle
- The esophagus proper
- LES, which is the entrance into the stomach
- Pressures generated by the UES, esophagus, and LES

Functionally the UES is a 2 to 6 cm high-pressure zone that relaxes early in the swallow sequence. Hyolaryngeal elevation and anterior motion is equally important to its opening. The UES is innervated centrally while the esophagus is primarily controlled by the enteric nervous system. Control of peristalsis in the upper esophagus is coordinated by the brainstem swallow center while the local enteric nervous system is responsible for peristalsis in the smooth muscle portion of the esophagus. The LES relaxes when the bolus approaches the smooth muscle portion of the esophagus and returns to its pre-swallow pressure five seconds after the bolus has entered the stomach.

It is imperative that the speech-language pathologist appreciates the importance of anterior and superior motion of the hyolaryngeal complex during the pharyngeal phase on the opening of the UES at the beginning of the esophageal phase. If this motion is diminished it may result in a secondary UES dysfunction with reduced opening. While the UES is no longer tonically closed once the swallow response has been triggered it does remain shut until traction opens it. Primary UES dysfunction, where other dynamic components of the swallow response are intact, must be carefully differentiated from secondary UES dysfunction. Lack of UES relaxation needs to be documented manometrically prior to medical or surgical interventions aimed at improving UES opening to reduce dysphagia. Appreciation for the likelihood of age and sex differences in normal pressure values must be factored into diagnostic decision making.

STUDY QUESTIONS

1. Explain the physiology of the UES opening sequence.
2. Name three main divisions of blood supply to the esophagus.
3. What is the difference between primary and secondary peristalsis?
4. Provide two similarities and two differences between the anatomy and physiology of the UES and LES.

5. Respond to a physician who says to you, "We are going to schedule a cricopharyngeal myotomy on Mr. Smith. Pooling in the pyriform sinuses indicates poor UES function. By surgically opening the UES I am sure he will swallow more easily."

REFERENCES

Bhatnagar, S. C., & Andy, O. J. (1995). *Neuroscience for the study of communicative disorders*. Baltimore: Williams & Wilkins.

Biancani, P., & Behar, J. (1995). Esophageal motor function. In T. Yamada (Ed.), *Textbook of gastroenterology* (2nd ed.). Philadelphia: J. B. Lippincott.

Boyce, G. A., & Boyce, Jr., H. W. (1995). Esophagus: Anatomy and structural anomalies. In T. Yamada (Ed.), *Textbook of gastroenterology* (2nd ed.). Philadelphia: J. B. Lippincott.

Brok, H. A. J., Copper, M. P., Stroeve, R. J., Ongerboer de Visser, B. W., Venker-van Haagen, A. J., & Schouwenburg, P. F. (1999). Evidence for recurrent laryngeal nerve contribution in motor innervation of the human cricopharyngeal muscle. *The Laryngoscope, 109*(5), 705–708.

Christensen, J. (1997). Mechanisms of secondary esophageal peristalsis. *The American Journal of Medicine, 103*(5A), 44S–46S.

Conklin, J. L., & Christensen, J. (1994). Neuromuscular control of the oropharynx and esophagus in health and disease. *Annual Review of Medicine, 45*, 13–22.

Diamant, N. E. (1997). Neuromuscular mechanisms of primary peristalsis. *The American Journal of Medicine, 103*(5A), 40S–43S.

Dodds, W. J., Hogan, W. J., Reid, D. P., Stewart, E. T., & Arndorfer, R. C. (1973). A comparison between primary esophageal peristalsis following wet and dry swallows. *Journal of Applied Physiology, 35*(6), 851–857.

Furness, J.B., & Bornstein, J.C. (1995). The enteric nervous system and its extrinsic connections. In T. Yamada (Ed.), *Textbook of gastroenterology* (2nd ed.). Philadelphia: J. B. Lippincott.

Jacobs, J. R., Logemann, J., Pajak, T. F., Pauloski, B. R., Collins, S., Casiano, R. R., & Schuller, D. E. (1999). Failure of cricopharyngeal myotomy to improve dysphagia following head and neck cancer surgery. *Archives of Otolaryngology—Head and Neck Surgery, 125*(9), 942–946.

Kahrilas, P. J. (1997). Upper esophageal sphincter function during antegrade and retrograde transit. *The American Journal of Medicine, 103*(5A), 56S–60S.

Kahrilas, P. J., Dodds, W. J., Dent, J., Logemann, J. A., & Shaker, R. (1988). Upper esophageal function during deglutition. *Gastroenterology, 95*(1), 52–62.

Lang, I. M., & Shaker, R. (1997). Anatomy and physiology of the upper esophageal sphincter. *The American Journal of Medicine, 103*(5A), 50S–55S.

Low, V. H., & Rubesin, S. E. (1993). Contrast evaluation of the pharynx and esophagus. *Radiologic Clinics of North America, 31*(6), 1265–1291.

Miller, A. J. (1999). *The neuroscientific principles of swallowing and dysphagia.* San Diego, CA: Singular.

Mu, L., & Sanders, I. (1996). The innervation of the human upper esophageal sphincter. *Dysphagia, 11*(4), 234–238.

Orr, W. C. (1986). *Esophageal motility techniques and clinical applications.* Littleton: Sandhill Scientific, Inc.

Pope, II, C. E. (1997). The esophagus for the nonesophagologist. *American Journal of Medicine, 103,* 19S–22S.

Sears, V. W., Jr., Castell, J. A., & Castell, D. O. (1990). Comparison of effects of upright versus supine body position and liquid versus solid bolus on esophageal pressures in normal humans. *Digestive Diseases and Sciences, 35*(7), 857–864.

Shaker, R., Dodds, W. J., Ren, J., Hogan, W. J., & Arndorfer, R. C. (1992). Esophagoglottal closure reflex: A mechanism of airway protection. *Gastroenterology, 102*(3), 857–861.

Shaker, R., & Lang, I. M. (1997). Reflex mediated airway protective mechanism against retrograde aspiration. *American Journal of Medicine, 103*(5A), 64S–73S.

Triadafilopoulos, G., Hallstone, A., Nelson-Abbott, H., & Bedinger, K. (1992). Oropharyngeal and esophageal interrelationships in patients with nonobstructive dysphagia. *Journal of Digestive Diseases and Sciences, 37*(4), 551–557.

Van Herwaarden, M. A., Katz, P. O., Gideon, R. M., Barrett, J., Castell, J. A., Achem, S., & Castell, D. O. (2003). Are manometric parameters of the upper esophageal sphincter and pharynx affected by age and gender? *Dysphagia, 18*(3), 211–217.

CHAPTER 4

Control of
the Normal Swallow

LEARNING OBJECTIVES

After completing the chapter and reviewing the study questions, you should be able to:

- Appreciate the limitations and benefits of a stage-model of swallowing

- Define the term *motor equivalence* and appreciate its importance to swallow physiology

- Understand the physiologic differences in swallow function between single bolus ingestion and meal-time eating

- List the bolus characteristics that may influence swallow physiology

- List the swallower characteristics that may influence swallow physiology.

INTRODUCTION

The systematic study of swallowing disorders is a relatively new endeavor that has been driven largely by the entry of speech-language pathology into dysphagia diagnosis and treatment. Because this research is in its infancy, we need to appreciate the fact that our understanding of dysphagia and normal swallowing is in a state of constant revision. As practicing dysphagia clinicians, we must be sensitive to the evolutionary nature of our field and poised to incorporate the most recent information into our daily practice. Even as the chapters of this book are written, new research will prove and disprove the information contained herein. It is the responsibility of the clinician to be vigilant in revising his or her knowledge base as the progression of the field of dysphagia continues to unfold.

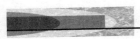

MODELING SWALLOWING AND DYSPHAGIA

The purpose of this chapter is to provide a current and complete conceptualization of normal swallowing. It may surprise you that we must begin by scrutinizing the very framework that we used to organize the first three chapters of this book: the four-phase model of deglutition physiology. Almost 150 years after the French scientist, Magendie, described an oral-pharyngeal-esophageal model of swallowing (Magendie, 1836), Logemann published an expansion of this model in her classic text (Logemann, 1983). This model subdivides the oral phase into preparatory and transport components to capture the two distinct functions of this phase. The heuristic and intuitive appeal of this model was (and is) so profound, that it became the organizational scheme for the diagnosis and treatment of dysphagia and for the exploration of normal deglutition. But, models, by their very nature, are imperfect, and the four-phase model of deglutition is no exception. Indeed, Robbins and her colleagues stated that "The division of oropharyngeal swallowing into stages is an artificial conceptualization of a functionally integrated and dynamic system" (Robbins, Hamilton, Lof, & Kempster, 1992). The artificial boundaries of the phases are neither recognized nor obeyed by the nervous system. Perhaps more perilous, the model does not accommodate all we know about the variation that occurs in the course of normal, meal-time eating and drinking. This variation is due to, minimally, three interrelated factors: **motor equivalence, bolus characteristics**, and individual **swallower variables**. We do not mean to suggest that we abandon the four-phase model. It remains a useful organizational scheme. However, we must recognize its limitations and refine it as we continue to discover the complexity of the unified physiologic activity that is swallowing.

Motor Equivalence

As a point of historical fact, swallowing has been viewed as a relatively rigid and fixed motor activity, mediated primarily by lower-level neural reflexes and control centers. Because of this, scientists have devoted energy to discovering the immutable or stable components of the swallow. They have attempted to find patterns of muscle activation and structural synergies that characterize the classic divisions of the swallow. Results to date suggest that some aspects of the swallow are more stable than others across people and swallowing conditions. These stable aspects are thought to be controlled by lower brain regions that are mediated by central pattern generators located mainly in the brainstem. However, even these relatively stable aspects have been shown to vary in form, either by peripheral sensory input or by input from higher brain regions (see, for example, Gay, Rendell, & Spiro, 1994; & Kendall, Leonard, & McKenzie, 2003). Therefore, it appears that many of the swallow components are rather *softly assembled*, allowing for great flexibility of function.

Flexibility in motor function is a highly adaptive and positive developmental phenomenon. Any motor goal can be accomplished in a multitude of different ways depending on the number and combination of joints and muscles available to move the relevant structures. This ability is commonly referred to in the motor control literature as motor equivalence. We alluded to the notion of motor equivalence in deglutition several times throughout the first three chapters of this book. For example, recall that chewing involves the rhythmic, rotary opening and closing of the jaw. The movement itself is quite stereotyped. However, when all of the muscles responsible for this movement are sampled, only the masseter shows fairly predictable activation patterns over cycles of chewing. This means that the other muscles act in concert with the masseter to accomplish the goal but that there are relatively loose constraints on how the nervous system activates them to get the job done. As a result, though the effectors may be the same, there is no immutable pattern of coordinative behavior for the muscles across (or even within) individuals. The benefit of motor equivalence in any motor system is the ability to accommodate perturbations or variations in ambient conditions. This is especially important because of the variety of food and liquid we enjoy and the circumstances under which we enjoy them. Table 4-1 summarizes the muscles that contribute to the various goals of the swallow mechanism.

A number of investigations have attempted to uncover the flexibility of the swallow mechanism by evaluating function during nondiscrete tasks such as *normal eating* or *sequential swallowing* from a cup. Dua, et al. (1997) used videoendoscopic and videofluoroscopic studies of fifteen subjects during a session of *normal mealtime eating*. They documented a number of events that challenged the facts derived from studies of discrete swallows. First, 76% of solid bolus and 60% of liquid bolus swallows were preceded by the bolus dwelling in the pharynx before the onset of the swallow response. That is to say, the bolus entered and remained in the pharynx during the oral phase of deglutition in the majority of cases. Such a finding among healthy adults is at odds with common clinical practice that regards entry of the bolus into the pharynx prior to the pharyngeal swallow response as potentially pathological. Second, the entry of the bolus into the pharynx was associated with partial adduction of the vocal folds, again occurring during the oral phase. This observation supports the existence of a pharyngoglottic closure reflex (Flaherty, Seltzer, Campbell, Weisskoff, & Gilbert, 1995; Ren, et al., 1994) in which the entry of material into the pharynx

Table 4-1. Muscle activity related to deglutition events.

SWALLOW ACTIVITY	MUSCLE	ACTION	INNERVATION
Bolus containment	Orbicularis oris (superior and inferior) Incisivus labii (superior and inferior)	Provide anterior seal of lips, especially for larger boluses; highly active during straw suck	VII
Bolus control	Buccinator Risorius	Provide cheek tension to keep bolus between occlusal surfaces of the teeth; reduce area of lateral sulci	VII
	Genioglossus Intrinsic tongue muscles	Anterior depression of tongue tip; creation of midline depression or channel	XII
Mastication	Masseter Medial pterygoid Temporalis	Raise mandible	V
	Lateral pterygoid Anterior belly digastric	Lower mandible	V
	Geniohyoid, mylohyoid	Lower mandible	XII
	Levator anguli oris Depressor anguli oris Levator labii superioris Depressor labii inferioris Zygomaticus Mentalis	Collectively move lips in coordination with jaw and tongue during chewing	VII
Oral bolus propulsion	Orbicularis oris (superior and inferior)	Press lips together and obliterate anterior labial sulcus during onset of bolus transport	VII
	Buccinator	Tense cheeks and obliterate lateral sulci during onset of bolus transport	V
	Intrinsic lingual muscles Genioglossus	Create channel in midline of tongue; progressive and sequential pressing of tongue against palate	XII
Velopharyngeal closure	Levator veli palatini Musculus uvulae	Elevate velum	X
	Tensor veli palatini	Tense anterior velum and open auditory tube	V

(continued)

Table 4-1. (*continued*)

SWALLOW ACTIVITY	MUSCLE	ACTION	INNERVATION
	Superior constrictor Horizontal fibers of palatopharyngeus	Move lateral pharyngeal walls medially; create Passavant's pad on posterior pharyngeal wall	IX, X
	Palatoglossus	Perhaps provide initial anterior depression of velum as *set up* response	IX, X
Hyolaryngeal elevation	Mylohyoid Geniohyoid Cervical plexus Anterior belly digastric	Elevate and anteriorly displace hyoid	XII
		V	
Laryngeal protection	Interarytenoids Lateral cricoarytenoid Thyroarytenoid	Adduct vocal folds	X
	Thyrohyoid Aryepiglottic(?)	Invert epiglottis	
Pharyngeal elevation and constriction	Superior, middle, and inferior constrictors, stylopharyngeus, salpingopharyngeus	Progressive contraction and elevation of pharynx	X IX, X X

triggers reflexive glottic closure; however, it is not easily resolved with the traditional view that glottal closure is linked with hyolaryngeal elevation. Third, vocal fold adduction almost always preceded submental muscle activity in these subjects. The activation of submental muscles is traditionally thought to be part of the *leading complex* of the swallow response as it occurs first in discrete swallows. Finally, this investigation found that the most common trigger site for the swallow response was the epiglottis. Subjects showed much variation in this regard, however, and the authors concluded that, "the summation of the afferent signals for the entire oropharyngeal sensory field will determine the onset of the spontaneous swallow" (Dua, et al., 1997, p. 80).

Similar findings were reported in a more recent study which showed that the dynamics of a single swallow cannot be extended to multiple swallows in straw drinking. Daniels and Foundas (2001) reported that multiple swallows over a 10-second interval revealed that the swallow response was triggered from multiple sites in the pharynx, including the valleculae, the epiglottis, and the pyriform sinuses. Further, they described three different patterns of hyolaryngeal movement. Type I movement was defined as repetitive swallows where the epiglottis returned to its upright position and the laryngeal vestibule opened following each swallow. Type II hyolaryngeal movement consisted of a continuously inverted epiglottis and closed laryngeal vestibule between consecutive swallows. Type III movement was classified as a combination of Type I and II patterns within the same individual during the 10-second straw drinking task. During this study, the investigators found that bolus material collected in the pharynx, often at the level of the pyriform sinuses, prior to swallow initiation in these healthy young-adult men. While data are preliminary with a small sample size, we can conclude that there is far more flexibility within and among individuals in how a swallow is performed. This is further supported by studies that have identified bolus aggregation in the pharynx during solid bolus swallows in normal healthy adults (Palmer, Rudin, Lara, & Crompton, 1992; Hiiemae & Palmer, 1999; Palmer, 1998) and by EMG and EEG studies that show differences in muscle activation patterns depending on swallow task (Ding, Larson, Logemann, & Radmaker, 2002).

Although these studies highlight the flexibility of the swallow mechanism, a study of sequential swallowing revealed that tongue activity during posterior propulsion of the bolus is among the more stable components of swallowing. Chi-Fishman and her colleagues reported distinct similarities between lingual action in normal discrete swallows and in sequential swallowing as subjects drank continuously from a cup (Chi-Fishman, Stone, & McCall, 1998). Despite the task differences and variations in bolus size, the lingual movement pattern was simple and invariant: the tongue raised sequentially from front to back in posterior propulsion of the bolus. Only the timing of the movement components differed between the two tasks, suggesting that lingual control has variant as well as invariant components.

In contrast, the differences in other swallowing parameters in discrete versus sequential swallowing are much more profound. Chi-Fishman and Sonies (2000) reported great variability in standard duration measures of oral and pharyngeal events between tasks and among individuals. The most stunning differences are those that challenge our classic understanding of the airway protection mechanism. Recall that studies of discrete swallows described the pharyngeal phase as fixed and involuntary, and triggered by the presence of the bolus, particularly in the area of the anterior faucial pillars. This stimulation was thought to mandate an involuntary sequence of events for airway protection: closure of the true and false vocal folds, elevation of the larynx, and inversion of the epiglottis over the laryngeal aditus. Chi-Fishman and Sonies found that this was not the case for sequential swallowing. The bolus frequently accumulated deep in the pharynx before the swallow response was initiated and, although the entryway to the airway was closed, the larynx did not completely elevate. Moreover, 30% of their subjects evidenced penetration of the bolus into the laryngeal vestibule, which cleared when the sequential swallowing was complete. This reinforces the suggestion of previous reports that laryngeal penetration and expulsion occurs regularly and without consequence in normal subjects. These important differences between discrete and sequential swallows reveal that the components of the pharyngeal phase of the normal swallow are not as hard-wired as we previously believed (also see Kendall, et al., 2003). The pharyngeal phase is not truly *involuntary* because it can be influenced by cortical messages associated with volitional swallow maneuvers. Thus, just as with the oral phase, the construct of motor equivalence must be recognized as operative in the pharyngeal phase of the swallow.

Studies such as these demonstrate the flexibility of control in swallowing and how the tenets of the four-phase model must be viewed in the appropriate context. Although there may be some hard-wired (invariant) components such as the pharyngoglottal closure reflex, the majority of components combine to achieve goals in a variety of ways, necessarily infringing on the boundaries of the four-phase model. In the next section, we will see how the characteristics of the bolus play into this complex equation.

Bolus Characteristics

Much of what we know about the four-phase model of swallowing has been gleaned from the observation of discrete swallows of barium material on videofluoroscopic examination. Recently, Kendall and her colleagues published a series of studies on the timing of events in normal swallowing and structural displacements associated with the discrete swallows of liquid barium (Kendall, McKenzie, Leonard, Goncalves, & Walker, 2000; Leonard, Kendall, McKenzie, Goncalves, & Walker, 2000; Kendall, et al., 2003). Their data support and extend previous reports and offer a normal basis of comparison for the diagnosis of dysphagia. Moreover, their study represents one of a growing number of investigations on how bolus characteristics influence swallow parameters. Referring to our discussion of motor equivalence, the normal swallow mechanism must be able to accommodate food that varies along a number of continua:

1. Bolus volume (size)
2. Consistency/viscosity
3. Temperature
4. Taste

Table 4-2 summarizes the current literature on how these bolus characteristics influence the pattern of normal swallowing. Keep in mind that these findings relate to isolated, discrete swallows.

Table 4-2. Effects of various bolus characteristics on swallowing.

VARIABLE	SUMMARY OF CURRENT FINDINGS
Bolus size (volume)	*Increase in bolus size is associated with:* • Decrease in oral and pharyngeal transit times • Earlier onset of anterior tongue base movement • Earlier onset and longer duration of palatal elevation • Earlier elevation of hyolaryngeal complex • Earlier UES opening and increase in both the duration and diameter of UES opening • Earlier elevation of the aryepiglottic folds • Longer swallowing apnea duration • Greater reconfiguration of the oral cavity and pharynx to accommodate the larger bolus • Higher lingual and pharyngeal propulsive pressures such that the expulsion of a large bolus takes the same amount of time as the expulsion of a smaller bolus (0.13 seconds) • Increase in thyroarytenoid contraction duration • Greater extent of hyoid elevation
Consistency/Viscosity	*Solid or semisolid bolus (as compared to liquid) results in:* • Longer stage transition durations • Longer duration of velar excursion • Longer pharyngeal transit duration • Shorter duration of UES opening • Food traveling in a single column through the pharynx down over the midline of the larynx during normal eating (does not split as does a liquid bolus) *Higher viscosity results in:* • Longer duration of pharyngeal contraction waves • Increase in the number of multiple swallows to clear bolus from mouth and pharynx • Increased oral and pharyngeal transit time (potentially) • Increased lingual force needed to initiate bolus transport and driving pressure
Temperature	• Contradictory evidence that cold affects timing of pharyngeal swallow response when it is applied to the anterior faucial pillars; it may quicken the response of subsequent swallows
Taste	• Sour bolus may enhance oral phase components in neurogenically dysphagic patients; its effect in normals is not established

(Information summarized from Chi-Fishman & Sonies, 2002; Dantas, Kern, Massey, et al., 1990; Ergun, Kahrilas, Lin, et al., 1993; Ertekin, Phelivan, et al., 1995; Hamlet, Choi, Zormeier, et al., 1996; Hiiemae & Palmer, 1999; Hiss, Treole, & Stuart, 2001; Kahrilas, Lin, Chen, & Logemann, 1996; Logemann, Pauloski, Colangelo, et al., 1995; Miller & Watkins, 1996; Perlman, VanDaele, & Otterbacker, 1995).

In general, a large bolus is associated with structures moving earlier and faster and traveling greater distances than is a smaller bolus. Swallowing a solid or semi-solid bolus is associated with longer latencies of swallow parameters, except for the duration of UES opening which is of a shorter duration than for liquid swallows. Material of high viscosity also increases latencies of swallow parameters and it is associated with higher propulsive forces than low viscosity material. The effects of variation in temperature and taste on swallowing are much less well understood. There is some evidence that application of cold to the anterior faucial pillars may enhance the pharyngeal swallow response, but this remains hypothetical. Insofar as a sour bolus increases salivary flow, there may be benefits to both oral and pharyngeal phase components, but this has not yet been studied systematically in healthy individuals.

The assessment of the effects of bolus characteristics on deglutition patterns further reveals the flexibility and *soft assembly* of the swallow physiology. This allows one to successfully process and ingest materials that vary along a continuum of dimensions without sacrificing airway protection. The final component of this neural control equation lies in characteristics of the person doing the eating. This is addressed in our next section.

Swallower Variables

The variables of age, sex, size, oro-pharyngeal-laryngeal morphology, and idiosyncratic motor control strategies surely contribute to individual variation in swallow patterns. Because these variables are so highly interrelated, it is difficult to study them separately. For example, men and their swallowing structures tend to be larger than women, thereby blurring the variables of sex and size. However, a growing number of studies have included observations about swallower variables. Of these, age has received the greatest attention to help clinicians discern between the pathology of dysphagia and the normal consequences of aging.

Aging is a complicated process, determined not only by the passage of years, but by genetic makeup and environmental factors. Despite wide variations in the physical manifestations of aging, some general principles of change apply to us all. Tissues that were once thin and supple tend to become thicker and harder. Tissue elasticity reduces over time and fat and connective tissue replace space once occupied by muscle. Sensory receptors reduce in number and change in morphology. Both sensory and motor nerve fibers exhibit slowed conduction velocities. Thus, the end result is a slowing and reduction in accuracy of motor performance and decreased acuity in the perception of sensory stimulation.

How do these general changes manifest in the swallowing mechanism? First, there are progressive changes in the oral environment. The oral mucosa becomes more **keratinized**. The tongue becomes smoother with atrophy of filiform and fungiform papillae. Although salivary secretion remains remarkably unchanged in the healthy aging individual, medication and diseases associated with aging frequently result in decreases in the amount and quality of salivary flow (Baum, 1989; Shipp, Pillemer, & Baum, 2002). There may be a loss or shift of dentition, along with commensurate changes in jaw and maxillary bone configuration. The temporomandibular joint (TMJ) may show degradation or reduced range of movement. There is a decrease in overall oral/pharyngeal/laryngeal sensation, as well as a decrease in the special sense of taste. The larynx, which continues to descend in the pharynx with age, becomes increasingly calcified and its mucosal surfaces become drier and less compliant.

Although not all studies have shown profound differences between young and elderly subjects, most report reductions in swallow efficiency. These changes are summarized in Table 4-3. As you examine this table, keep in mind that these changes are not severe enough to be classified as pathologic. Even though there is slowness, weakness, and decreased efficiency, swallowing usually occurs safely and without incident. However, nearly all of the age-related changes listed in this table are ones we associate with dysphagia. One can imagine that it would take very little impairment of the nervous system to create decompensation and, hence, dysphagia in an elderly person.

CLINICAL NOTE 4-1

Aging Versus Pathology

Normal aging results in many deglutition differences that, in the context of pathology, could be labeled as dysphagia. However, Kendall and Leonard (2001) reviewed over 1300 videofluorographic swallow studies on patients over 65 years of age and discovered that dysphagic patients, but not normal elderly controls, exhibited pharyngeal weakness. The implication is that, at least with respect to pharyngeal contraction, aging alone does not predispose one to develop a dysphagia. Instead, other etiological factors must come into play.

Although only a few studies have been devoted to identifying the effects of sex differences on swallowing patterns, the results have not been overwhelming. Most of the findings (Figure 4-1) appear to be traceable to differences in size, with men generally being larger than women. In studies that have examined bolus and task variables simultaneously, very few sex interactions were discovered.

Table 4-3. Effects of aging on various deglutition parameters.

AGING	SUMMARY OF CURRENT FINDINGS
Oral phases	• Slowing and decreased efficiency of tongue movement • Reduced strength of masticatory muscles • Increased oral transit times • Bolus positioned more posteriorly in the oral cavity • Decreased suction pressures through straw with repetitive swallows; while swallow pressures remain similar over the lifespan, stamina declines
Pharyngeal phase	• Swallow response triggered low in pharynx • Larger bolus volumes required to trigger pharyngeal swallow • Rate of spontaneous swallowing is less frequent • Delayed anterior hyoid movement • Reduced anterior excursion of hyolaryngeal complex • Increased duration of velar elevation • Increased pharyngeal transit duration • Progressive pharyngeal contraction is slowed • More swallows required to clear oral and pharyngeal cavities; increased post-swallow residue • Increased frequency of polyphasic extraneous laryngeal movements • Three times more likely than younger individuals to inhale after swallowing • Longer swallowing apnea duration • Increased frequency of coughing after swallow • Reduced pharyngeal and laryngeal sensitivity
UES	• Decreased amplitude of esophageal peristalsis • Decreased UES opening size, but preserved intrasphincter flow rate due to increase in hypopharyngeal intrabolus pressure • Delayed UES opening/relaxation, related to increased oral transit times • Reduced UES flexibility

(Information summarized from Aviv, 1997; Aviv, Martin, Keen, Debelt, & Blitzer, 1993; Baum, 1989; Calhoun, Gibson, Hartley, Minton, & Hokanson, 1992; Caruso & Max, 1997; Feldman, Kapur, Alman, & Chauncey, 1980; Heeneman & Brown, 1986; Hiss, Treole, & Stuart, 2001; Kendall & Leonard, 2001; Kendall, Leonard, & McKenzie, 2003; Leonard, et al., 2000; Logemann, 1990; Logemann, Pauloski, Rademaker, et al., 2000; Nilsson, et al., 1996; Robbins, et al., 1992; Plant, 1998; Rademaker, Pauloski, Colangelo, & Logemann, 1998; Shaker, Ren, Zamir, Sarna, Liu, & Sui, 1994; Shipp, Pillemer, & Baum, 2002.)

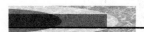

SUMMARY

The swallowing process is substantially more flexible (and, therefore, more complicated) than the four-phase model implies. It is a unified physiologic system whose components blend in a multitude of ways to accomplish the

Figure 4-1. Effects of sex on swallowing variables.

- Submental muscle activation occurs earlier in men than women
- UES opening longer for women than for men
- Hyoid elevation greater in men than women (likely related to the extraneous third variable of swallower height)
- Larynx-to-hyoid approximation greater in men than women (contributing to closer approximation of the epiglottis to the arytenoid cartilages as the larynx is elevated farther under the tongue base)
- Pharyngeal area (expressed as a ratio between pharyngeal area at maximum constriction to pharyngeal area during bolus hold) greater for men than women
- Swallowing apnea period greater for women than men

(Information summarized from Logemann, Pauloski, Rademaker, et al., 2000; Rademaker, Pauloski, Colangel, & Logemann, 1998.)

goal of safe ingestion. Some components of deglutition may be invariant (or less variant), but the majority are influenced by task, bolus, and swallower variables. Discrete swallows differ from continuous swallows. Swallowing a small bolus differs from swallowing a large bolus. Swallow function will differ between men and women and young and elderly individuals. The critical task for the clinician is to understand the domain of normal so that pathologic swallowing may be accurately diagnosed.

STUDY QUESTIONS

1. Summarize the differences in findings between studies of discrete bolus ingestion and those of mealtime or sequential swallows.
2. Define motor equivalence and give an example.
3. What are the bolus characteristics most closely related to changes in deglutition parameters?
4. Describe the effects of age on the swallow mechanism.
5. Does swallowing a large bolus, as compared to a small bolus, affect physiology? If so, how?

REFERENCES

Aviv, J. (1997). Effects of aging on sensitivity of the pharyngeal and supraglottic areas. *American Journal of Medicine, 103*(5A), 74S–76S.

Aviv, J. E., Martin, J. H., Keen, M. S., Debell, M., & Blitzer, A., (1993). Air pulse quantification of supraglottic and pharyngeal sensation: A new technique. *Annals of Otology, Rhinology, and Laryngology, 102,* 777–780.

Baum, B. J. (1989). Salivary gland secretion during aging. *Journal of the American Geriatric Society, 37*(5), 453–458.

Calhoun, K. H., Gibson, B., Hartley, L., Minton, J., & Hokanson, J. A. (1992). Age-related changes in oral sensation. *Laryngoscope, 12*, 109–116.

Caruso, A. J., & Max, L. (1997). Effects of aging on neuromotor processes of swallowing. *Seminars in Speech and Language, 18*(2), 181–192.

Chi-Fishman, G., & Sonies, B. (2000). Motor strategy in rapid sequential swallowing: New insights. *Journal of Speech, Language, and Hearing Research, 43*, 1481–1492.

Chi-Fishman G., & Sonies, B. C. (2002). Effects of systematic bolus viscosity and volume changes on hyoid movement kinematics. *Dysphagia, 17*(4), 278–287.

Chi-Fishman, G., Stone, M., & McCall, G. (1998). Lingual action in normal sequential swallowing. *Journal of Speech, Language, and Hearing Research, 41*, 771–785.

Dantas, R., Kern, M., Massey, B., Dodds, W., Kahrilas, P., Brasseur, J., Cook, L., & Lang, I. (1990, May). Effect of swallowed bolus variables on oral and pharyngeal phases of swallowing. *American Journal of Physiology*, G675–G681.

Dejaeger, E., Pelemans, W., Ponette, E., & Vantrappen, G. (1994). Effect of body position on deglutition. *Digestive Diseases and Sciences, 39*(4), 762–765.

Ding, R., Larson, C. R., Logemann, J. A., & Rademacker, A. W. (2002). Surface electromyographic and electroglottographic studies in normal subjects under two swallow conditions: Normal and during the Mendelsohn maneuver. *Dysphagia, 17*(1), 1–12.

Dua, K., Shaker, R., Ren, J., Podvrsan, B., & Trifan, A. (1997). Coordination of deglutitive glottal function and pharyngeal bolus transit during eating and drinking. *Gastroenterology, 112*, 73–83.

Ergun, G., Kahrilas, P., Lin, S., Logemann, J., & Harig, J. (1993, November). Shape, volume and content of the deglutive pharyngeal chamber imaged by ultrafast computerized tomography. *Gastroenterology*, 1396–1403.

Ertekin, C., Pehlivan, M., Aydogdu, I., Ertas, M., Uludag, B., Celebi, G., Colakoglu, Z., Sadguyu, A., & Yuceyar, N. (1995). An electrophysiological investigation of deglutition in man. *Muscle & Nerve, 18*, 1177–1186.

Feldman, R. S., Kapur, K. K., Alman, J. E., & Chauncey, H. H. (1980). Aging and mastication: Changes in performance and threshold with natural dentition. *Journal of the American Geriatrics Society, 28*, 97–103.

Flaherty, R., Seltzer, S., Campbell, T., Weisskoff, R., & Gilbert, R. (1995, September). Dynamic magnetic resonance imaging of vocal cord closure during deglutition. *Gastroenterology*, 843–890.

Gay, T., Rendell, J. K., & Spiro, J. (1994). Oral and laryngeal muscle coordination during swallowing. *Laryngoscope, 104*, 341–349.

Hamlet, S., Choi, J., Zormeier, M., Shamsa, F., Stachler, R., Muz, J., & Jones, L. (1996). Normal adult swallowing of liquid and viscous material: Scintigraphic data on bolus transit and oropharyngeal residues. *Dysphagia, 11*(1), 41–47.

Heeneman, H., & Brown, D. H. (1986). Senescent changes in and about the oral cavity and pharynx. *Journal of Otolaryngology, 15*, 214–216.

Hiiemae, K. M., & Palmer, J. B. (1999). Food transport and bolus formation during complete feeding sequences on foods of initial different consistencies. *Dysphagia, 14*(1), 31–42.

Hiss, S. G., Treole, K., & Stuart, A. (2001). Effects of age, gender, bolus volume, and trial on swallowing apnea duration and swallow/respiratory phase relationships of normal adults. *Dysphagia, 16*(2), 128–135.

Kahrilas, P. J., Lin, S., Chen, J., & Logemann, J. A. (1996). Oropharyngeal accommodation to swallow volume. *Gastroenterology, 111,* 297–306.

Kendall, K. A., & Leonard, R. J. (2001). Pharyngeal constriction in elderly dysphagic patients compared with young and elderly nondysphagic controls. *Dysphagia, 16*(4), 272–278.

Kendall, K. A., Leonard, R. J., & McKenzie, S. W. (2003). Sequence variability during hypopharyngeal bolus transit. *Dysphagia, 18*(2), 85–91.

Kendall, K. A., McKenzie, S., Leonard, R. J., Goncalves, M. I., & Walker, A. (2000). Timing of events in normal swallowing: A videofluoroscopic study. *Dysphagia, 15*(2), 74–83.

Leonard, R. J., Kendall, K. A., McKenzie, S., Goncalves, M. I., & Walker, A. (2000). Structural displacements in normal swallowing: A videofluoroscopic study. *Dysphagia, 15*(3), 146–152.

Logemann, J. A., (1983). *Evaluation and treatment of swallowing disorders.* Austin, TX: Pro-Ed.

Logemann, J. A. (1990). Effects of aging on the swallowing mechanism. *Otolaryngologic Clinics of North America, 23,* 1045–1056.

Logemann, J. A., Pauloski, B. R., Colangelo, L., Lazarus, C., Fujiu, M., & Kahrilas, P. J. (1995). Effects of a sour bolus on oropharyngeal swallowing measures in patients with neurogenic dysphagia. *Journal of Speech, Language, and Hearing Research, 38,* 556–563.

Logemann, J. A., Pauloski, B. R., Rademaker, A. W., Colangelo, L. A., Kahrilas, P. J., & Smith, C. H. (2000). Temporal and biomechanical characteristics of oropharyngeal swallow in younger and older men. *Journal of Speech, Language, and Hearing Research, 43*(5), 1264–1274.

Miller, J. L., & Watkin, K. (1996). The influence of bolus volume and viscosity on anterior lingual force during the oral stage of swallowing. *Dysphagia, 11*(2), 117–124.

Nilsson, H., Ekberg, O., Olsson, R., & Hindfelt, B. (1996). Quantitative aspects of swallowing in an elderly nondysphagic population. *Dysphagia, 11*(3), 180–184.

Palmer, J. B. (1998). Bolus aggregation in the pharynx does not depend on gravity. *Archives of Physical Medicine and Rehabilitation, 79,* 691–696.

Palmer, J. B., Rudin, N. J., Lara, G., & Crompton, A. W. (1992). Coordination of mastication and swallowing. *Dysphagia, 7*(4), 187–200.

Perlman, A., VanDaele, D., & Otterbacher, M. (1995). Quantitative assessment of hyoid bone displacement from video images during swallowing. *Journal of Speech and Hearing Research, 38,* 579–585.

Plant, R. L. (1998). Anatomy and physiology of swallowing in adults and geriatrics. *Otolaryngology Clinics of North America, 31*(3), 477–488.

Rademaker, A. W., Pauloski, B. R., Colangelo, L. A., & Logemann, J. A. (1998). Age and volume effects on liquid swallowing function in normal women. *Journal of Speech, Language, and Hearing Research, 41,* 274–284.

Ren, J., Shaker, R., Dua, K., Trifan, A., Podvrsan, B., & Sui, Z. (1994). Glottal adduction response to pharyngeal water stimulation: Evidence for a pharyngoglottal closure reflex (abstr.). *Gastroenterology, 106,* A558.

Robbins, J., Hamilton, J. W., Lof, G., & Kempster, G. B. (1992). Oropharyngeal swallowing in normal adults of different ages. *Gastroenterology, 103,* 823–829.

Shaker, R., Ren, J., Zamir, Z., Sarna, A., Liu, J., & Sui, Z. (1994). Effect of aging, position, and temperature on the threshold volume triggering pharyngeal swallows. *Gastroenterology, 107,* 396–402.

Shipp, J. A., Pillemer, S. R., & Baum, B. J. (2002). Xerostomia and the geriatric patient. *Journal of the American Geriatrics Association, 50*(3), 535–543.

CHAPTER 5

Direct and Indirect Oropharyngeal and Esophageal Imaging

LEARNING OBJECTIVES

After completing the chapter and reviewing the study questions, you should be able to:

- Recognize the anatomical plane of examination when viewing diagnostic images

- Recognize the type of image (endoscopic, fluoroscopic) and identify basic landmarks in the oropharyngeal and esophageal regions

- Understand the rationale for the type of testing conducted for individual patients depending on signs and symptoms

- Understand and follow the physician's diagnosis based on your knowledge of diagnostic tests, the patient's clinical signs and symptoms, and findings of studies

- Apply understanding of test findings to discussion of therapeutic implications with physicians and patient/family members.

INTRODUCTION

Anatomy and physiology can be observed up close and personal through diagnostic imaging. As you would expect, the structures look much different depending upon the visualization method used and orientation of the image (think frontal view versus coronal or axial view of your own head). As well, information about the structure and function of the upper digestive tract may be gleaned in an indirect manner such as measuring pressure at a specific location or recording the number of reflux occurrences as measured by a sensor located within the system of interest. Physiology may be inferred from these indirect measures.

This chapter provides an overview of anatomical planes of examination and the different imaging methodologies as they pertain to the evaluation of deglutition function. Both direct and indirect measurement methodologies of the upper aerodigestive tract are covered. Methodologies discussed are only those that are used clinically on a regular basis given that the focus of this text is clinical in nature. Speech-language pathologists will want to be familiar with these methodologies, their purpose, and expected type of information from the test outcome, when speaking with medical personnel.

ANATOMICAL PLANES OF VIEW

The diagnostic imaging views obtained may be oriented in a number of planes including lateral, anterior-posterior, superior, oblique, and axial (cross-sectional) views. Cross-sectional axial images are viewed from the foot of the patient by radiologists. Figure 5-1 shows the various names for the anatomical planes used when describing structures of swallow during diagnostic imaging. Speech-language pathologists usually view swallowing dynamics in the lateral and anterior-posterior (A-P) planes during a modified barium swallow study. Fiberoptic endoscopic examination of swallow (FEES) provides a view from the superior perspective of the dynamic structures of swallow. Oblique views are more often used when examining velopharyngeal port dynamics and the esophagus.

Because cross-sectional views are so different from what the speech-language pathologist is used to seeing, we will begin this section by briefly addressing cross-sectional images of the gastroesophageal junction and the stomach.

Cross-Sectional Anatomy

The gastroesophageal junction is difficult to visualize because of its location and the fact that the esophagus takes a curving path through the lower chest and abdominal cavity to reach the stomach. Let us review major landmarks and the path taken by the esophagus before discussing what the structures look like in cross-section. The thoracic portion of the esophagus lies anterior to the aorta. Its path brings it through the diaphragm (hiatus) on the right side. The esophagus then courses to the left in an anterior direction for approximately 2 cm before attaching to the stomach. In the abdominal cavity, the esophagus lies posterior and to the left of the liver, anterior to the aorta, and to the right side of the stomach fundus or center (Deyoe & Balfe, 1995). This gives the gastroesophageal junction an offset appearance with a seemingly off-center stomach. An axial (cross-sectional) view of a CT (computed tomography) at the level of the gastroesophageal junction is provided in Figure 5-2a. As you can see, the oval-shaped esophagus is in the posterior mediastinum with the stomach to the person's left and the liver taking up most of the right side. (You view these images as though looking directly at the individual—so the stomach is on

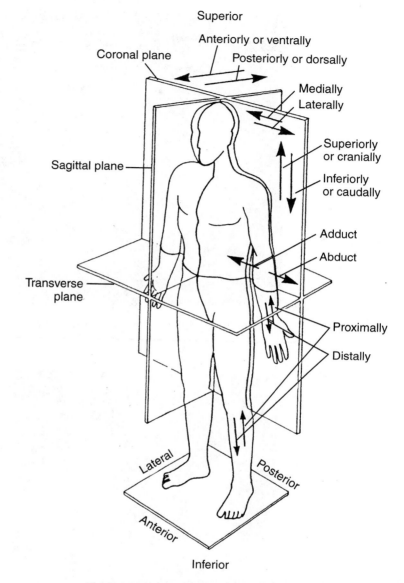

Figure 5-1. Anatomical planes of dissection.

the right side of your image and the liver appears on the left.) The anatomic level of the *slice* being viewed will influence the appearance of the structures (see Clinical Note 5–1 for explanation of anatomical slices). Figure 5-2b shows a more distal view of the same structures. This type of axial view is used by radiologists to examine the thickness of the gastric wall and to look for epigastric tumors (outside but in the region of the stomach).

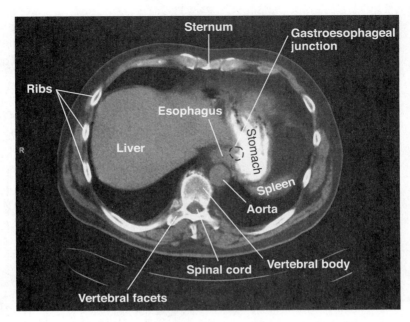

Figure 5-2a. Cross-sectional CT image of gastroesophageal junction.

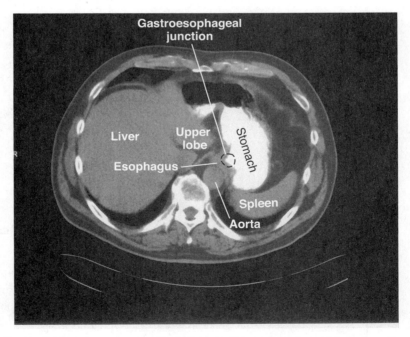

Figure 5-2b. Cross-sectional CT image of gastroesophageal junction distal to 5-2a.

CLINICAL NOTE

5-1

What is an Anatomical Slice and When Would I See One?

In any type of imaging procedure that uses many sectional views of structures, one plane or *slice* will be in focus at any given time. The radiologist can view these multiple slices on a computer to examine different structures that are positioned at different levels in the body. Conceptually, it is like viewing a specific slice or plane at any given location in the body. You would view an anatomical slice in CT, PET, or MRI scans. A CT (computed tomography) scan takes multiple X-rays in the cross-sectional plane and then computer synthesizes the images. A PET (positron emission tomography) scan provides an image of local metabolic function in tissue (like uptake of biochemicals) that have positron-emitting radionuclides mixed into the material given to the patient. A computer synthesizes the data. In magnetic resonance imaging (MRI) a patient is placed in a magnetic field and the body's nuclei are excited by radiofrequency pulses. The measured signal strength from the body's hydrogen ions varies within the body according to hydrogen concentration in the tissue. Again, the signals are computer processed (McDonough, 1994).

A CT axial view may also be used to view the thoracic cavity when assessing pneumonia. Figure 5-3 is an axial CT image of a right lobe aspiration pneumonia.

Lateral Plane Anatomy

The lateral plane is one of two views most trained speech-language pathologists are used to seeing during diagnostic imaging of swallow. It is most often used for radiographic (X-ray) studies. Care must be taken in patient positioning prior to radiographic lateral view imaging in order to see only the structures of interest. As you sit in your chair reading, scrunch your shoulders up toward your ears and slump forward slightly. Now think about a lateral radiographic beam aimed at your neck at the level of your larynx. What structures will the beam pass through? Most likely, the upper pectoral girdle will be superimposed on the structures you are trying to view. Now straighten into an upright, seated posture and again imagine the lateral beam. It will have access to structures down to the base of the neck at approximately the level of the larynx and UES. Any structure inferior to this region will not be seen independently from the pectoral girdle or ribs and thoracic cavity.

Figure 5-4 shows the oropharyngeal areas of interest in the lateral view. The anterior boundary is the lips and includes all structures in the oral cavity. Any metal such as dental fillings, caps, or dentures will appear very light and opaque on X-ray. Or appearances may be the exact opposite. Fluoroscopy is often viewed in positive mode where dense tissue, such as bone or dental fillings, appears dark and air spaces, such as the pharynx, are white. If earrings are worn they may appear to

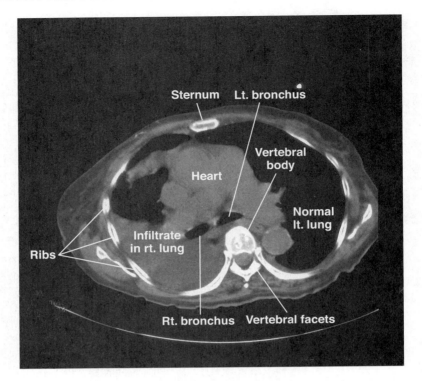

Figure 5-3. Axial view CT of right lobe pneumonia.

be located in the oral cavity because this view does not account for the three-dimensional nature of the head. As well, slight lateral tipping of the head will reveal what appears to be an extra set of teeth, maxilla, or mandible but is, in reality, the other side of the facial arch.

The nasopharynx provides the uppermost boundary of interest so that the soft palate can be observed during velopharyngeal closure. In the lateral view, the soft palate looks very different at rest (Figure 5-4) than during velopharyngeal closure (Figure 5-5). The cervical and thoracic vertebrae are the posterior limit of the area of interest in the pharyngeal cavities and are included in the radiographic field in order to allow examination for skeletal abnormalities that may impair swallow function. In the pharyngeal cavity, recesses of interest include the valleculae and pyriform cavities. The valleculae are easily visible in the lateral view with or without material present. Keep in mind that in the lateral view you are seeing one vallecula superimposed on the other. The pyriform sinus is only appreciated when filled with radiopaque material since the space formed by the pharyngeal constrictor fibers attaching to the thyroid cartilage is not visible in the lateral view unless filled as in Figure 5-6. Notice in this figure that the valleculae are outlined with barium. At the inferior most point of the pharynx, the UES is viewed laterally as a local constriction (Figure 5-7). In

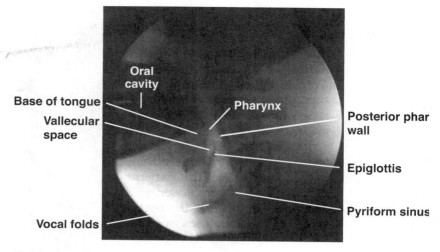

Figure 5-4. Lateral view of oral cavity, pharynx, and esophagus from nasopharynx to UES.

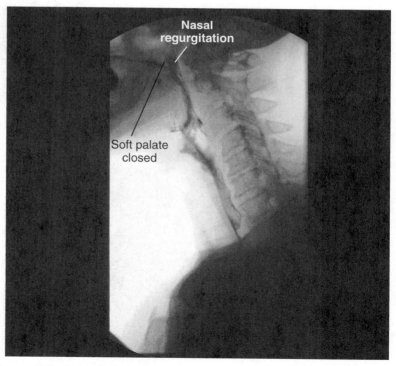

Figure 5-5. Lateral view of oropharyngeal region showing velopharyngeal closure.

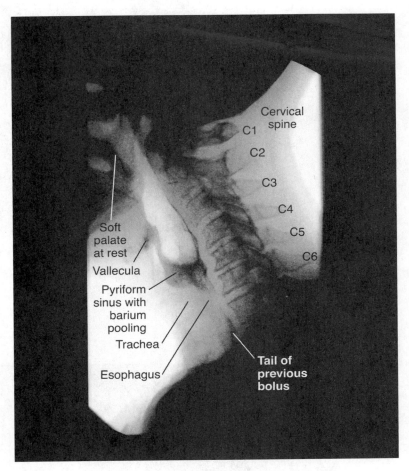

Figure 5-6. Lateral view showing vallecula outlined and pyriform sinus filled with barium.

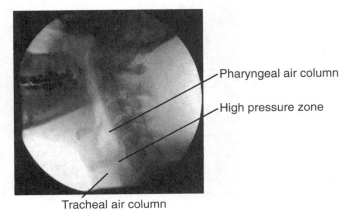

Figure 5-7. Lateral view showing UES high pressure zone.

the image, you can see the tail of the previous bolus in the esophagus. This delineates the high pressure zone of the UES. The constriction and subsequent opening of this valve moves during the swallow when the hyolaryngeal complex elevates during the swallow response.

The lateral view is also used with chest X-rays when diagnosing, among other things, aspiration pneumonia. Aspiration pneumonia may occur with numerous injuries or diseases that affect level of consciousness, neurological integrity, and gastroesophageal function (Falestiny & Yu, 1999). Regardless of the cause, the end result is material in the airway and lungs that cannot be cleared by the individual. A normal lateral view chest X-ray is shown in Figure 5-8. Notice that you are able to see the inferior-most lobes of the lung as points, with the two sides superimposed on each other in this lateral view.

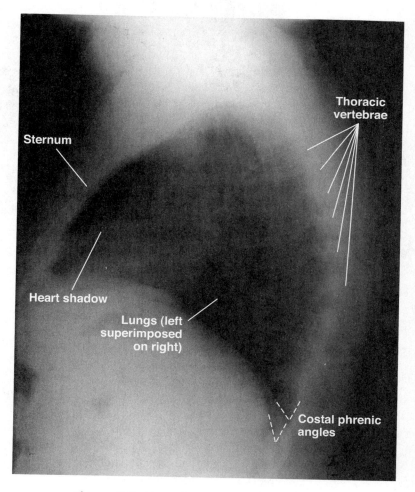

Figure 5-8. Lateral view, normal chest X-ray.

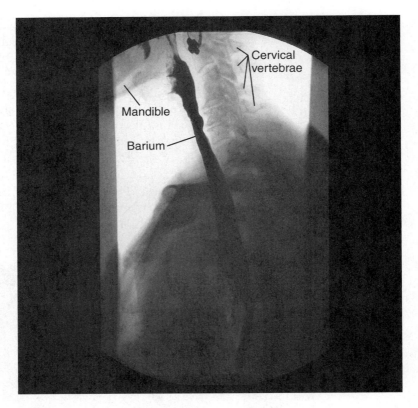

Figure 5-9. Lateral view, fluoroscopic image during esophagram.

The lateral view is also shown on esophagrams as in Figure 5-9 which depicts contrast material in the esophagus during a pharyngeal swallow response.

Anterior-Posterior Plane Anatomy

The anterior-posterior (A-P) plane allows a complete view of both sides of the oropharyngeal cavities and provides a midline dynamic view of the proximal esophagus. During swallow, this view is noted for allowing assessment of symmetry between the right and left sides of structures of interest. The most prominent difference between this view and the lateral view is in the pharynx where the pharyngeal recesses are much more visible as separate entities. The valleculae appear as paired, medially placed indentations above the larynx. The pyriform sinuses can be seen laterally in the inferior portion of the pharynx. These recesses are most easily viewed when coated with radiopaque material (Figure 5-10).

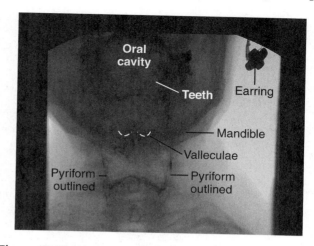

Figure 5-10. A-P view of valleculae and pyriform sinuses.

During a fluoroscopic imaging study, a bolus is followed through the length of the esophagus in the A-P plane down to the LES, which serves as the lower limit to the area of interest. While the speech-language pathologist does not have responsibility for diagnosis of esophageal disorders, the radiologist does and will often do a brief scan from the UES to the LES at the end of a modified barium swallow. This is particularly important if the cause of symptoms reported is not identified in the oropharynx. An informed speech-language pathologist should recognize normal structure and function in this region. Figure 5-11a shows an A-P view during an esophagram. The swallowed bolus in Figure 5-11b contained effervescent crystals—notice the distended appearance of the espohagus and the bubbles in the stomach. Notice the offset appearance of the stomach.

An A-P chest X-ray is used, in conjunction with other tests, to diagnose pneumonia. When associated with dysphagia, the radiologist is trying to rule out an aspiration pneumonia. Figures 5–12a and 5–12b are examples of a normal chest X-ray and a right lobe aspiration pneumonia, respectively.

Superior Plane Anatomy

Superior plane views are often observed during various endoscopic procedures, anywhere from the nasopharynx to the stomach. At the initiation of an upper gastrointestinal endoscopy, the physician will often look at the laryngeal vestibule for signs of mucosal irritation, inflammation, or irregularities with a superior view as shown in Figures 5-13a

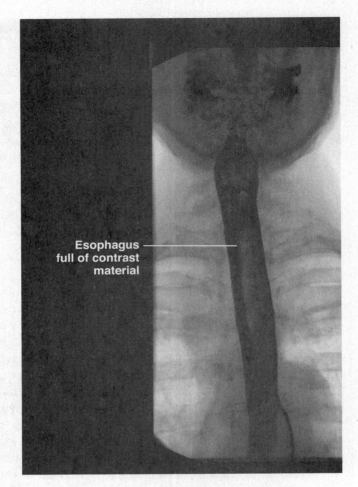

Esophagus
full of contrast
material

Figure 5-11a. A-P view of fluoroscopic esophagram image.

and 5–13b. In color, the images are strikingly different with severe redness observed in Figure 5-13b. Keep in mind, however, that from a
superior vantage point, what is viewed depends on where the tip of the
endoscope is placed. If the endoscope is in the nasopharnx, the view of
the oropharynx and laryngopharynx will be obstructed by the closed
velopharyngeal port if the person is phonating or swallowing. A superior plane view will be obstructed by any and all closed valves if the
endoscope is positioned above the valve. So endoscopic positioning will
depend on the structures being examined.

Within the esophagus, the superior view on endoscopy appears to
be peering down an oval tunnel that gradually twists and turns leading

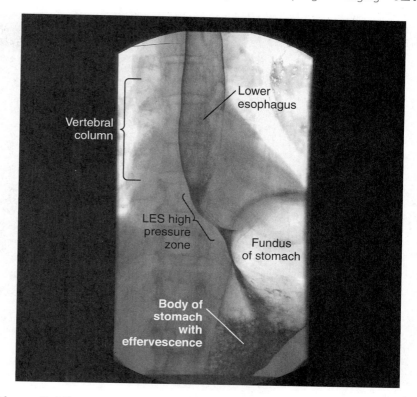

Figure 5-11b. A-P view of fluoroscopic esophagram image using effervescent crystals.

to the LES and stomach. The mucosal surface, viewed endoscopically, is similar from the cervical esophagus to the LES.

Oblique Plane Anatomy

The oblique view of the oropharyngeal region can be obtained by either aiming the X-ray beam from under the chin in an oblique angle or doing the same from behind the head near the occiput. This plane allows the dynamic assessment of velopharyngeal port activity during speech and swallow. It is not a frequently used view for oropharyngeal swallow function but is for esophageal views when the fluoroscope is aimed at the chest obliquely. The view used may be either anterior or posterior oblique. This angling prevents the view of the esophagus from being superimposed on the vertebral column behind it (Figure 5-14).

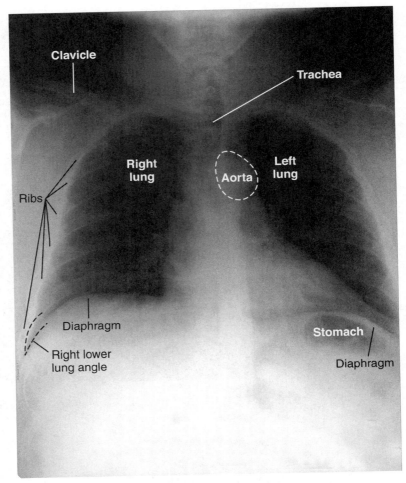

Figure 5-12a. A-P view, normal chest X-ray.

DIAGNOSTIC IMAGING METHODOLOGIES

The upper gastrointestinal tract may be visualized using numerous methods—from a direct view of the structures (as in **endoscopy**) to **contrast radiography** (as in an esophagram or modified barium swallow), **nuclear medicine** (scintigraphy), **computed tomography** (CT scan), or **magnetic resonance imaging** (MRI). The method chosen by the physician is determined based on the patient's symptoms, the location of the suspected problem, and the information needed to rule out, confirm, or grade specific diseases. A number of methods provide complementary information as when **manometry** (which can measure

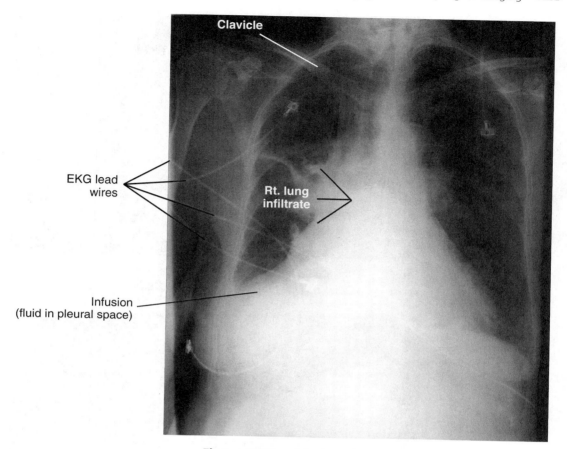

Figure 5-12b. A-P view, chest X-ray of pneumonia.

pressure in the pharynx, at the UES, through the esophagus, and at the LES) is combined with an esophagram viewed fluoroscopically (**manofluorography**). This provides the physician with information about pressures generated within the digestive tract at the same time bolus transit is observed. One particular imaging method is no better than another—it all depends on the purpose of the study and the information sought. Often, weaknesses inherent in one method can be improved upon by combining techniques, such as adding contrast to a CT scan, to provide a maximum amount of diagnostic information. The type of examination will likely be determined by the referring physician and radiologist. The speech-language pathologist is responsible for informing that decision by communicating the type of information needed for clinical management decisions.

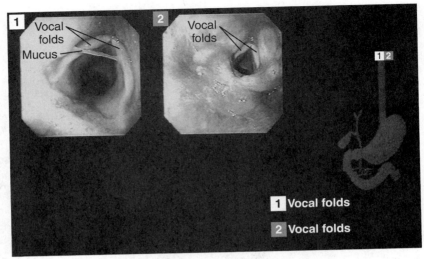

Figure 5-13a. Superior endoscopic view of larynx during upper GI endoscopy—normal vocal folds. (*Courtesy of V. Duane Bohman.*)

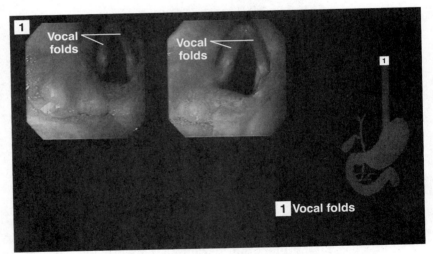

Figure 5-13b. Superior endoscopic view of larynx during upper GI endoscopy—erythematous vocal folds. (*Courtesy of V. Duane Bohman.*)

Endoscopy

Most endoscopic procedures use a flexible fiberoptic endoscope to directly visualize structures of interest and are recorded to videotape or, most currently, digitally. These procedures may be conducted under sedation by a gastroenterologist using a large-diameter endoscope passed through the mouth (for what is typically called an upper gas-

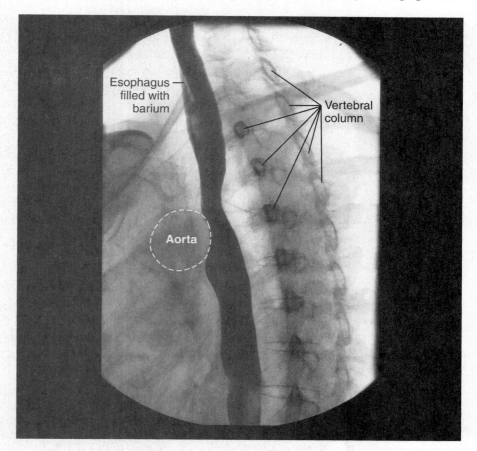

Figure 5-14. Oblique view of the esophagus on esophagram.

trointestinal endoscopy) or they may be done using either no anesthetic or a topical anesthetic by a speech-language pathologist using a small-diameter endoscope passed through the nose, as in a flexible fiberoptic examination of swallow (FEES). Use of topical anesthetics must be weighed for patient comfort against the importance of maintaining the sensory integrity of the pharynx. Recent research suggests that there is minimal difference in comfort between use or non-use of topical anesthetic during FEES (Leder, et al., 1997; Singh, Brockband, & Todd, 1997).

Endoscopic exams allow for the evaluation of tissue appearance—its color, whether blood vessels are apparent, and the quality of tissue, or whether it is irritated or friable (easily torn or made to bleed). Within the digestive tract, normal tissue appearance and color varies depending on the location within the pharynx or esophagus—proximal or distal. Endoscopy also allows for medical/surgical procedures, such as biopsy, to be conducted through a separate channel of the endoscope. A second channel in the scope used during FEES allows for sensory testing with calibrated puffs of air aimed at the mucosa of the supraglottal region to establish a baseline for sensation. When sensory testing is conducted in this fashion the test is called fiberoptic examination of swallow with sensory testing, or FEESST. As fiberoptics improve in small bore (diameter) endoscopes, such as those used during FEEST, decreased light penetration resulting from the space occupied by the channel to deliver the air puffs will be less of a drawback.

Endoscopes vary in length and diameter. Figure 5-15a shows a small-diameter, flexible fiberoptic endoscope used to visualize the nasal, pharyngeal, and laryngeal cavities. Endoscopes used to examine the esophagus, stomach, and duodenum are longer and have a wider diameter as seen in Figure 5-15b.

Upper Gastrointestinal Endoscopy

Endoscopy of the upper gastrointestinal (GI) tract includes imaging the hypopharynx, esophagus, stomach, and duodenum using a flexible fiberoptic endoscope paired with a cold light source, camera, and video or digital recording system. The scope will often have an opening for air insufflation and a water jet to clear mucus from the viewing end of the

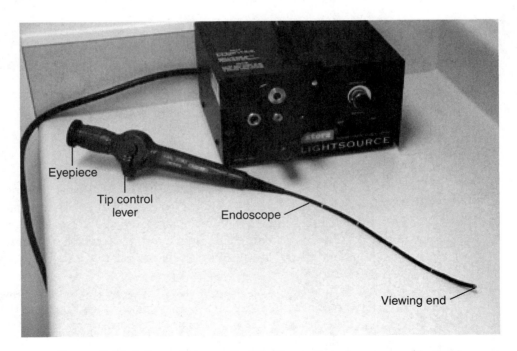

Figure 5-15a. 4 mm diameter flexible fiberoptic endoscope used in FEES.

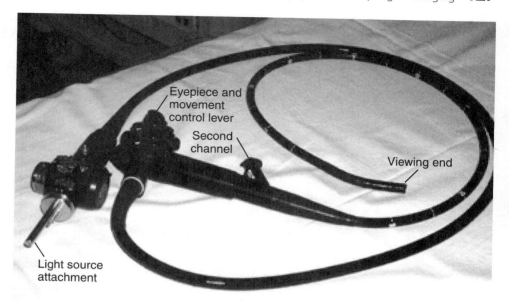

Figure 5-15b. 11 mm diameter two-channel flexible fiberoptic endoscope used in upper gastroesophageal endoscopy.

scope. Suction is available through the scope to remove both liquids and gases. A separate channel allows instruments to be passed to either collect tissue for biopsy, to give injections, or to remove foreign objects. An array of probes for Doppler, pH, and electrical activity as well as biopsy forceps (with different cutting tools) and cytology brushes (to collect cell samples from the lumen walls) may be passed through this additional channel of the scope. In order to accommodate these extra channels, the endoscope is of a larger diameter than that used during FEES by a speech-language pathologist. Upper GI endoscopy is performed by a gastroenterologist in a medical office, outpatient facility, or hospital setting. It may be the first examination of choice or may follow such exams as a pharyngoesophagogram or modified barium swallow study. Most often, patients are sedated prior to the examination with a combination of procedural sedation and antianxiety medications such as Valium (diazepam) and Versed (midazolam). While not asleep, they are in a *twilight* condition. This also is referred to as *conscious sedation*. When smaller bore scopes are used sedation is minimal, if used at all. A bite guard holds the patient's mouth open and prevents injury to the endoscopist should fingers be used to guide the scope. The scope is passed through the mouth and into the pharynx. At the level of the UES the patient is instructed to swallow and the scope enters the esophagus.

The entire length of the esophagus is examined for mucosal abnormalities, structural defects, or neoplasms. At approximately 40 cm from the UES, the patient is asked to sniff and movement of the diaphragm can be observed. This is one way to test for a hiatal hernia where stomach tissue may invert up through the LES (Tytgat, 1995). The stomach and duodenum may be examined. The viewing end, or lens, of the scope is controlled with a knob near the eyepiece that the endoscopist turns. Rotation of the scope is also used to move the scope lens and view structures.

A number of therapeutic techniques may be implemented during diagnostic endoscopy. Upper GI endoscopy can be used to dilate esophageal strictures by sending a guidewire with a spring tip or a catheter with a balloon tip down to the level of constriction. When the spring tip is activated, or the balloon inflated, the fibers of the stricture are broken and the diameter of the tube is increased. This allows passage of food boluses without impedance. Bleeding vessels in the upper gastrointestinal tract may be treated with **sclerotherapy**, injection of a chemical agent into the problem vein. Bleeds may also be sealed with **electrocoagulation** that burns tissue with an electric current. A method also exists for attaching a band or ligature to a varix (dilated vein) using the endoscope.

Fiberoptic Endoscopic Examination of Swallow

FEES is an endoscopic examination of the velopharynx, oropharynx, pharynx, and larynx. Oral and esophageal phases of swallow are not evaluated with this procedure (ASHA, 2002). FEES allows bedside documentation of dysphagia symptoms (penetration or aspiration). It was developed by Langmore and colleagues in 1988 for the assessment of dysphagia (Langmore, Schatz, & Olson, 1988; Langmore, Schatz, & Olson, 1991). A narrow, flexible, fiberoptic endoscope, such as the one in Figure 5-15a, is inserted into the nasal passage and advanced to the level of the larynx. Topical anesthetic in the nose may or may not be used depending on scope diameter, patient tolerance, and clinician experience. The *Manual of Dysphagia Assessment in Adults* (Murray, 1999), part of the Dysphagia series, is an excellent resource that describes each step of this exam (as well as the clinical bedside and videofluoroscopic exam)—conducting an endoscopic procedure, interpreting the findings, and communicating the results.

FEES is particularly useful for patients who cannot be transported to radiology for a modified barium swallow, who have significant positioning problems, who are severely medically compromised and could not handle aspiration, or when direct visualization of the larynx is desirable following surgery that may compromise the recurrent laryngeal nerve. This test does not provide a view of the entire pharyngeal phase during the act of swallowing—a *white out* of the endoscopic image results when the pharynx closes around the scope during the swallow response. Anatomy of oral, pharyngeal, and laryngeal structures can only be observed before and after the swallow response, not during the swallow. While inferences can be made about airway protection, all three levels of protection (true vocal fold, ventricular fold, and aryepiglottic fold and epiglottic closure) cannot be observed endoscopically at the same time. FEES does provide a better view than fluoroscopy when trying to quantify amount of pooled secretions, assess accumulation of residue, test for pharyngeal and laryngeal sensation, and measure the number of spontaneous swallows over a period of minutes (Murray, Langmore, Ginsberg, & Dostie, 1996; Langmore & McCulloch, 1997). Given the association of pooled material in the laryngeal vestibule with an increased risk of aspiration (Murray, Langmore, Ginsberg, & Dostie, 1996), FEES is able to provide clinically significant information quickly and efficiently. Fluoroscopy provides more information about oral-phase dynamics, coordination of oropharyngeal movements, posterior tongue movement and apposition with the posterior pharyngeal wall, hyolaryngeal elevation, aspiration during swallow, UES opening, esophageal phase dynamics, and evaluation of the effortful swallow technique and Mendelsohn maneuver (Langmore & McCulloch, 1997).

FEESST is a variant on FEES that includes sensory testing of the pharyngeal and laryngeal mucosa with calibrated air puffs to establish a discrimination threshold and/or evaluate the presence or absence of a laryngeal adductor reflex (LAR) (Aviv, 1997; Aviv, 2000; Aviv, Kim, Sacco, Kaplan, Goodhart, Diamond, & Close, 1998; Aviv, Martin, Keen, Debell, & Blitzer, 1993; Aviv, Martin, Kim, Sacco, Thomson, Diamond, & Close, 1999). The endoscope used has an extra channel for delivery of air puffs. Results provide information about the integrity of the superior laryngeal nerve (SLN) responsible for afferent information from the epiglottal region, pharyngeal, and laryngeal mucosa. The addition of sensory testing to FEES is based on the premise that reduced afferent information likely plays a role in many dysphagia symptoms (Aviv, 2000). Early indications are that patients with impaired laryngopharyngeal sensation, indicated by an absent LAR, are at a statistically significant increased risk for penetration and aspiration (Aviv, Spitzer, Cohen, Ma, Belafsky, & Close, 2002). A study of 500 patients evaluated the safety of the procedure and found no airway compromise, no significant heart rate alteration before or after the exam, and no significant nose bleeds. The test was judged safe with only mild discomfort (Aviv, Kaplan, Thomson, Spitzer, Diamond, & Close,

2000). Continued research is examining the affect of age-related changes to sensory functioning which is commonly believed to decrease with increased age.

Contrast Radiography

Contrast radiography is a broad term that includes a number of radiographic or X-ray studies. These procedures are most often conducted in a Diagnostic Imaging or Radiology department. The type of equipment used may vary (see Clinical Note 5–2). *Contrast radiography* is a general term which simply means that a radiopaque material, a contrast material that X-ray cannot penetrate, is used to highlight and view anatomical structures and motility through structures.

CLINICAL NOTE 5-2

Types of X-ray Equipment

Medical facilities use different types of X-ray equipment and speech-language pathologists need to familiarize themselves with the specific radiology suite in which they will conduct modified barium swallow (MBS) studies. Room setup will vary, even within a particular facility. Often, a designated room with recording capabilities will be assigned for the MBS. Some rooms have a standard table that can be positioned vertically with the patient placed, either standing or seated, in the narrow space between the table and the fluoroscope arm. Other rooms may use a C-arm machine (which looks like a giant C that can be rotated in multiple directions) that can be positioned flexibly around the seated patient. Portable systems with additional space between the arm and the main unit of the machine allow for positioning of large chairs (such as *geri-chairs*, a reclining chair found in many hospital rooms). Audio and video may be recorded as an analog signal or digital signal.

Contrast radiographic techniques may be used to examine the entire length of the gastrointestinal tract, literally from top to bottom. Where the contrast is introduced (through which orifice) simply depends on what structure(s) or where motility is to be examined. The thickness and coating ability of the contrast material used will depend on what is being visualized and how clearly defined surfaces need to be. When looking at swallow anatomy and physiology the barium contrast will be introduced into the oral cavity. When soft palate function is being evaluated, a small amount of barium will be introduced into the nasal cavity through the nostrils. The amount of barium ingested will vary according to the type and purpose of the study being conducted. Herein lies the rub. While a traditional esophagram (discussed in detail below) does send the radiopaque barium contrast through the oral and pharyngeal cavities, the amount of contrast swallowed may be very large. This allows excellent visualization of motility but pretty well obliterates the view of anatomical structures of interest in the oral and pharyngeal phases of swallow. *An esophagram or barium swallow and a modified barium swallow (MBS) or videofluoroscopic swallow study (VFSS) are not the same examination.* Many speech-language pathologists in the medical setting must artfully deal with confusion of the two studies when the MBS is first introduced to a diagnostic imaging department. For this reason alone, it is important for the speech-language pathologist to know what the different radiographic exams assess and how the examinations are conducted. This section of the chapter will review the most common radiographic procedures used to assess the upper gastrointestinal tract.

Pharyngoesophagram

Typically, for a complete examination of the pharynx and esophagus, a radiologist will videotape a **pharyngoesophagram**, most commonly known as an *esophagram, upper gastrointestinal series,* or *barium swallow,* to assess motility and also take still X-rays to assess anatomy. The terms are pretty generic, often loosely used, and not always descriptive of the exact structures viewed. The term *esophagram* is often substituted for *pharyngoesophagram.* In the field of radiology the term *barium swallow* is somewhat obsolete and has been replaced by the term *esophagram.* Strictly speaking, a pharyngoesophagram, or esophagram, will image the structures between the oropharynx to the gastric cardia (the part of the stomach where the esophagus connects). Figure 5-16 shows an A-P view with barium in the esophagus.

An upper gastrointestinal series will include all the structures viewed in an esophagram with the addition of the stomach and duodenum, the top part of the small intestine. The type of contrast used in these studies and order of presentation may vary (see Clinical Note 5–3). Barium may be thin or thick. A thin barium (considered light or heavy by volume weight) is presented to the patient in a large container or cup. The radiologist provides specific directions on the number of swallows he wants the patient to take. The patient is instructed to swallow sequentially as well as discretely with single swallows. Patient position, upright or supine, is controlled during or just following ingestion of the contrast material to thoroughly coat the structure of interest, such as the stomach. Images may be fluoroscopic, and therefore moving, or static (still). The still X-ray shots taken after a swallow of barium suspension are called *spot films* and refer to a still photograph taken at a specific location at one point in time. Spot films are designed to provide documentation about structural integrity.

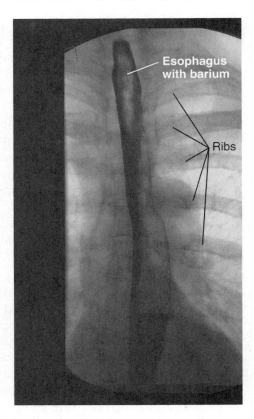

Figure 5-16. A-P view, fluoroscopic image during esophagram.

Barium

Barium is the typical contrast material used for an esophagram. A single contrast study will use thin barium (either light or heavy by volume weight) and fill up the structure of interest, such as the esophagus or stomach. In a double contrast study, a thick barium will be used to coat the structure of interest. A second step requires introducing air into the structure to distend it in order to view surface contours. Effervescent crystals may be used or the straw the person is drinking from will have a hole placed above the liquid line so that air is swallowed along with the barium. Examples of double contrast use includes visualization of tears in the mucosal surface of the esophagus or fungal infections that cause esophageal plaques (like cadidiasis).

A number of Diagnostic Imaging Centers will add powdered Kool-Aid or drink mix crystals to thin barium in order to flavor the chalky white mixture, especially when large quantities must be ingested as during an esophagram. This improves the taste (somewhat) while not affecting consistency.

Views are typically lateral and frontal or A-P (anterior-posterior) depending on the structure wanted for a view. Oblique views are often used to best visualize the esophagus without the image being superimposed against the vertebral column.

An esophagram requires numerous swallows to evaluate different structures and different movement patterns. In order to view certain structures or movements best, the patient's position is varied and the bolus type and amount is specified. Table 5-1 provides a summary of the position and bolus type/amount typically used. Keep in mind that in individual facilities there may be numerous variations depending on the individual radiologist conducting the study. The radiologist's goal is to visualize structural or motility disorders best depending on the symptoms reported by the patient. Protocols are not rigid standardized tests that must be followed in a specified way for each individual examined.

Modified Barium Swallow

The modified barium swallow (MBS), also known as a videofluoroscopic swallow study (VFSS), continues to be the most frequently used test when examining anatomy and physiology of the swallow mechanism. It remains the pre-eminent method to view the oral, pharyngeal, and early esophageal phase in real time and to diagnose the underlying cause(s) for the symptoms of aspiration and penetration. Also it allows visualization of the pharyngeal phase while compensatory strategies are tested for their ability to increase swallow safety and efficiency. Currently, no other technology has this versatility. The speech-language pathologist should be aware of current research that continues to support the efficacy of the MBS and its overall cost efficiency against inpatient hospital costs for the management of pneumonia or pulmonary complications secondary to aspiration. Clinical research continues to indicate that up to a third of dysphagic patients who aspirate do so silently, without coughing, as seen on a fluorographic lateral view in Figure 5-17 (Aviv, Martin, Sacco, Zagar, Diamond, Keen, & Blitzer, 1996; Horner & Massey, 1988; Lazarus & Logemann, 1987).

And at least preliminary data suggests that patients who demonstrate laryngeal penetration and aspiration on MBS, compared to those with dysphagia but no penetration/aspiration, are up to 10 times more likely to develop pneumonia. In the same study, a small group of silent aspirators were shown to be at an even greater risk—up to 13 times more likely to develop pneumonia (Pikus, Levine, Yang, Rubesin, Katzka, Laufer, & Gefter, 2003). An MBS is the only current clinical method that allows uninterrupted visualization of the pharyngeal phase during the act of swallowing for the purpose of observing physiology. That being said, it continues to have poor interrater reliability on all

Table 5–1. Contrast radiographic examination protocols (based on Low & Rubesin, 1993).

BODY POSITION	FILM	VIEW	ANATOMICAL LEVEL	BOLUS TYPE	AMOUNT	MANEUVER	STRUCTURES VIEWED
Upright	Videofluoroscopy	Lateral	Oropharyngeal	High density	8 to 10 ml	Swallow	Epiglottis & laryngeal vestibule
Upright	Videofluoroscopy	Lateral	Oropharyngeal	High density	15 to 20 ml	Swallow	UES
Upright	Double contrast spot film	Lateral	Oropharyngeal	High density	Residual contrast from previous high density liquid barium bolus	*say /i/*	Soft palate; tonsillar fossae, posterior pharyngeal wall; base of tongue;va lleculae; epiglottis; aryepiglottic folds
Upright	Videofluoroscopy	Frontal	Oropharyngeal	High density	8 to 10 ml	Swallow	Surface of tongue base; tonsillar fossae contours; valleculae, lateral walls of hypopharynx in profile
Upright	Spot	Frontal	Oropharyngeal			Modified valsalva by creating intraoral air pressure	All pharyngeal structures previously listed
Upright	Spot	Oblique	Oropharyngeal			Head tilt to enlarge spaces	Epiglottis; anterior walls of valleculae; pyriform sinuses
Upright	Double contrast		Esophageal	High density barium and effervescent agent	Rapid drinking to distend esophagus		Multiple consecutive swallows GERD; tumors of gastric cardia

(*continues*)

Table 5–1. (*continued*)

BODY POSITION	FILM	VIEW	ANATOMICAL LEVEL	BOLUS TYPE	AMOUNT	MANEUVER	STRUCTURES VIEWED
Prone	Single contrast	Right anterior oblique	Esophageal	Low density	8 to 10 ml	Single swallow	Esophageal motility
Prone	Single contrast	Right anterior oblique	Esophageal	Low density	Full cup	Continuous drinking	Able to identify esophageal webs, aortic arch anomalies, hiatal hernias, strictures, rings
Recumbent	Double contrast	Right lateral	Esophageal	High density barium and effervescent agent	Rapid drinking to distend esophagus	Multiple, consecutive swallows	GERD; tumors of gastric cardia

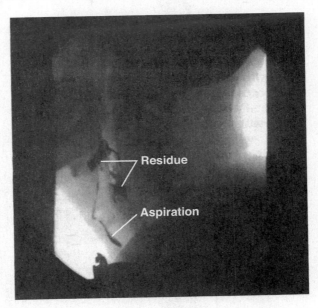

Figure 5-17. Lateral view, fluorographic image of aspiration.

swallow parameters (such as lip closure, delayed pharyngeal response, soft palate elevation, etc.) except whether the patient aspirates or not. This has been documented even among experienced raters from internationally recognized swallow centers (Stoeckli, Thierry, Huisman, Seifert, & Martin-Harris, 2003). Stoekli, et al., concluded that swallow parameters need to be defined with a greater degree of specificity (as in the definition of aspiration) and a consensus among raters must be obtained (Kuhlemeier, Yates, & Palmer, 1998; Ott, 1998; Scott, Perry, & Bench, 1998; Stoeckli, et al., 2003; Wilcox, Liss, & Siegel, 1996).

In Chapter 4 you discovered that bolus properties contribute substantially to the specific parameters of the swallow. It follows, then, that bolus properties will be among the manipulated variables during a diagnostic evaluation of swallow, such as in the MBS. But truly manipulating bolus properties is a bit more complicated than the *thin, thick, paste,* and *solid* hierarchy suggests. Important factors include the bolus **density** (weight), **viscosity** (thickness), and **yield stress** (difficulty to propel fluid). To further complicate matters, viscosity is influenced by temperature. These terms fall within the scope of **rheology** and fluid characterization factors—the study of properties associated with flow and deformation of a substance. Fluid can also be classified based on whether it is Newtonian or non-Newtonian. This refers to Newton's Law in physics, which states that the force applied to make something move is directly proportional to its flow. Many fluids we ingest are Newtonian—

things like water, juice, milk, honey, maple syrup. As you see from those examples, they may be thin or thick. But when fluids require more or less force applied than the resulting flow, they are considered non-Newtonian substances which include such food items as custards, yogurt, and baby food, or barium suspension used during videofluoroscopic exams. It is likely that barium-impregnated foods, used to make diagnostic and management decisions, do not have the same rheologic characteristics as their non-barium-impregnated versions. One recent, small study indicated that mealtime fluids are less dense and viscous than those fluids used during videofluoroscopy (Cichero, et al., 1997). It is easy to see how judgments made from the MBS may be flawed in estimating oral intake safety in real-world, mealtime eating situations. For example, a person with poor oral control may have done well in handling a *thin* barium bolus, not because of appropriate oral motor control skills for thin liquids, but because the increased viscosity of the test material made it easier to hold together prior to swallow response. This individual may continue to have problems handling a morning cup of *thin* coffee since the level of *thinness* varies from real-life to test situation. Currently, there is no easy way around this difficulty. It has been suggested that how a substance *looks* or *seems to pour* is far less accurate than the liquid's sensation in the mouth (referred to as *mouthfeel*). If two liquids do not move or feel the same in your mouth, it is likely that the rheological properties are not the same (Cichero, et al., 1997). Our clinical decision-making should be tempered by these concerns with test materials. Current research is calling for the establishment of a standard for the rheologic measurement of foods, nomenclature used, and interrater agreement between clinicians (Steele, Van Lieshout, & Goff, 2003). A commercial company in the US, EZ-EM, has responded to this need. EZ-EM produces the Varibar® line specifically for diagnostic use in the MBS without the need to dilute or thicken the products (Figure 5-18).

In the past, SLPs have added barium to thin liquids, nectars, or puddings in an effort to simulate normal foods more naturally. This does not improve standardization across tests or among clinics. Currently, the Varibar line is standardized for viscosity and yield stress in four consistencies: thin liquid, nectar, honey, and pudding (Figure 5-19). The four consistency categories have been designed so that the viscosity values do not overlap. As well, the viscosity and yield stress values approach those of actual food consistencies. The barium is apple flavored for the three liquid consistencies and vanilla flavored for the pudding consistency, in an effort to make the contrast material more palatable. Perhaps most importantly, the material has been designed to clear following normal deglutition rather than tenaciously coat structures, as do most commercial barium products designed for imaging of the gastroesophageal tract (e.g., esophagrams).

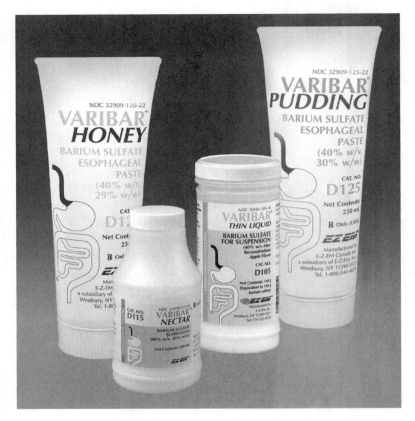

Figure 5-18. EZ-EM Varibar® barium products. (*Courtesy of EZ-EM, Inc. Used with permission.*)

For an MBS the patient is seated. Adaptive seating or careful positioning may be needed for individuals with motor disorders or structural problems of the head and neck to facilitate best swallow performance (see Clinical Note 5–4).

CLINICAL NOTE
5-4

Adaptive Seating Devices

Since posture and head and neck alignment during swallow is important for adequate function, as well as good fluoroscopic visualization, some medical centers will use a special, narrow patient chair to conduct the MBS (as shown in Figure 5-20). These types of specially designed chairs are mobile, can be tilted forward or backward, and allow lateral and A-P viewing without disrupting the image as some wheelchairs are prone to do. An adaptive seating chair is especially helpful when conducting an MBS on a patient who is motorically impaired.

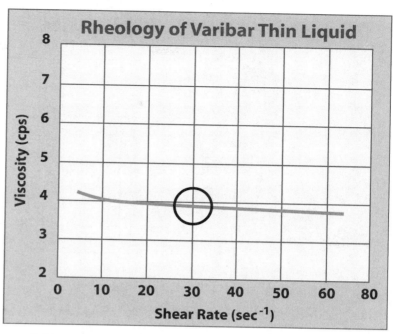

Figure 5-19a. Viscosity and yield stress graph for Varibar® thin liquid barium contrast. (*Courtesy of EZ-EM, Inc. Used with Permission.*)

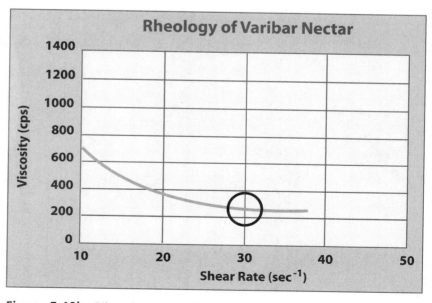

Figure 5-19b. Viscosity and yield stress graph for Varibar® nectar barium contrast. (*Courtesy of EZ-EM, Inc. Used with Permission.*)

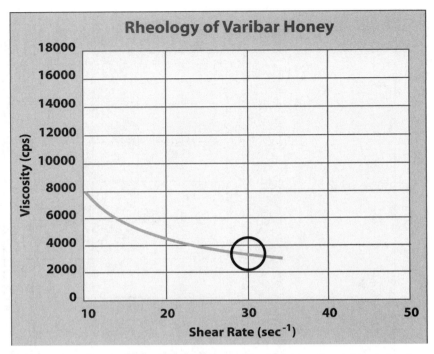

Figure 5-19c. Viscosity and yield stress graph for Varibar® honey barium contrast. (*Courtesy of EZ-EM, Inc. Used with Permission.*)

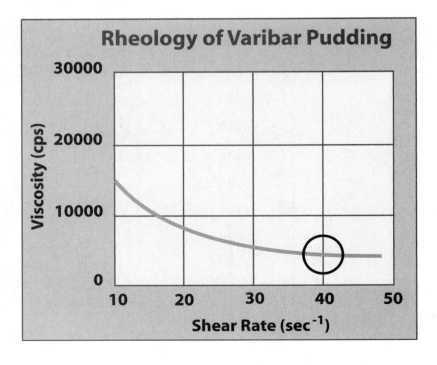

Figure 5-19d. Viscosity and yield stress graph for Varibar® pudding barium contrast. (*Courtesy of EZ-EM, Inc. Used with Permission.*)

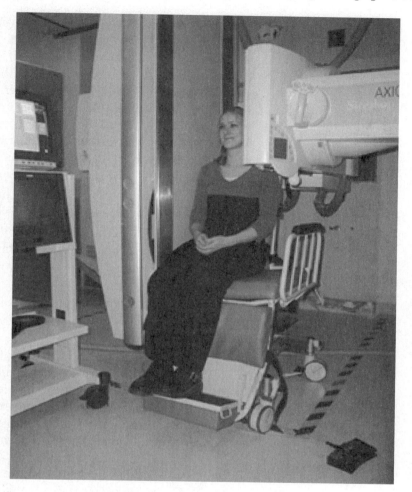

Figure 5-20. Patient in Hausted chair.

During an MBS, the speech-language pathologist provides the patient with differing amounts of thin and thick liquids, semisolid and solid foods, while the radiologist or radiology technician is responsible for controlling the fluoroscope. Food presentation may be by spoon, fork, cup, or straw and may be controlled by either the patient or the speech-language pathologist, depending upon the patient's ability. Procedures vary across settings and facilities but should follow some basic principles.

1. The purpose of the study is to examine oropharyngeal and upper esophageal anatomy and identify the physiological cause of dysphagic symptoms.

2. The food consistency thought to be swallowed most safely by the patient should be presented first during the MBS. This allows observation of the patient's best performance first.

3. If gross aspiration of the bolus occurs without reflexive or voluntary airway clearing the study should be terminated. While barium is considered to be relatively inert, a large quantity in the respiratory system is not a good idea and can compromise people with respiratory or systemic diseases. A recent report suggests the possibility that aspiration of barium may cause mild, long-term fibrosis (Voloudaki, Ergazakis, & Gourtsoyiannis, 2003).

4. A minimum of two to three boluses each of graded amounts of liquids should be presented—typically 1 ml, 3 ml, 5 ml, 10 ml, and normal mouthfuls (20 to 60 ml) from a cup (Logemann, 1998).

5. Semisolid and solid boluses may be small initially—approximately 1/3 teaspoon—then gradually increased to patient's normal bolus size.

6. Once the cause(s) of the symptoms is determined, strategies to improve function should be implemented and evaluated during the MBS.

Different facilities and settings will use various foods to mix with barium. Remember that the purpose of the study is to reflect the normal mealtime behaviors and difficulties best with the intent to improve swallow safety and efficiency. The closer you are able to simulate mealtime eating, the more realistic and generalizable your MBS results may be for that particular individual. Strategies such as baking barium right into bread (Gantz, 1997) or using minimal amounts of contrast in favored foods may yield better diagnostic and therapeutic results (see Clinical Note 5-5). An important caveat is that interrater reliability on the qualitative judgments made while reviewing the videofluoroscopic examination is notoriously low among experienced clinicians even when a rigid protocol of the same materials is used for all patients and decisions are binary (such as *yes/no* or *present/absent*) (Stoeckli, Seifert, & Martin-Harris, 2003). Making the examination more reflective of normal mealtime ingestion may increase these difficulties.

Clinical Note 5-5

Barium Bread

Baking barium into bread has been found to maintain a normal mouthfeel when used as a solid food during a modified barium swallow and avoids the problem of two consistencies, presented simultaneously (cookie plus paste), representing a solid food. Radiopacity was examined by a radiologist and found to be evenly distributed within the bread slice and functionally opaque for an MBS. EZ-EM, the manufacturer of the powdered barium, was contacted and they reported

continues

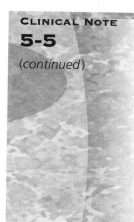

that baking temperatures (and freezing temperatures for storage) would not alter the composition of the barium. Powdered barium, incorporated into bread dough, did not sink to the bottom of loaves during baking. The taste was judged unaltered compared to regular bread by a group of speech-language pathologists (Gantz, 1997).

Recipe

Using a standard white bread recipe from a hospital dietetics department, add one and a half (1 ½) cups of barium powder (60% wt/vol) per two loaves of bread. Mix in a non-metal bowl to avoid barium residue. Bread can be sliced and frozen for individual use. Warm to room temperature 30 minutes before needed.

Nuclear Medicine—Scintigraphy

Scintigraphy is not used routinely in the diagnosis of aspiration in the adult population but has been used with some frequency in the pediatric population. A brief description of the technique is provided for general background knowledge. This methodology can be conceptualized as the opposite of a traditional X-ray. Rather than having the radiographic beams aimed at the individual, with the resulting image recorded on film as in an X-ray, scintigraphy relies on the transmission from an ingested radionuclide that can be detected by a special camera, called a gamma camera.

When used to diagnose aspiration, a radionuclide such as technetium-99m sulfur colloid, is mixed into the ingested material. Following ingestion, the patient is placed in a supine position under a gamma camera for imaging. The camera picks up the transmitted image from the radionuclide in the system. Imaging may continue for up to two hours post-ingestion of the radionuclide. A second imaging session may take place two hours later or, in the case of adults, the next morning, if used to detect aspiration during sleep. The images are captured at a frame rate of 15 seconds per frame and computer manipulated to provide *loops* for viewing. This methodology allows for quantification of aspirated material. Radionuclide studies are considered to be more sensitive to identifying aspiration than traditional barium studies but do expose patients to radiation through ingestion of the radionuclide (Collier, 1997).

Computed Tomography and Magnetic Resonance Imaging

Currently, CT scans and MRI of the oropharyngeal and esophageal structures are typically not used as primary diagnostic tools for oropharyngeal and esophageal problems. They may be used to stage diagnosed diseases, such as cancer, or to delineate masses found through other imaging techniques such as chest X-rays (Baron, 1995). Recent reports have outlined the use of CT in helping to determine the extent of esophageal infection (by actinomycosis) in AIDS patients (Arora, et al., 2003). Current clinical diagnosis and management of dysphagia rarely includes use of these images taken of the oropharyngeal and esophageal structures. However, different MRI methodologies have been explored in the search for non-invasive methods, without radiation exposure or risk of aspirating contrast materials, of studying individuals with dysphagia. The main difficulty has been in the trade-off between temporal and spatial resolution. Techniques that provide good time resolution (and can therefore capture very fast events like swallowing) have had poor spatial resolution—the ability to see structures differentiated from other structures. Single-shot, fast spin, echo dynamic MRI has sacrificed temporal resolution for improved spatial resolution that enables measurement of laryngeal elevation, oropharyngeal diameter, and tongue base and soft palate displacement (Hartl, Albiter, Kolb, Luboinski, & Sigal, 2003). Temporal measures cannot be made. No contrast material is needed. Normal foods can be used; however, solids provide a less intense signal than water and are difficult to identify if they fragment in the mouth or when they incorporate saliva. There remain a number of technical difficulties with this technique but it may hold clinical potential.

Pharyngeal Manofluorography

The combination of videofluoroscopy and manometry, also known as videomanometry, is beginning to emerge as a clinical tool. Recall that manometry was described in Chapter 3. Manometry alone is unable to inform the practitioner about pressures generated in the oropharyngeal and esophageal regions in relation to the bolus of food moving through the system. On the other hand, fluoroscopy alone cannot address incomplete UES relaxation even when the timing of opening is within normal limits. By combining the two types of studies, dynamic patterns may be quantified in terms of distance from anatomic structures and across duration as measured in milliseconds or seconds (Salassa, 1997). The timing and extent of sphincteric function and intrabolus pressures can be quantified. This information helps in assigning severity, directing treatment decisions, and evaluating treatment efficacy, and may provide needed information when deciding on medical-surgical intervention or behavioral treatment.

It is important to remember that manometry measures pressure within a cavity—it cannot measure the propulsive force applied to a bolus. A 100 cm catheter, 1.5 × 3 mm or 2 × 4 mm, containing three or four pressure-sensitive transducers, spaced out along its length, is most often used. Current improvements in types of sensors include the use of circumferential transducers and balloon sensors (van Herwaarden, Katz, Gideon, Barrett, Castell, Achem, & Castell, 2003; Matttioli, Lugaresi, Zannoli, Brusori, & d'Ovidio, 2003; Matttioli, Lugaresi, Zannoli, Brusori, d'Ovidio, & Braccaioli, 2003). Positioning of the catheter is important because the pharynx and esophagus produce pressure waves that are different in the A-P direction and the superior-inferior direction. Like the UES, more pressure is generated anterior-to-posterior than by lateral or side-to-side force (Sears, Castell, & Castell, 1991). The spacing of the transducers corresponds to the location of the tongue base, hypopharynx, UES, and esophagus. The types of pressures recorded by the catheter include resting, prebolus, intrabolus, and postbolus pressures measured in mm Hg (Salassaa, 1997). After topical anesthetic is administered the catheter is passed through the most patent nostril and advanced 27 cm. Sensors are located and checked for position. After the catheter is placed and secured, the MBS protocol, as described earlier in the chapter, is conducted. Specific information from the manometric portion of the study includes the timing of the lowest UES sensor pressure reading in relation to the location of the head of the bolus. This is a measure of UES relaxation and laryngeal elevation. It is most often a negative number, −2 to −6 mm Hg, in normal cricopharyngeal function, indicating that the relaxation/elevation occurred before the head of the bolus arrived. Post-swallow clearing waves can be used to quantify pharyngeal strength. Salassa (1997) suggests that clearing waves of 80 to 120 mm Hg are normal; 60 to 75 mm Hg are mildly impaired; 40 to 60 mm Hg are moderate; and less than 35 mm Hg are severely impaired.

MANOMETRY AND pH STUDIES

The most common test for diagnosis of gastroesophageal reflux disease (GERD) remains manometry and pH testing. Because speech-language pathologists frequently deal with the dysphagia and dysphonia associated with GERD, and provide input to the physician for medical management, this test will be explained in detail.

These studies are often conducted to confirm or rule out GERD, noncardiac chest pain, or motor disorders affecting the esophagus such as **scleroderma** (Nostrant, 1995). The four main regions explored manometrically include the LES, smooth muscle portion of the esophageal body, the striated portion of the esophagus, and the UES.

This procedure involves inserting the catheter into the nasopharynx and then gently guiding it through the UES, esophagus, and LES into the stomach. The catheter is then retracted either steadily (rapid pull-through method) or stepwise (station pull-through method) while manometric readings are taken from transducers at intervals. Following each pull-through the catheter is repositioned in the stomach. This process is repeated at least three times to record pressure measurements. Next, measures of the smooth portion of the esophagus are made on approximately 10 water swallows. The striated muscle portion of the esophagus can be targeted by using a station pull-through method with additional wet swallows. UES measurements of pressure and relaxation are made last. The process used at the LES is repeated here at the UES.

A standard manometric assessment provides information on amplitude of contraction and temporal measures (durations). Simultaneous contractions (also called common body contractions) in different segments of the esophagus, contractions initiated without a swallow or repetitive waves, are all considered pathological. Approximately 15% of wet swallows fail to initiate esophageal peristalsis (Wiley, Nostrant, & Owyang, 1995). Peristaltic failure on wet swallows is age-sensitive and is less prevalent in younger adults than the elderly.

pH studies are designed to see how well the esophagus clears acid, how long clearance takes, whether symptoms differ between acid or saline exposure, and whether gastroesophageal reflux is likely present. The test generally follows the manometric examination. The patient is given a 15 ml bolus of hydrochloric acid through the catheter, placed approximately 5 cm above the LES. Instructions request that the patient dry swallow every 30 seconds until the pH level returns to baseline level. Any disorder that disturbs peristalsis or reduces saliva availability may reduce acid clearance ability of the esophagus. Normal findings are considered pH values above four. Values below four are considered indicative of reflux.

Another component to pH testing is called the Bernstein examination. While no longer used routinely, it can be helpful in diagnosing chest pain. This portion of the testing is designed to elicit the reported symptoms of pain. First, saline is infused for five minutes. Then hydrochloric acid is infused in the same manner for a maximum of 30 minutes, or until symptoms are reported. A positive test for reflux would be pain with acid, but not saline, infusion. Conversely, no pain elicited by the acid infusion is negative for reflux. A positive test for a hypersensitive esophagus would be pain elicited on both saline and acid infusions. If the Bernstein exam was positive for reflux, the test would further try to simulate increased gastric pressure by infusing acid while placing the person in prone and supine positions on the right and left sides. Readings are taken throughout the exam. This is considered standard acid reflux testing (Wiley, Nostrant, & Owyang, 1995).

A related procedure is called ambulatory, 24-hour pH testing. This test does what its name implies—the catheter placed into the esophagus is left there for 24 hours and readings are made periodically and stored in a portable microcomputer that a person can carry around or wear with a belt. This is most commonly done when reflux symptoms are laryngopharyngeal in nature and treatment-resistant, or pre- and post-operatively for fundoplication (antireflux surgery). This is currently the most widely-used, single test for diagnosis of laryngopharyngeal and gastroesophageal reflux.

In the first three days following esophagectomy and gastric pull-up procedures, aspiration of stomach contents is difficult to diagnose and may lead to serious complications such as pneumonia. Intratracheal, long-term pH monitoring to detect aspiration was reported for a small group of patients and found to identify aspiration episodes. A drop in the pH to less than four was defined as an episode of aspiration. Statistical analysis showed that aspiration occurred most often in the first postoperative day, compared to the two following days (Stein, Bartels, & Siewert, 2003).

SUMMARY

This chapter addressed both direct and indirect measures of the upper digestive tract used to identify both structural and functional problems during swallow. We have approached diagnostic imaging of the oropharyngeal and esophageal regions by first discussing the various planes of examination used clinically. Speech-language pathologists rely heavily on superior, lateral, and A-P views when conducting or participating in endoscopic or videofluorographic procedures. Specific methodologies used by speech-language pathologists, as part of multidisciplinary teams, were described and included modified barium swallow studies—the most widely used test for observation of system physiology—and FEES, which may provide complementary information. The speech-language pathologist may or may not be present for an esophagram, conducted by the radiologist, which is used to diagnose gross anatomical defects and motility. Indirect methods from identifying problems, such as gastroesophageal reflux disease—including pharyngeal manofuorography, manometry, and pH testing—were described.

STUDY QUESTIONS

1. What plane of view best shows symmetry during swallow physiology on a modified barium swallow?

2. What is the medical "gold standard" for diagnosis of laryngopharyngeal reflux?

3. What is the difference between an *esophagram* and a *modified barium swallow* study?

4. Respond to the statement, *Thin barium is the same as most thin liquids we eat at mealtime.*

5. What is the best imaging technique for evaluating swallow function?

REFERENCES

American Speech-Language-Hearing Association. (2002). Knowledge and skills for speech-language pathologists performing endoscopic assessment of swallowing functions. *ASHA Supplement 22*, 107–112.

Ashoni, A. K., Nord, J., Olofinlade, O., & Javors, B. (2003). Esophageal actinomycosis: A case report and review of the literature. *Dysphagia, 18*(1), 27–31.

Aviv, J. E. (1997). Sensory discrimination in the larynx and hypopharynx. *Otolaryngology, Head and Neck Surgery, 116*(3), 331–334.

Aviv, J. E. (2000). Clinical assessment of pharyngolaryngeal sensitivity. *American Journal of Medicine, 108* (supplement 4a), 68S–72S.

Aviv, J. E., Kaplan, S. T., Thomson, J. E., Spitzer, J., Diamond, B., & Close, L. G. (2000). The safety of flexible endoscopic evaluation of swallowing with sensory testing (FEESST): An analysis of 500 consecutive evaluations. *Dysphagia, 15*(1), 39–44.

Aviv, J. E., Kim, T., Sacco, R. L., Kaplan, S., Goodhart, K., Diamond, B., & Close, L. G. (1998). FEESST: A new bedside endoscopic test of the motor and sensory components of swallowing. *Annals of Otology, Rhinology, and Laryngology, 107*(5 Pt 1), 378–387.

Aviv, J. E., Martin, J. H., Keen, M. S., Debell, M., & Blitzer, A. (1993). Air pulse quantification of supraglottic and pharyngeal sensation: A new technique. *Annals of Otology, Rhinology, and Laryngology, 102*(10), 777–780.

Aviv, J. E., Martin, J. H., Sacco, R. L., Zagar, D., Diamond, B., Keen, M. S., & Blitzer, A. (1996). Supraglottic and pharyngeal sensory abnormalities in stroke patients with dysphagia. *Annals of Otology, Rhinology, and Laryngology, 105*(2), 92–97.

Aviv, J. E., Martin J. H., Kim, T., Sacco, R. L., Thomson, J. E., Diamond, B., & Close, L. G. (1999). Laryngopharyngeal sensory discrimination testing and the laryngeal adductor reflex. *Annals of Otology,. Rhinology and Laryngology 108*(8), 725–730.

Aviv, J. E., Spitzer, J., Cohen, M., Ma, G., Belafsky, P., & Close, L. G. (2002). Laryngeal adductor reflex and pharyngeal squeeze as predictors of laryngeal penetration and aspiration. *Laryngoscope, 112*(2), 338–341.

Baron, R. L. (1995). Applications of computed tomography to the gastrointestinal tract. In T. Yamada (Ed.), *Textbook of gastroenterology* (2nd ed.). Philadelphia: J. B. Lippincott.

Cichero, J. A. Y., Hay, G., Murdoch, B. E., & Halley, P. J. (1997). Videofluoroscopic fluids versus mealtime fluids: Differences in viscosity and density made clear. *Journal of Medical Speech-Language Patholgy, 5*(3), 203–215.

Collier, B. D. (1997). Detection of aspiration: Scintigraphic techniques. *American Journal of Medicine, 103*(5A), 135S–137S.

Deyoe, L. A., & Balfe, D. M. (1995). Cross-sectional anatomy. In T. Yamada (Ed.), *Textbook of gastroenterology* (2nd ed.). Philadelphia: J. B. Lippincott.

Falestiny, M. N., & Yu, V. L. (1999). Aspiration pneumonia. In R. L. Carrau & T. Murry (Eds.), *Comprehensive management of swallowing disorders*. San Diego, CA: Singular.

Gantz, K. S. (1997). *Use of barium bread in the videofluoroscopic evaluation of swallowing*. Poster presented at the American Speech-Language-Hearing Association Conference, Boston, MA.

Hartl, D. M., Albiter, F., Kolb, F., Luboinski, B., & Sigal, R. (2003). Morphologic parameters of normal swallowing events using single-shot fast spin echo dynamic MRI. *Dysphagia, 18*(4), 255–262.

Kauer, W. K., Stein, H. J., Bartels, H., & Siewert, J. R. (2003). Intratracheal long-term pH monitoring: A new method to evaluate episodes of silent acid aspiration in patients after espohagectomy and gastric pull up. *Journal of Gastrointestinal Surgery, 7*(5), 599–602.

Kuhlemeier, K. V., Yates, P., & Palmer, J. B. (1998). Intra- and interrater variation in the evaluation of videofluorographic swallowing studies. *Dysphagia, 13*(3), 142–147.

Langmore, S. E., & McCulloch, T. M. (1997). Examination of the pharynx and larynx and endoscopic examination of pharyngeal swallowing. In A. L. Perlman & K. Schulze-Delrieu (Eds.), *Deglutition and its disorders*. San Diego: Singular.

Langmore, S. E., Schatz, K., & Olsen, N. (1988). Fiberoptic endoscopic examination of swallowing safety: A new procedure. *Dysphagia, 2*(4), 216–219.

Langmore, S. E., Schatz, K., & Olsen, N. (1991). Endoscopic and videofluoroscopic evaluations of swallowing and aspiration. *Annals of Otology, Rhinolgy & Laryngology, 100*(8), 678–681.

Leder, S. B., Ross, D. A., Briskin, K. B., & Sasaki, C. T. (1997). A prospective, double-blind, randomized study on the use of a topical anesthetic, vasoconstrictor, and placebo during transnasal flexible fiberoptic endoscopy. *Journal of Speech-Language Hearing Research, 40*(6), 1352–1357.

Low, V. H., & Rubesin, S. E. (1993). Contrast evaluation of the pharynx and esophagus. *Radiologic Clinics of North America, 31*(6), 1265–1291.

Mattioli, S., Lugaresi, M., Zannoli, R., Brusori, S., & d'Ovidio, F. (2003). Balloon sensors for the manometric recording of the pharyngoesophageal tract: An experimental study. *Dysphagia, 18*(4), 249–254.

Mattioli, S., Lugaresi, M., Zannoli, R., Brusori, S., d'Ovidio, F., & Braccaioli, L. (2003). Pharyngoesophageal manometry with an original balloon sensor probe for the study of oropharyngeal dysphagia. *Dysphagia, 18*(4), 242–248.

McDonough, J. T., Jr. (Ed.). (1994). *Stedman's Concise Medical Dictionary* (2nd ed.). Philadelphia: Williams & Wilkins.

Murray, J. 1999 *Manual of dysphagia assessment in adults.* Clifton Park NY: Delmar Thomson Learning.

Murray, J., Langmore, S. E., Ginsberg, S., & Dostie, A. (1996). The significance of accumulated oropharyngeal secretions and swallowing frequency in predicting aspiration. *Dysphagia, 11*(2), 99–103.

Nostrant, T. T. (1995). Evaluation of gastrointestinal motility: Methodologic considerations. In T. Yamada (Ed.), *Textbook of gastroenterology* (2nd ed.). Philadelphia: J. B. Lippincott.

Ott, D. J. (1998). Observer variation in evaluation of videofluoroscopic swallowing studies: A continuing problem. *Dysphagia, 13*(3), 148–150.

Pikus, L., Levine, M. S., Yang, Y. X., Rubesin, S. E., Katzka, D. A., Laufer, I., & Gefter, W. B. (2003). Videofluoroscopic studies of swallowing dysfunction and the relative risk of pneumonia. *American Journal of Roentgenology, 180*(6), 1613–1616.

Scott, A., Perry, A., & Bench, J. (1998). A study of interrater reliability when using videofluoroscopy as an assessment of swallowing. *Dysphagia, 13*(4), 223–227.

Sears, V. W., Castell, J. A., & Castell, D. O. (1991). Radial and longitudinal asymmetry of human pharyngeal pressures during swallowing. *Gastroenterology, 101*(6), 1559–1563.

Singh, V., Brockband, M., & Todd, G. (1997). Flexible transnasal endoscopy: Is local anesthetic necessary? *Journal of Laryngology & Otology, 111,* 616–618.

Steele, C. M., Van Lieshout, P. H. H. M., & Goff, H. D. (2003). The rheology of liquids: A comparison of clinicians' subjective impressions and objective measurement. *Dysphagia, 18*(3), 182–195.

Stoeckli, S. J., Huisman, T. A. G. M., Seifert, B., & Martin-Harris, B. J. W. (2003). Interrater reliability of videofluoroscopic swallow evaluation. *Dysphagia, 18*(1), 53–57.

Tytgat, G. N. (1995). Upper gastrointestinal endoscopy. In T. Yamada (Ed.), *Textbook of gastroenterology* (2nd ed.). Philadelphia: J. B. Lippincott.

Van Herwaarden, M. A., Katz, P. O., Gideon, R. M., Barrett, J., Castell, J. A., Achem, S., & Castell, D. O. (2003). Are manometric parameters of the upper esophageal sphincter and pharynx affected by age and gender? *Dysphagia, 18*(3), 211–217.

Voloudaki, A., Ergazakis, N., & Gourtsoyannis, N. (2003). Late changes in barium sulfate aspiration: HRCT features. *European Radiology, 13*(9), 2226–2229.

Wilcox, F., Liss, J. M., & Siegel, G. M. (1996). Interjudge agreement in videofluoroscopic studies of swallowing. *Journal of Speech and Hearing Research, 39*(1), 144–152.

CHAPTER 6

Physiological Bases of Neurogenic Dysphagia and Treatment Strategies

LEARNING OBJECTIVES

After completing the chapter and reviewing the study questions, you should be able to:

- Understand normal cortical, subcortical, and peripheral connections involved in sensory and motor control of swallow function

- Understand the complexity of neural disruption in neurogenic dysphagia

- Recognize co-occurrence of neurogenic-based dysphagia in neurodegenerative disease processes

- Understand the role of individual variability and presentation of neurogenic dysphagia

- Appreciate the anatomic and physiologic rationale for treatment strategies.

INTRODUCTION

Information in Chapter 4 indicates that deglutition is an extraordinarily flexible event, whose specific characteristics are determined by both bolus and swallower variables. At the core of this flexibility are the sensory-motor loops through the brain. These loops allow us to make a startling number of decisions and on-line adjustments in movement patterns, typically without any conscious contributions on our part. All of the movements are orchestrated by the central nervous system, in response to sensory information provided by peripheral receptors, and executed by the drive of nerves to the muscle tissue. Clinical populations have shown that damage anywhere along these vast swallow pathways can cause deficits in swallowing, some so severe as to completely preclude oral feeding. The purpose of this chapter is to explore the types of dysphagia symptoms and patterns associated with damage to these intricate neural pathways.

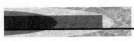

NEUROLOGICAL PATHOLOGY

Although the tissue of the central nervous system is encased in the protective bones of the skull and vertebral column and cushioned by cerebrospinal fluid, it is still very vulnerable to injury and disease. The major categories and types of neurological pathology, along with typical patterns of disability associated with each, are summarized in Table 6-1.

NEURAL REGULATION OF SWALLOWING

Previous chapters stressed the importance of peripheral sensory receptors and their communication with motor nuclei in the brainstem for swallowing. However, this critical loop (between peripheral receptors projecting to the nucleus tractus solitarius and motor commands emanating from the nucleus ambiguus) is only part of the story of the neural control of swallowing. Recent imaging studies, and a history of clinical evidence, have converged to confirm that the cerebral cortex and subcortical structures play a crucial role in both automatic and volitional swallowing (Martin, Goodyear, Gati, & Menon, 2001). We now believe that the cortical representation for swallowing is multifocal and bilateral, but with hemispheric dominance for at least some swallow tasks (Mosier, Liu, Maldjian, Shah, & Modi, 1999). Critical swallow regions have been identified in the cerebral cortex, basal ganglia and thalamus, and the cerebellum. Collectively, these swallow regions are thought to be instrumental in swallow initiation and fine-tuning movement parameters associated with deglutition by way of sensorimotor integration. Functional loops or *modules* among these higher structures supply their information to the nuclei in the brainstem for the accomplishment of safe and efficient swallows (Mosier & Bereznaya, 2001). Table 6-2 provides a summary of the most current supranuclear (above the brainstem) sites reported in the literature, along with their proposed contributions to swallow control.

NEUROGENIC DYSPHAGIA

With the vast neural system underlying swallow control, it is no wonder that dysphagia is a common feature of many neurological insults or diseases. Any pathology in the nervous system that affects critical tissue or pathways for the neural control of swallowing will produce neurogenic dysphagia. However, the relationship between site of lesion and dysphagia is not as distinct as that of site of lesion and speech/language-disorders. Perhaps because of the complexity of the interconnected cortical and subcortical loops, patients with similar lesions in terms of

Table 6–1. Summary of neurological etiologies often associated with the symptom of dysphagia.

ETIOLOGY	PATHOLOGY	IMPAIRMENT
Cerebrovascular accident (CVA)	Interference of blood supply to brain either by blockage of the blood vessel (thrombo-embolic event), or by hemorrhage (aneurysm); and subsequent tissue death (ischemia)	Determined by location and extent of lesion
Traumatic brain injury	Neural damage that results from an abrupt external event	Diffuse impairment, sensorimotor, affective, cognitive deficits
	Closed head injury: cranial impact or violent movement resulting in diffuse and widespread injury, edema, hematoma, axonal shearing	
	Penetrating head wound: entry of object through the skull that causes focal injury, bleeding, tissue damage	Impairment determined by location and extent of injury
Neoplasm	Growth of tumor in central or peripheral nervous system that impinges on normal function of the associated brain regions; benign or cancerous, proliferating or static, operable or inoperable	Impairment determined by location, extent, and variety of neoplasm
Infection	Infection introduced through the blood stream to the brain, its meningeal layers, and cerebrospinal fluid; diffuse damage that may be reversible or irreversible	Diffuse symptoms including sensorimotor and cognitive impairment
Toxins	Reversible or irreversible neural damage resulting from the introduction of toxins through the blood-brain barrier	Symptoms dependent on type and extent of damage
Degenerative diseases	Any pathological process that affects the central and/or peripheral nervous system; typically progressive; pattern of neural degeneration defines the disease	Dependent on etiology
Metabolic disorders	Rare occurrence of a metabolic disorder due to absence of a specific enzyme	May relate to several disease processes of the esophagus
Collagen vascular diseases (rheumatoid arthritis, lupus erythematosus, Sjögren's syndrome, scleroderma, dermatomyisitis, polymyositis)	Chronic degeneration of connective tissue components produced by a variety of autoimmune mechanisms; also called connective tissue disease	May involve the esophagus and predispose to reflux esophagitis and, in some patients, the development of esophageal strictures; periodontitis as a consequence of xerostomia may result from these diseases

Table 6–2. Supranuclear regions and pathways associated with swallow control and their hypothesized roles.

STRUCTURE	REGION	ROLE
Cerebral cortex	Lateral precentral gyrus	Primary motor representation for the oral, pharyngeal, and esophageal musculature
	Lateral postcentral gyrus	Processing of sensory information from the face including taste sensation; likely important for monitoring salivary accumulation or aspects of liquid bolus; sensation from oropharynx during oral stage manipulations
	Insula	Mediates sensory input and motor output from oropharynx and esophagus; contains at least part of the "gustatory cortex" mediating taste; anterior insula particularly linked with swallow control
	Frontal operculum	May play a role in orofacial sensorimotor behaviors
	Anterior cingulate cortex	May be important for attention allocation for volitional swallowing; selection of the sensorimotor plan
	Premotor cortex-parietal cortex loop	Planning swallow movement sequence among oral, pharyngeal, laryngeal, and esophageal structures
	Occipitoparietal cortex	Important for processing and integrating sensory and motor information; selecting appropriate motor plans based on nature of sensory input
	Periventricular white matter	Particularly linked with lingual coordination in swallowing
Basal ganglia	Loop of Broca's area, sensory cortex, corpus callosum, basal ganglia, and thalamus	Integrates sensory information about the bolus properties with the internal representation of swallow movements for an appropriate match

(Summarized from work presented by the following authors: Daniels & Foundas, 1999; Daniels, Brailey, & Foundas, 1999; Kern, et al., 2001; Martin, et al., 2001; Mosier & Brereznaya, 2001.)

territory, size, side, and acuteness often exhibit very different swallowing patterns (Alberts, Horner, Gray, & Brazer, 1992). For example, one patient with a left hemisphere stroke may have dysphagia characterized by oral phase disruption. A second patient with a left hemisphere stroke may have dysphagia characterized by pharyngeal stasis and aspiration after the swallow. And another patient with a left hemisphere stroke may not have dysphagia at all. The overlap of dysphagia symptoms in patients with neurological diseases and the lack of homogeneity amongst patients with similar neurological etiologies present a challenge for the speech-language pathologist. Nonetheless, the clinical examination will often reveal clusters of symptoms or hallmark features that are associated with a particular disease process or site of lesion. Although it functions as an integrated and dynamic system, oropharyngeal swallowing is divided into oral, pharyngeal, and esophageal stages when pathology is present in order to more effectively discuss where the breakdown in the system occurs. Oral, pharyngeal, and esophageal stage symptoms in neurogenic dysphagia are discussed in the following sections. Keep in mind that many disease processes affect more than one stage of swallowing.

Oral Stage Symptoms in Neurogenic Dysphagia

Weakness, paralysis, and/or incoordination of oral stage structures may result in inefficient preparation and/or transit of the bolus. These types of difficulties are common symptoms of cranial nerve lesions, particularly damage to the hypoglossal (CN XII) and facial (CN VII) nerves, and central nervous system damage to the cortex, periventricular white matter, or basal ganglia circuitry that is responsible for oral structure coordination. Some common examples of dysphagic symptoms of the oral stages include: drooling, pocketing of food in the buccal or labial sulci, difficulty manipulating the bolus, difficulty chewing, prolonged oral preparation time, and loss of control of the bolus. Patients who have unilateral peripheral facial paralysis, with intact pharyngeal and laryngeal musculature, cough and choke on solids and liquids during the acute stages of their disorder (De Swart, Verheij, & Beurskens, 2003). These pharyngeal stage symptoms may result from problems with motor, sensory, taste, and parasympathetic innervation (Secil, Aydogdu, & Ertekin, 2002). Another possible explanation for isolated facial paralysis to cause pharyngeal stage problems is that the highly automatic swallowing process is disrupted due to the lack of oral coordination and compensatory strategies that are applied by the patient (De Swart, et al., 2003). Table 6-3 summarizes common oral preparation and oral stage disorders along with possible motor/sensory sources.

Pharyngeal Stage Symptoms in Neurogenic Dysphagia

Recall the array of bolus-propulsive and airway-protective events that comprise the pharyngeal stage of deglutition. Damage that affects any aspect of this coordinative event may result in dysphagia. Because pharyngeal stage deficits increase the risk of choking and aspiration, sufficient clinical measures must rule out this component for the patient's safety.

Table 6–3. Common oral preparation and oral stage symptoms of swallowing disorders and possible motor and sensory mechanisms that should be assessed on examination.

SYMPTOM	MOTOR DYSFUNCTION	SENSORY DYSFUNCTION	OTHER
Drooling	Orbicularis oris	Disordered sensation in anterior oral cavity and/or lower face	Lack of initiation of pharyngeal phase; inefficient and infrequent swallowing
Pocketing of food in lateral sulci	Cheek muscles (buccinator and risorius); tongue musculature	Disordered sensation between the periodontal structures and mucosa of the cheek	
Pocketing of food in anterior sulci	Orbicularis muscle; tongue musculature	Disordered sensation in anterior oral cavity	
Difficulty manipulating the bolus	Cheek muscles; tongue musculature	Disordered sensation throughout oral cavity	
Difficulty chewing	Tongue muscles; muscles of mastication	Disordered proprioception in temporomandibular joint; disordered sensation of periodontal structures	
Excessive gagging	Hyperactive velopharyngeal closure	Oral hypersensitivity	Gastroesophageal reflux
Prolonged oral preparation time	Tongue musculature; facial muscles; muscles of mastication	Decreased oral sensation	Swallowing apraxia; xerostomia
Loss of control of the bolus	Tongue musculature; facial muscles; velopharyngeal musculature	Decreased oropharyngeal sensation	

Careful examination and visualization techniques are particularly important because many of these patients suffer sensory and motor deficits that suppress signs of dysphagia. Patients with severely diminished laryngopharyngeal sensation are at high risk of aspirating thin liquids even when pharyngeal motor function is intact (Setzen, Cohen, Perlman, Belafsky, Buss, Mattucci, & Ditkoff, 2003). If both laryngopharyngeal sensation and pharyngeal motor function are discovered to be impaired during clinical examination, the risk for aspiration is very high (Setzen, et al., 2003). It is estimated that a third of patients with neurogenic pharyngeal stage deficits aspirate silently, without any outward signs of difficulty such as coughing or choking (Aviv, et al., 1996; Horner & Massey, 1988; Lazarus & Logemann, 1987).

Neurophysiology of Silent Aspiration

Silent aspiration is defined as the entrance of food, liquid, or secretions below the vocal folds without any outward sign of difficulty. The normal physiological response to aspiration of material is a forceful cough. There are many reasons why this normal cough response is absent in many patients following a neurological event. The laryngeal mucosa has many receptors that are sensitive to chemical stimulation. These receptors are innervated by afferent fibers of the superior laryngeal nerve. A reflexive cough occurs when these chemoirritant receptors are stimulated (Addington, Stephens, Gilliland, & Rodriguez, 1999). Following neurological injury, the cough reflex may be weakened or absent up to a month or longer; in some cases it may remain impaired indefinitely (Kobayashi, Hoshino, Okayama, Sekizawa, & Sasaki, 1994). Damage to this normal physiological response increases the risk of aspiration, which may lead to the development of pneumonia.

Identification of Silent Aspiration

How is silent aspiration identified? Traditionally, silent aspiration has been identified during instrumental examination of swallowing using videofluoroscopy or videoendoscopy. If the patient aspirates during the examination, the clinician notes whether or not the patient showed any signs of feeling the aspiration such as coughing, choking, throat clearing, eyes watering, etc. If the patient does not show any of these signs, he or she is labeled a *silent aspirator* and the patient is identified to be at risk for development of aspiration pneumonia. What if, however, the patient *does not* aspirate during this brief examination? How can one be certain that the patient has adequate airway protection based on several swallows conducted in a rigidly controlled setting?

Addington and colleagues (1999) developed a way to test the integrity of the laryngeal cough reflex. The laryngeal cough reflex is critical to airway protection and the prevention of aspiration pneumonia. In this bedside test, subjects inhale a nebulized mix of tartaric acid and water as a microaerosal. This mixture causes cough stimulation in normal subjects. A weak or absent involuntary cough following inhalation shows that the neurological protection of the airway is impaired. This test appears to reliably identify stroke patients at risk of developing aspiration pneumonia (Addington, et al., 1999; Addington, Stephens, & Gilliland, 1999; Stephens, Addington, & Widdicombe, 2003). The reflex cough test is another clinical tool available for assessing the risk of developing aspiration pneumonia in neurologically impaired patients by identifying those at risk for inadequate airway protection and silent aspiration.

Pharyngeal stage deficits are common in diseases and injuries that affect large, multiple, or diffuse regions of the brain, and in degenerative diseases that impact muscle tone or coordination. Pharyngeal stage problems may also occur with peripheral nerve lesions, particularly of the vagus nerve (CN X). Examples of dysphagic symptoms that occur in the pharyngeal stage of deglutition include: delay in triggering the pharyngeal swallow, penetration, aspiration, reduced hyolaryngeal elevation, vallecular stasis, pyriform sinus stasis, and pharyngeal stasis. Table 6-4 summarizes common pharyngeal stage disorders along with possible motor and sensory sources.

Table 6–4. Common pharyngeal stage symptoms and possible motor and sensory sources that should be assessed on examination.

SYMPTOM	MOTOR DYSFUNCTION	SENSORY DYSFUNCTION	OTHER
Delay in triggering the pharyngeal swallow	Oral, pharyngeal, laryngeal, and/or esophageal musculature	Oropharynx and/or laryngopharynx	Swallowing apraxia
Laryngeal penetration	Hyolaryngeal elevation; laryngeal closure	Mucosa of larynx	
Aspiration	Hyolaryngeal elevation; laryngeal closure	Mucosa of larynx	Stasis aspirated after the swallow
Reduced hyolaryngeal elevation	Anterior belly of digastric, mylohyoid, geniohyoid, and thyrohyoid		
Vallecular stasis	Tongue base retraction; hyolaryngeal elevation	Valleculae and epiglottis sensation	
Pyriform sinus stasis	Hyolaryngeal elevation; cricopharyngeus muscle relaxation; pharyngeal constrictor function	Mucosa of pyriform sinuses	
Pharyngeal stasis	Superior constrictor; middle constrictor; inferior constrictor; hyolaryngeal elevation; cricopharyngeus muscle relaxation	Mucosa of pharynx	Xerostomia
Nasal regurgitation	Incomplete or mistimed velopharyngeal closure	Reduced sensation of posterior tongue, faucial pillars, velum, and/or posterior pharyngeal wall	Pharyngeal pooling

Botox for Spasmodic Dysphonia and Dysphagia as a Complication

Botulinum toxin (Botox) is used as a neuromuscular treatment that causes temporary paralysis in muscles by blocking the presynaptic release of acetylcholine at the neuromuscular junction. Botox has been used in the treatment of a variety of neurological disorders associated with inappropriate muscular contractions. These disorders as a group are called **dystonias**. Examples of dystonia include blepharospasm (uncontrolled eye blinking), torticollis (spasms twisting the neck), and spasmodic dysphonia (spasms affecting the larynx). Spasmodic dysphonia (SD), or focal laryngeal dystonia, is a condition in which the muscles of the larynx intermittently contract too strongly during vocalization. There are several types of laryngeal dystonia, including adductor, abductor, and mixed. In adductor SD, the vocal fold muscles close too tightly causing a strain-strangled, rough voice quality and decreased loudness. In abductor SD, the posterior cricoarytenoid muscle that opens the vocal folds intermittently contracts too tightly creating a breathy voice quality with sudden, intermittent voice arrests.

Botox has been used in the treatment of SD since the 1980s. The purpose of Botox is to treat the symptoms of SD by weakening the injected laryngeal muscles. Immediately following the injection of Botox into the laryngeal muscles, the patient often has a whispered or high-pitched voice quality and may aspirate liquids. The patient is taught the supraglottic swallow in order to temporarily protect the airway. Normal swallowing function typically returns within a couple of weeks. The effect of the Botox injection is short-term and needs to be repeated every three to five months.

Botox also has been used in the treatment of patients with dysphagia caused by dysfunction of the upper esophageal sphincter (Alberty, Oelerich, Ludwig, Hartmann, & Stoll, 2000; Blitzer & Sulica, 2001; Shaw & Searl, 2001). Patients with problems of the UES musculature have difficulty passing a bolus into the esophagus resulting in hypopharyngeal retention of the bolus with consequent penetration and/or aspiration. Historically, this problem has been treated with mechanical dilation and/or cricopharyngeal myotomy. More recently, investigators have injected Botox into the UES causing a temporary weakness. While early reports on this treatment have claimed efficacy for those patients with underlying muscle spasm, or hypertonicity of the UES musculature, long-term data with large sample size are not yet available (Ahsan, Meleca, & Dworkin, 2000; Alberty, et al., 2000; Blitzer & Sulica, 2001; Shaw & Searl, 2001). Some proponents of the treatment believe that a positive response to Botox can confirm the diagnosis of criocopharyngeal muscle spasm (Ahsan, Meleca, & Dworkin, 2000), although this seems a rather drastic method for diagnostic use.

Esophageal Stage Symptoms in Neurogenic Dysphagia

Esophageal motility is dependent on fully functioning, striated and smooth muscle as well as intact central and local neural mechanisms (refer to Chapter 3). There are a number of neuromuscular problems in the upper digestive tract (below the level of the UES) that can result in symptoms of oropharyngeal dysphagia in adults. Any disease process that threatens the integrity of muscle or neural control of striated or smooth muscle has the potential to impair esophageal motility. The most common symptom of a motility disorder is dysphagia and **odynophagia** (pain during swallowing). Discomfort arises because, quite literally, food gets stuck somewhere in the system. While not amenable to behavioral treatment provided by speech-language pathologists, an understanding and recognition of the disorders and symptomatology is necessary in order for the speech-language pathologist to effectively communicate with the patient and physician.

CLINICAL NOTE 6-4

Botox Treatment for LES Dysfunction

Botulinum toxin has also been used in the treatment of **achalasia** (failure of the lower esophageal sphincter to relax). This therapy involves injection of Botox into each of the four quadrants of the LES. This treatment often has successful results initially; however, long-term results continue to be studied (D'Onofrio, Annese, Miletto, Leandro, Marasco, Sodano, & Iaquinto, 2000; Neubrand, Scheurlen, Schepke, & Sauerbruch, 2002). Botox treatment for achalasia does not have serious adverse effects and has been most successful in elderly patients and in patients with less severe lower esophageal sphincter pressure (D'Onofrio, et al., 2000; Neubrand, et al., 2002). Patients who do not benefit from Botox injection into the LES may be candidates for dilation or myotomy.

A number of the disorders discussed below are observable on videofluoroscopic swallow studies and endoscopic examinations. While there are numerous disease processes that may result in motility dysfunction, some of the more common, or potentially disruptive, ones are described here. Prior to dysphagia evaluation, speech-language pathologists are strongly encouraged to carefully research any diagnosed systemic disease process. Often, collagen vascular diseases, endocrine, and metabolic disorders will have associated esophageal motility disturbances. Awareness of the pathophysiology of the disease may assist in diagnosis and management decisions.

Diffuse Esophageal Spasm and Nutcracker Esophagus

Diffuse esophageal spasm is a motor disorder in which the smooth muscle fibers of the esophagus contract in large amplitude, long duration, multiple contractions. Often, the contractions are spontaneous. The contractions often are painful and the multiple, simultaneous contractions often impair bolus movement during ingestion of food (Goyal, 2001). The underlying pathophysiology is not well understood. Reduction in enteric motor neurons as seen in achalasia is not present.

Nutcracker esophagus is a descriptive term for the presence of extremely high amplitude pressure waves in patients with non-cardiac chest pain or dysphagia. The criterion varies among gastroenterologists, but the range of pressures fall between 150 and 200 mm Hg (Richter, 1995).

Achalasia

The term achalasia means *failure to relax*. Achalasia is a motor disorder of the esophagus that results when smooth muscle fibers of the lower esophageal sphincter (LES) do not relax during swallowing-induced peristalsis. Normal peristaltic waves are replaced by asynchronous, low amplitude waves. The net result is a relatively adynamic esophagus that provides poor bolus transport. The motor disorder is the result of enteric nerve dysfunction in which the number of myenteric neurons is drastically reduced (Goyal, 2001). Symptoms of achalasia may include dysphagia accompanied by chest pain and regurgitation of food that is trapped in the esophagus. Regurgitation of food can lead to coughing or breathing problems. Achalasia is definitively diagnosed by manometry (Richter, 1995). Esophageal manometry can specifically demonstrate the abnormalities of muscle function that are characteristic of achalasia. Treatments include oral medications (nitrates and calcium-channel blockers), dilation of the esophagus, surgery (myotomy), and injection of muscle-relaxing medicines (botulinum toxin) directly into the esophagus.

Failure of the UES to relax properly is sometimes referred to as cricopharyngeal achalasia. The term achalasia, however, is reserved for the smooth muscle of the LES. *Cricopharyngeal dysfunction* better describes failed relaxation of the cricopharyngeal muscle. Cricopharyngeal dysfunction is identified during radiographic study by a prominent bar on the posterior wall of the pharynx at the level of the cricopharyngeus during the swallow. Manometric measurements are necessary to properly diagnose cricopharyngeal dysfunction. Treatments for cricopharyngeal dysfunction are based on severity and may include changes in diet, swallow behavior modification strategies, muscle strengthening exercises, dilation, myotomy, and injection of botulinum toxin (see discussion: Botulinum toxin [Botox] in the treatment of spasmodic dysphonia, upper esophageal dysfunction, and achalasia).

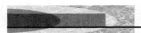

CLINICAL PRESENTATION OF NEUROGENIC DYSPHAGIA

Brief descriptions of the most common forms of neurogenic dysphagias encountered in clinical practice will be presented under the following headings:

- Disorders of the Cerebral Hemispheres and Brainstem
- Demyelinating Diseases
- Disorders of Movement: Extrapyramidal and Cerebellar Disorders
- Motor Unit Abnormalities
- Muscular Dystrophies and Other Myopathies
- Connective Tissue Disease

Proposed rationale for certain anatomic-physiologic based treatment strategies will then be presented.

Disorders of the Cerebral Hemispheres and Brainstem

Cortical structures influence swallow function and may be interrupted by numerous factors such as stroke, disease processes, injury, or congenital defects.

Cerebrovascular Accident

Stroke is the number one neurologic cause of dysphagia. Approximately 160,000 to 573,000 (or 42 to 75 percent) stroke patients are affected by dysphagia each year (Agency for Health Care Policy and Research, 1999). Many patients who suffer a cerebrovascular accident (CVA) have swallowing difficulty initially and then gradually improve with time, with the majority experiencing no major dysfunction after six months (Smithard, et al., 1997; Nilsson, Eckberg, Olsson, & Hindfelt, 1998). The severity and duration of impairment has been found to vary depending on the location of the stroke along with the presence of other risk factors such as being dependent for feeding, being dependent for oral care, number of decayed teeth, tube feeding, more than one medical diagnosis, number of medications, smoking, chronic airway disease, hypertension, and diabetes (Langmore, et al., 1998; Ding & Logemann, 2000). Multiple strokes, large strokes, and brainstem strokes have long been known to have the most devastating results on swallowing function (Horner, Massey, & Brazer, 1988; Horner, Buoyer, Alberts, & Helms, 1991; Ding & Logemann, 2000). It is also well established that unilateral strokes of the cerebral cortex, right and left hemisphere, can also result in dysphagia (Veis & Logemann, 1985; Robbins, Levine, Maser, Rosenbek, & Kempster, 1993). Although attempts have been made to correlate symptoms of dysphagia to the left or right hemisphere, results have not been consistent (Veis & Logemann, 1985; Johnson, McKenzie, Rosenquest, Lieberman, & Sievers, 1992; Robbins, Levine, Maser, Rosenbek, & Kempster, 1993; Daniels & Foundas, 1999). Possible explanations of this inconsistency are: (1) the level (cortical or subcortical) and location (anterior or posterior) of the lesion *within* the hemisphere is the important variable; and/or (2) there is asymmetrical motor representation of pharyngeal function in the cerebral cortex. Daniels and Foundas (1999) found that if the lesion is located in the anterior insular cortex or in the subcortical periventricular white matter, the patient is at a greater risk for aspiration than if the lesion is located in the posterior insular cortex or in the subcortical gray matter. Conversely, Hamdy and colleagues have shown repeated evidence that there is a dominant cortical hemisphere for pharyngeal motor representation, irrespective of handedness (Hamdy, et al., 1997; Hamdy, et al., 1998). The latter finding helps explain how swallowing function can recover following a unilateral hemisphere stroke. The undamaged hemisphere takes over the pharyngeal representation over time (Hamdy, et al., 1998). Dysphagia symptoms associated with CVA include reduced lingual control, slow oral transit, delayed triggering of the swallow response, reduced pharyngeal wall contraction, increased pharyngeal transit time, reduced laryngeal sensitivity, reduced laryngeal elevation, valleculae and pyriform sinus stasis, penetration, and aspiration.

Wallenberg's Syndrome, or Lateral Medullary Syndrome

Wallenberg's syndrome is a neurological disorder characterized by dysphagia and dysphonia. The cause of Wallenberg's syndrome is usually the occlusion of the posterior inferior cerebellar artery (PICA) or one of its branches supplying the lower portion of the brainstem, resulting in cerebellar and pyramidal tract signs. There is often partial involvement of the fifth, ninth, tenth, and eleventh cranial nerves (CN V, IX, X, XI). The pharyngeal stage of swallowing is typically impaired.

Brainstem Lesions

CVA, neoplasm, congenital defects, and traumatic brain injury all may affect the swallowing centers in the brainstem. Consequences range from mild impairment to the complete inability to swallow (Vigderman, Chavin, Kososky, & Tahmoush, 1998). Dysphagia symptoms will vary according to where the damage occurs; however, the following swallowing symptoms have been reported in patients who have suffered brainstem damage: oral manipulation and transit difficulty, pharyngeal asymmetry, unilateral laryngeal paresis or paralysis resulting in dysphonia, reduced duration and extent of laryngeal elevation, reduced cricopharyngeal opening, valleculae and pyriform sinus stasis, penetration, and aspiration (Horner, et al., 1991; Crary, 1995; Huckabee & Cannito, 1999). Despite the high incidence of dysphagia in this population, the long-term outcomes are favorable for over 80 percent of patients who receive aggressive intervention (Horner, et al., 1991; Crary, 1995; Huckabee & Canito, 1999; Meng, Wang, & Lien, 2000). Examples of intervention that have proven successful for this population include the use of surface electromyography to provide biofeedback on the use of maneuvers designed to enhance the duration and extent of laryngeal elevation, the use of head postures, thermal stimulation, and alteration of diet viscosity (Horner, et al., 1991; Crary, 1995; Huckabee & Canito, 1999).

Traumatic Brain Injury

In traumatic brain injury (TBI) the brain may be injured in a specific location or the injury may be diffused to many different parts of the brain. It is this indefinite nature of brain injury that makes treatment unique for each patient. Deficits to cognition, motor function, perception, speech, language, and social skills may all affect the ability to eat normally. Severity of the dysphagia in head injury patients increases in those who are comatose and increases with longer duration of the coma (Lazarus & Logemann, 1987). Delayed pharyngeal swallow response, reduced lingual control, and silent aspiration are among the dysphagia signs exhibited by TBI patients (Lazarus & Logemann, 1987).

Demyelinating Diseases

Any disease that damages the insulating tissue of nerve axons subserving muscles to structures involved in swallow may result in dysphagia.

Multiple Sclerosis

While the precise causes of multiple sclerosis (MS) are not yet known, much scientific research indicates that a number of factors in combination, including immunologic, environmental, viral, and genetic, are probably involved. It is now generally accepted that MS involves an autoimmune process involving an abnormal immune response directed against the central nervous system (CNS) that leads to the destruction of myelin (the fatty sheath that surrounds and insulates the nerve fibers). This demyelinization causes the nerve impulses to be slowed or halted and produces the symptoms of MS. Spasticity and incoordination of the oropharyngeal and respiratory muscles create functional problems with speech and deglutition. Dysphagia is common in MS due to disordered brainstem/cerebellar function, overall disability, depressed mood, and low vital capacity (Thomas & Wiles, 1999). Physiological function of the larynx and pharynx may be affected in patients with MS with the symptom of dysphagia (Abraham & Yun, 2002). Specific areas to examine in MS patients include the delay and incoordination of laryngeal movements and pharyngeal constrictor dysmotility (Abraham & Yun, 2002). The leading causes of morbidity and mortality in patients with MS are complications of dysphagia including dehydration, malnutrition, and aspiration pneumonia (Abraham, 1994).

Disorders of Movement: Extrapyramidal and Cerebellar Disorders

These motor disorders are associated with pathology that lies outside the pyramidal tracts, involving the basal ganglia and cerebellum. Disturbances in the function of neurotransmitters may result in hyperkinesia that occurs in disorders such as the **chorea**s (e.g., Huntington's disease) or may result in hypokinetic rigid disorders (e.g., Parkinsonism). Dysphagia often occurs at some stage in these disease processes.

Huntington's Disease

Huntington's disease (HD) is a hereditary, degenerative brain disease. Usually beginning in mid-life, cells in the caudate nucleus of the basal ganglia begin to die, causing a relentless deterioration of intellectual ability, emotional control, balance, and speech. Chorea, or involuntary movements, is usually a symptom. Dysphagia signs stem from the oral and pharyngeal stage disorders of lingual chorea and **tachyphagia** (abnormally rapid eating or bolting of food). This leads to other signs such as oral bolus retention or *squirreling*, impaired bolus formation, impaired voluntary swallow initiation, delayed pharyngeal swallow, laryngeal vestibule penetration/aspiration, and pooling in the pyriform sinuses (Leopold & Kagel, 1985; Kagel & Leopold, 1992). Hyperextension of the head and neck during the swallow contributes to these observed problems (Leopold & Kagel, 1985; Kagel & Leopold, 1992). Compensatory techniques such as reducing hyperextension, ingesting a lemon ice bolus prior to introducing food, placement of textured food on the lateral molars, verbal cuing on position and mastication, and reducing bolus amounts have been found to benefit the HD patient (Kagel & Leopold, 1992). These techniques should be taught to the patient's caregivers due to the cognitive disabilities that accompany advanced disease.

Parkinson's Disease

Parkinson's disease (PD) is a slowly progressive disease that affects a small area of cells in the midbrain known as the substantia nigra. Gradual degeneration of these cells causes a reduction in the neurotransmitter, dopamine. When dopamine depletion reaches a critical threshold, patients exhibit a resting tremor on one side of the body; generalized slowness of movement initiation (bradykinesia); stiffness of limbs (rigidity); and gait or balance problems (postural dysfunction). Dysphagia has been demonstrated in 63 to 81 percent of patients with PD (Agency for Health Care Policy and Research, 1999). Patients with PD often deny dysphagia symptoms despite distinct abnormalities (Robbins, Logemann, & Kirshner, 1986; Bushmann, Dobmeyer, Leeker, & Perlmutter, 1989). One of the striking features of the motor disability in patients with PD is bradykinesia (prolonged reaction time to initiate a movement). Rigidity and bradykinesia underlie the disordered volitional stage of deglutition (Robbins, et al., 1986). Impaired lingual movement, minimal jaw opening, abnormal head and neck posture, and impulsive eating behavior have been found to lead to the following oral and pharyngeal stage disorders: delayed oral transit time (characterized by tongue pumping and piecemeal deglutition), impaired sensorimotor integration, delayed pharyngeal swallow, pooling in the valleculae, pooling in the pyriform sinuses, reduced pharyngeal contraction, and silent aspiration (Bushmann, et al., 1989; Leopold & Kagel, 1996; Leopold & Kagel, 1997; Robbins, et al., 1986). Some PD patients demonstrate improved deglutition following use of the drug levodopa (Bushmann, et al., 1989). Coordination of drug therapy with mealtimes should therefore be clinically attempted in patients with PD while monitoring for improvement. PD patients who have received dysphagia therapy (range of tongue motion exercises, tongue resistance exercises, exercises to increase the adduction of the vocal folds, the Mendelsohn maneuver, and range of motion exercises in the neck, trunk, and shoulder joints) have demonstrated a quicker initiation of the swallow response (Sharkawi, Ramig, Logemann, Pauloski, Rademaker, & Smith, et al., 2002; Nagaya, Kachi, & Yamada, 2000).

Pseudobulbar Palsy

Pseudobulbar palsy is a syndrome characterized by spastic weakness of the pharyngeal musculature causing dysphagia, dysarthria, and dysphonia. Emotional lability is often a part of the syndrome. Pseudobulbar palsy results from diseases affecting the cerebral hemispheres and/or the corticobulbar tracts, including multiple sclerosis, amyotrophic lateral sclerosis, and cerebrovascular disorders.

Motor Unit Abnormalities

Disorders of the motor unit are classified according to the segment that is selectively affected. Any disease that affects the motor unit may result in dysphagia.

Amyotrophic Lateral Sclerosis

Amyotrophic lateral sclerosis (ALS), known as *Lou Gehrig's disease*, is a progressively neurodegenerative disease of unknown etiology that attacks brain and spinal cord nerve cells that control voluntary movement, affecting both upper and lower motor neuron systems to varying degrees. The loss of motor neurons causes the muscles under their control to weaken and atrophy, leading to paralysis. The pattern of dysphagia symptoms rather closely reflects the location of degenerative changes. Dysphagia eventually occurs in all types of ALS, although the clinical course and time of onset differs (Kawai, Tsukuda, Mochimatsu, Enomoto, Kagesato, & Hirose, et al., 2003). The degeneration of upper motor neurons results in symptoms that include increased deep tendon reflexes and a demonstration of pathologic reflexes. When lower motor neurons in the brainstem (bulbar neurons) are affected, the muscles responsible for speech, chewing, and deglutition atrophy. Patients with bulbar ALS present with oral and pharyngeal dysphagia, characterized by reduction in tongue mobility and oral-bolus control, delay in triggering the pharyngeal swallow response, reduced pharyngeal contraction, reduced laryngeal elevation, stasis in the valleculae, stasis in the pyriform sinuses, residue on the pharyngeal walls, penetration, and aspiration (Logemann, 1998). Many of these patients develop malnutrition and weight loss as a result of their progressive dysphagia, accelerating their muscle weakness (Kirshner, 1989). Behavioral management to improve dysphagic symptoms includes the use of compensatory procedures such as postures, tactile-thermal stimulation, and modification of diet. Exercises are contraindicated with ALS patients because they cause further fatigue of the musculature (Logemann, 1998). Medical management to improve dysphagic symptoms includes: percutaneous gastrostomy (PEG), removal of submaxillary glands, tracheostomy, and salivary diversion (Hillel, Dray, Miller, Yorkston, Konikow, Strande, & Browne, 1999). Nutritional and respiratory failure occurs in most patients with ALS.

Guillaine-Barre Syndrome

Guillaine-Barre syndrome (GBS) is an acute disease of the peripheral nerves. The rapid onset of weakness and often, paralysis of the legs, arms, muscles of respiration, and face characterize it. Abnormal sensations often accompany the weakness. The cause is unknown. Approximately 50 percent of cases occur shortly after a viral infection with symptoms that may include a sore throat or diarrhea. Some theories suggest an autoimmune mechanism, in which the patient's defense system of antibodies and white blood cells is triggered into damaging the nerve covering or insulation, leading to weakness and abnormal sensation. If the muscles of mastication and deglutition are involved, the patient may be completely unable to eat by mouth. GBS improves spontaneously and most patients experience total recovery. The patients may temporarily be treated with alternative feeding until adequate recovery allows for return to safe oral feeding. Dysphagia signs have been reported in both the oral and pharyngeal stages of swallowing and vary according to the cranial nerves that are involved (Chen, Donofrio, Frederick, Ott, & Pikna, 1996).

Myasthenia Gravis

Myasthenia gravis (MG) is a disease that affects how nerve impulses are transmitted to muscle at the neuromuscular junction. It is an *autoimmune* disease in which the body generates an immune system attack against its own skeletal muscles. Although people with MG virtually always do very well when treated properly, MG can be life-threatening when muscle weakness interferes with respiration. MG is characterized by fluctuating ocular or bulbar weakness and often with limb weakness that becomes progressively fatigued with repeated use. MG often affects the muscles innervated by the bulbar nuclei (face, lips, eyes, tongue, throat, and neck). Sudden inability to swallow or to breathe may occur at any time (Nishino, 1993). Dysphagia symptoms often appear after the musculature is fatigued; therefore, it is recommended that the MBS study be conducted before and after a meal in order to evaluate the disorder when symptoms are present. Dysphagia is caused by weakness of the striated muscles in the pharynx and esophagus. Dysphagia signs that have been described in patients with MG include: decreased pharyngeal motility, valleculae and pyriform sinus stasis, laryngeal penetration, aspiration, and impaired esophageal transit (Linke, Witt, & Tatsch, 2003; Kluin, Bromberg, Feldman, & Simmons, 1996). Pharmacological treatment positively affects striated muscles in the pharynx and upper esophagus (Linke, et al., 2003). Due to fatigability of the musculature, it is recommended that patients with MG be taught to use compensatory strategies such as postures, modification of diet, and eating several small meals a day (Logemann, 1998).

Lambert-Eaton Myasthenia Syndrome

A less common autoimmune disease of the neuromuscular junction is Lambert-Eaton (myasthenia) syndrome (LEMS). LEMS patients typically have weakness in pelvic, thigh, shoulder, and arm muscles. However, cranial nerves may be affected, causing muscle weakness that may result in dysphagia and aspiration (Nishino, 1993). LEMS can be life-threatening when muscle weakness interferes with respiration.

Muscular Dystrophies and Other Myopathies

Muscular dystrophy and other myopathies such as polymyositis and dermatomyositis have progressive muscle weakness in common. Decreasing muscle strength can compromise the person's ability to swallow normally, thus leading to dysphagia.

Muscular Dystrophy

There are nine muscular dystrophies (MD) each with its own set of signs and symptoms. Infantile myotonic dystrophy may cause severe dysphagia, which may lead to aspiration and disruption of normal feeding in children (Brin & Younger, 1988). Adult-onset myotonic dystrophy is characterized by hyperexcitability of the skeletal muscle (myotonia) and muscle degeneration (**myopathy**). Patients with MD often experience pharyngeal and esophageal dysphagia characterized by incomplete upper esophageal sphincter relaxation and a hypotonic or atonic esophagus (Costantini, et al., 1996; Marcon, et al., 1998). These esophageal problems may result in bolus transport problems with food getting stuck at the UES or within the esophagus itself. Oculopharyngeal muscular dystrophy (OPMD) is an adult-onset muscular dystrophy associated with swallowing problems, articulation problems, resonance problems, ptosis, trunk limb weakness, and difficulty with breath support. Dysphagia signs of OPMD include reduced or absent pharyngeal peristalsis, reduced opening of upper esophageal sphincter, valleculae and pyriform sinus stasis, penetration, aspiration, pneumonia, and weight loss (Perie, Eymard, Laccourreye, Chaussade, Fardeau, & Lacau-St. Guily, 1997). Dysphagia in OPMD patients is often managed surgically with an upper esophageal sphincter myotomy with good initial results in patients with adequate pharyngeal contraction (Perie, et al., 1997; Fradet, Pouliot, Robichaud, St. Pierre, & Bouchard, 1997). Patients with Duchenne's muscular dystrophy (DMD) often experience dysphagia due to esophageal motility alterations and delayed gastric emptying resulting in regurgitation, epigastric pain, constipation, and distention (Camelo, Awad, Madrazo, Aguilar, & Awad, 1997). Patients in the later stages of DMD often have **macroglossia** (large tongue) and may experience difficulties in the oral phase of deglutition (Willig, Paulus, Lacau-St. Guily, Beon, & Navarro, 1994).

Inflammatory Myopathies

Polymyositis (PM) and dermatomyositis (DM) are two forms of inflammatory myopathies which are diseases of muscle caused by an immune response; muscle weakness is their major sign. Dermatomyositis also causes a skin rash. Both are thought to be autoimmune diseases in which the body's immune system attacks the muscles. The main features of dysphagia in PM and DM are dryness of the mouth (xerostomia), decreased pharyngeal contraction, and decreased upper esophageal sphincter opening (Willig, Paulus, Lacau-St. Guily, Beon, & Navarro, 1994; Lacau-St. Guily, Perie, Willig, Chaussade, Eymard, & Angelard, 1994). Pharmacological and surgical intervention include the use of steroids and immunoglobin and cricopharyngeal myotomy respectively (Lacau-St. Guily, et al., 1994; Dalakas, 1998; Marie, et al., 1999). Marie, et al. (1999) treated steroid-resistant PM/DM patients, who presented with severe dysphagia requiring gastric tube feeding, with intravenous immunoglobin therapy. Dysphagia was effectively treated with the immunoglobin therapy and the patients were able to return safely to oral feeding.

Connective Tissue Disease

Connective tissue disease, also referred to as collagen vascular disorders and autoimmune disease, is characterized by widespread inflammatory damage to connective tissues and blood vessels. These changes often lead to dysphagia.

Scleroderma, or Progressive Systemic Sclerosis

Scleroderma or PSS is a relatively rare autoimmune disease, diagnosed most often in middle-aged women, that targets blood vessels and connective tissues of the body. The fibrous changes associated with scleroderma affect the skin, lungs, esophagus, digestive tract, and kidneys. This systemic disease affects the esophagus by causing atrophy of smooth muscle fibers in the esophagus, weak contractions of the lower esophagus during peristalsis, and an incompetent LES. Fibrosis may occur in the esophageal walls. The net result is dyspagia for liquids and solids and a predisposition to reflux esophagitis particularly in the supine position due to the incompetent LES. Treatment is currently symptomatic with aggressive attention to reflux prevention (Goyal, 2001).

Sjögren's Syndrome

Sjogren's syndrome is an immune system disorder that results in severe dryness of mucous membranes in the mouth, eyes, pharynx, larynx, and digestive tract. Symptoms are the result of insufficient production of fluids by the lacrimal, salivary, and other glands in the body. It primarily affects middle-aged women. Treatment is symptomatic and directed at easing dryness of affected structures. Increased hydration is recommended to facilitate swallow and keep oral structures moist.

Treatment Considerations

The primary focus of this text is the anatomy and physiology of deglutition and dysphagia rather than clinical approaches to treatment; however, the majority of clinical approaches derive from the understanding of the neurology, anatomy, and physiology that underlies normal and disordered deglutition. In this spirit, an overview of the management of neurogenic dysphagia with underlying physiological bases is presented, and a summary is listed in Table 6-5.

The swallowing clinician has a number of management strategies to choose from and becomes a dysphagia detective when determining the best treatment choice for each unique patient. Often a combination of treatment strategies is necessary. When gathering information, the following variables help determine the proper course of treatment for dysphagia of neurological origin: 1) the clinical and instrumental examination results, 2) the neurological disease and expected course, 3) the patient's motivation, 4) the patient's cognitive abilities, 5) the patient's abilities to volitionally move the head, neck, and body, 6) the effects of fatigue on the musculature, and 7) the patient's support network. Prognosis depends on the etiology, pathophysiology of the disease process, and severity of the dysphagia. The rationale for deciding which treatment to try is based upon the attempt to find the least restrictive, easiest, and least fatiguing treatment that will allow safe swallowing. Ideally, the treatment chosen will be used on a temporary basis until the patient's swallow recovers. However, there are patients who can only swallow safely and efficiently using a treatment strategy permanently.

Logemann (1993) suggests introducing treatments in the following order: 1) postural techniques, 2) techniques to enhance oral sensation, 3) swallowing maneuvers, and 4) diet changes. Postural techniques are introduced first because they can be applied to a large variety of patients, require minimal learning, and have been reported to be effective in eliminating aspiration (Logemann, 1993; Rasley, Logemann, Kahrils, Rademaker, Pauloski, & Dodds, 1992; Horner, Massey, Riski, Lathrop, & Chase, 1988). Postural variations redirect food flow and change pharyngeal dimensions in systematic ways in order to facilitate safe passage of the bolus through a less functional physiology. Rasley and colleagues (1992) found that 77 percent of patients with oropharyngeal dysphagia benefited from postural changes. More specifically, aspiration was eliminated in all bolus volumes in 25 percent of the patients using postural changes. Postural adjustments include head back, chin tuck, head rotation, head tilt, and side lying.

Increasing sensory input is recommended for a patient with reduced recognition of food in the mouth, or for patients with a delayed/absent triggering of the pharyngeal swallow. Unfortunately, the

Table 6–5. Summary of treatment strategies, their underlying rationale, instructions to the patient, and desired swallow outcomes.

TREATMENT STRATEGY	WHY DO IT? (rationale based upon swallowing symptoms)	HOW TO DO IT?	WHAT DOES IT DO?	SUPPORTING EVIDENCE
Head back	Difficulty with oral control and bolus transport. Must have normal pharyngeal phase	Patient tilts head back during the swallow	Uses gravity to propel the bolus into the pharynx; duration of UES relaxation decreases with increased head extension	Rasley, Logemann, Kahrilas, Rademaker, Pauloski, & Dodds, 1993; Castell, Castell, Schultz, & Georgeson, 1993
Chin tuck	Lack of oral control resulting in premature spillage of the bolus into the pharynx; delay in triggering the pharyngeal swallow; reduced airway closure; reduced tongue-base retraction (vallecular stasis)	Patient tilts head forward, touching chin firmly to chest before the swallow	Keeps the bolus in an anterior position allowing better control and preventing premature spillage; widens the vallecula to prevent bolus from entering the airway; puts the epiglottis in a more protective position; narrows the airway entrance; pushes the tongue-base toward the pharyngeal wall	Lewin, Hebert, Putnam, & DuBrow, 2001; Bulow, Olsson, & Ekberg, 2001; Welch, Logemann, Rademaker, & Kahrilas, 1993
Head rotation to the weak side	Unilateral pharyngeal paralysis or paresis; unilateral vocal fold paralysis or paresis; reduced opening of the cricopharyngeal sphincter	Patient turns head fully to the weak side before the swallow	Directs the bolus down the stronger side closing the pyriform sinus on the damaged side; increases vocal fold closure by placing extrinsic pressure on the thyroid cartilage; increases the length of cricopharyngeal sphincter opening and decreases cricopharyngeal resting pressure, thereby reducing pyriform sinus stasis	Ohmae, Ogura, Kitahara, Karaho, & Inouye, 1998; Logemann, Kahrilas, Kobara, & Vakil, 1989

(continues)

Table 6–5. (*continued*)

TREATMENT STRATEGY	WHY DO IT? (rationale based upon swallowing symptoms)	HOW TO DO IT?	WHAT DOES IT DO?	SUPPORTING EVIDENCE
Head tilt to the stronger side	Unilateral pharyngeal paralysis or paresis	Patient tilts head to the stronger side prior to the swallow	Directs the bolus down the stronger side by utilizing the effects of gravity	
Side lying	Reduced pharyngeal contraction leading to pharyngeal residue and aspiration after the swallow	Patient lies down on side during eating and drinking	Eliminates gravitational effect on pharyngeal residue; reduces risk of aspiration by holding the bolus on the pharyngeal walls	Drake, O'Donoghue, Bartram, Lindsay, & Greenowood, 1997; Rasley, et al., 1993
Tactile thermal application (TTA)	Delayed swallow initiation; reduced sensory recognition of the bolus in the oral cavity	Clinician uses a small, long-handled laryngeal mirror held in ice water for several seconds and then lightly rubs up and down vertically along the anterior faucial arches; light contact is repeated 5 to 10 times and is followed by a trial of ice water; stimulation is repeated 4 to 5 times daily for 5 to 10 minutes each time for several weeks to a month (Logemann, 1983)	TTA has been used clinically to shorten the timing of the pharyngeal swallow response	Sciortino, Liss, Case, Gerritsen, & Katz, 2003; Lazzara, Lazarus, & Logemann, 1986; Rosenbek, Roeker, Wood, & Robbins, 1996
Cold, textured, and/or flavored bolus	Delayed swallow initiation; reduced sensory recognition of the bolus in the oral cavity	Present the patient with a cold, textured, or flavored bolus (e.g., sour)	These techniques have been used clinically to shorten the timing of the oral and pharyngeal swallow response	Hamdy, Jilani, Price, Parker, Hall, & Power, 2003; Pelletier & Lawless, 2003; Logemann, et al., 1995

(*continued*)

Table 6–5. (*continued*)

TREATMENT STRATEGY	WHY DO IT? (rationale based upon swallowing symptoms)	HOW TO DO IT?	WHAT DOES IT DO?	SUPPORTING EVIDENCE
Carbonated thin liquids	Delayed pharyngeal swallow resulting in penetration and aspiration and increased pharyngeal transit time; reduced pharyngeal wall contraction resulting in pharyngeal retention		Carbonated liquids have been shown to reduce penetration and aspiration compared to non-carbonated liquids; carbonated liquids showed reduced pharyngeal transit time and pharyngeal retention when compared to thickened liquids	Bulow, Olsson, & Ekberg, 2003
Supraglottic swallow*	Reduced or late vocal fold closure (aspiration during swallow); delayed pharyngeal swallow	Inhale and hold your breath; Swallow while holding your breath; cough; swallow again. (Use of FEES to provide biofeedback is recommended)	Protect airway before and during the swallow; improves coordination of the swallow	Martin, Logemann, Shaker, & Dodds, 1993
Super-supraglottic swallow*	Reduced or late vocal fold closure (aspiration during swallow); delayed pharyngeal swallow	Inhale; hold your breath and bear down hard; swallow while holding your breath hard; cough; swallow again	Bearing down helps tilt the arytenoids forward, close the false vocal folds, and close the entrance to the airway	Logemann, 1998; Logemann, Pauloski, Rademaker, & Colangelo, 1997
Effortful swallow	Reduced tongue-base retraction (vallecullar stasis)	Swallow hard; push and squeeze all of the muscles of your mouth and throat	Effort increases posterior tongue-base movement and thus improves clearance of bolus from valleculae	Logemann, 1998; Bulow, Olsson, & Ekberg, 2001

(*continued*)

Table 6–5. (*continued*)

TREATMENT STRATEGY	WHY DO IT? (rationale based upon swallowing symptoms)	HOW TO DO IT?	WHAT DOES IT DO?	SUPPORTING EVIDENCE
Mendelsohn maneuver	Reduced laryngeal elevation; reduced cricopharyngeal opening; discoordinated swallow	As you swallow and your voice box lifts up, hold it at the top with your muscles for several seconds (Logemann, 1998); use of surface EMG for biofeedback is recommended (Crary & Groher, 2000)	Increases the duration and width of cricopharyngeal augmentation reducing pyriform sinus stasis and eliminating aspiration; improves coordination and timing of swallowing events; strengthens and retrains the muscles of laryngeal elevation	Bartolome & Neumann, 1993; Kahrilas, Logemann, Krugler, & Flanagan, 1991; Lazarus, Logemann, & Gibbons, 1993; Kahrilas, et al., 1991
Oral-motor exercises	Weakness of the oral musculature results in drooling, loss of control of the bolus, inability to manipulate the bolus, difficulty chewing, and/or pocketing of food	See Chapter 7 for specific oral-motor exercises	Improve lip closure; extend vertical and antero-posterior range of motion of the tongue; improve chewing	Lazarus, Logemann, Huang, & Rademaker, 2003; Sharkawi, Ramig, Logemann, Pauloski, Rademaker, Smith, et al., 2002
Shaker exercises	Reduced cricopharyngeal opening (pyriform sinus stasis and aspiration)	Lay flat on your back and raise your head high enough to see your toes without raising your shoulders; hold your head in this position for one minute; rest one minute (3 times); now raise your head up and down repetitively (30 times)	Strengthens the suprahyoid muscles that open the upper esophageal sphincter, thus resulting in greater opening of the UES and decreasing pressure above the UES	Shaker, Easterling, Kern, Nitschke, Massey, Daniels, Gran, Kazandjian, & Dikeman, 2002; Shaker, et al., 1997; program has been effective in restoring oral feeding in some patients with abnormal UES opening (Shaker, et al., 2002)
Electrical simulation of the thyrohyoid musculature	Reduced laryngeal elevation	Synchronized electrical stimulation of the thyrohyoid muscles through electrodes placed on the neck; treatments may last up to 4 hours daily	Stimulating contraction of the thyrohyoid muscles during swallowing improves dysphagia resulting from reduced laryngeal elevation	Leelamanit, Limsakul, & Geater, 2002; Freed, Freed, Chatburn, & Christian, 2001

(continued)

Table 6–5. (*continued*)

TREATMENT STRATEGY	WHY DO IT? (rationale based upon swallowing symptoms)	HOW TO DO IT?	WHAT DOES IT DO?	SUPPORTING EVIDENCE
Thin liquid diet	Reduced tongue coordination; reduced tongue strength; reduced cricopharyngeal opening; reduced pharyngeal wall contraction		Easier to propel back through the use of gravity (head back); passes into esophagus more easily	Logemann, 1998
Thick diet	Delayed pharyngeal swallow; decreased laryngeal elevation; reduced vocal fold closure		Thin liquids flow quickly and are more difficult to control; thin liquids penetrate the larynx more easily	Bhattacharyya, Kotz, & Shapiro, 2003; Buklow, Olsson, & Ekberg, 2003; Robbins, Levine, Maser, Rosenbek, & Kempster, 1993
Pureed diet	Delayed pharyngeal swallow; reduced airway closure; reduced laryngeal elevation; chewing difficulty	Foods are blended to a pureed consistency	Do not flow as quickly as thin liquids; therefore easier to control; do not require chewing	
Mechanical soft diet	Difficulty chewing	Ground meat; fruits and vegetables are cooked until soft	Soft enough to be easily chewed	

*The supraglottic and super-supraglottic swallow maneuvers may be contraindicated for patients with a history of stroke or coronary artery disease due to demonstrated abnormal findings during swallowing training sessions (Chaudhuri, Hildner, Brady, Hutchins, Aliga, & Abadilla, 2002).

efficacy studies to date have not confirmed the utility and carry-over of these techniques. Techniques that may enhance oral sensation include thermal tactile application (TTA) and introduction of a cold, sour, textured, carbonated, or large bolus (Bulow, Olsson, & Ekberg, 2003; Logemann, 1998; Rosenbek, Robbins, Fishback, & Levine, 1991; Logemann, Paloski, Colangelo, Lazarus, Fujiu, & Kahrilas, 1995).

Swallow maneuvers require the patient to concentrate on swallowing and to perform multi-step directions involving increased muscular effort. Swallow maneuvers are designed to alter disordered swallowing physiology by improving range of motion and controlling the timing of an individual's response. Swallow maneuvers and exercises include supraglottic swallow, super-supraglottic swallow, effortful swallow, Mendelsohn maneuver, oral-motor exercises, and the Shaker exercise.

Information from Chapter 4 indicates that bolus characteristics are related to differences in swallow physiology. For this reason, diet modifications may facilitate a safer or more efficient swallow. Use of thin viscosity, thicker viscosity, thickened liquids, pureed foods, or mechanical soft foods are among the more common recommendations to try depending on the functional deficit.

Tables 6-6 and 6-7 contain summaries of common oral and pharyngeal symptoms, respectively, associated with neurogenic dysphagias, and the types of behavioral and/or medical therapies associated with each.

SUMMARY

Any alteration to the neurological system has the potential to cause dysphagia. It is important for the speech-language pathologist to explore the neuroanatomical level of the disease process by conducting both clinical and instrumental dysphagia examinations. By combining results from both examinations, the speech-language pathologist can determine the motor and sensory etiologies and signs and symptoms of the presenting dysphagia. These results will guide the choice of treatment strategies that are chosen according to anatomic/physiologic rationale.

STUDY QUESTIONS

1. Describe three common symptoms of dysphagia that occur in the oral stages of swallowing. List possible motor and sensory sources of each symptom.

2. Describe three common symptoms of swallowing disorders that occur in the pharyngeal stage of deglutition. List possible motor and sensory sources of each symptom.

3. What is the number one cause of neurogenic dysphagia?

4. What are some common neurological disease processes that may include dysphagia as one of its symptoms?

5. In what order should treatment strategies that can be applied to patients with dysphagia be introduced?

6. What is the physiological rationale for the head-turn posture that is used in dysphagia management?

Table 6–6. Behavioral and/or medical therapies associated with oral stage signs and symptoms in neurogenic dysphagia. *It should be noted that the efficacy of many of the therapies listed herein remains to be established.*

DISORDER	BEHAVIORAL THERAPY	MEDICAL THERAPY
Drooling	Use of cuing and self-monitoring to increase awareness of saliva, improve lip closure, and swallow more frequently (Dunn, Cunningham, & Backman, 1987)	Surgical: salivary gland excision/rerouting (Shott, Myer, & Cotton, 1989); correction of dental malocclusion (Shapira, Becker, & Moskovitz, 1999)
	Use of EMG to the orbicularis oris muscle to provide biofeedback on lip closure (Koheil, Sochaniwskyj, Bablich, Kenny, & Milner, 1987)	Pharmacological: atropine sulfate (Dworkin & Nadel, 1991); scopolamine (Brodtkorb, et al., 1988); glycopyrrolate (Neverlien, Sorumshagen, Eriksen, Grinna, Kvalshaugen, & Lind, 2000)
Pocketing of food in lateral sulci	Introducing food to the stronger/more sensitive side of the oral cavity (Larsen, 1973)	
	Head tilt to the stronger side	
	Range of motion exercises for the tongue, tongue coordination exercises with gauze, and bolus control exercises (Logemann, 1998)	
Pocketing of food in anterior sulci	Head back posture; oral-motor exercises	
Difficulty manipulating the bolus	Head back posture; oral-motor exercises	Intraoral prosthetics (see Chapter 7)
Difficulty chewing	Range of motion exercises for the tongue and jaw, tongue coordination and chewing exercises with the use of clinician-controlled gauze and bolus control exercises (Logemann, 1998)	
	Change to diet consistency that is more easily managed such as liquids, purees, or mechanical soft	
Excessive gagging	Desensitization through use of applied pressure, vibration, and ice	
Prolonged oral preparation time	Oral-motor exercises; change to diet consistency that is easier managed such as liquids, purees, or mechanical soft	
Loss of control of the bolus	Oral-motor exercises; tactile thermal application to increase oral sensitivity	

Table 6–7. Behavioral and/or medical therapies associated with pharyngeal stage signs and symptoms in neurogenic dysphagia. *It should be emphasized that the efficacy of many of the therapies listed herein remains to be established.*

DISORDER	BEHAVIORAL THERAPY	MEDICAL THERAPY
Delay in triggering the pharyngeal swallow	Chin tuck; tactile thermal application; cold, textured, and/or flavored bolus; (super) supraglottic swallow; thick or pureed diet	
Laryngeal penetration	Chin tuck; head rotation to the weak side; (super) supraglottic swallow; Mendelsohn maneuver; thick or pureed diet	
Aspiration	Chin tuck; head rotation to the weak side; (super) supraglottic swallow; Mendelsohn maneuver; thick or pureed diet	If due to unilateral vocal fold paralysis: vocal fold medialization surgically or with injection techniques
Reduced hyolaryngeal elevation	Mendelsohn maneuver; Shaker exercise; electrical stimulation of the thyrohyoid musculature	
Vallecular stasis	Chin tuck; effortful swallow	
Pyriform sinus stasis	Head rotation; Mendelsohn maneuver; Shaker exercise	Cricopharyngeal dilation, myotomy, Botox injection
Pharyngeal stasis	Head rotation to the weak side; head tilt to the stronger side; side lying posture; Mendelsohn maneuver; Shaker exercise; alternating thin and thick viscosity to clear stasis	
Nasal regurgitation	Avoid chin tuck position; thicken liquids	Prosthetics: palatal lift prosthesis Surgical: pharyngeal flap surgery or palatoplasty

REFERENCES

Abraham, S. (1994). Treating swallowing problems in MS patients. *Multiple Sclerosis, 13,* 4–5.

Abraham, S. S., & Yun, P. T. (2002). Laryngopharyngeal dysmotility in multiple sclerosis. *Dysphagia, 17*(1), 69–74.

Addington, W. R., Stephens, R. E., Gilliland, K., & Rodriguez, M. (1999). Assessing the laryngeal cough reflex and the risk of developing pneumonia after stroke. *Archives of Physical Medicine and Rehabilitation, 80*(2), 150–154.

Addington, W. R., Stephens, R. E., & Gilliland, K. A. (1999). Assessing the laryngeal cough reflex and the risk of developing pneumonia after stroke: An interhospital comparison. *Stroke, 30*(6), 1203–1207.

Agency for Health Care Policy and Research (AHCPR). (1999). Diagnosis and treatment of swallowing disorders (dysphagia) in acute-care stroke patients. Evidence report/technology assessment, number 8.

Ahsan, S. F., Meleca, R. J., & Dworkin, J. P. (2000). Botulinum toxin injection of the cricopharyngeus muscle for the treatment of dysphagia. *Otolaryngology Head and Neck Surgery, 122*(5), 691–695.

Alberts, M. J., Horner, J., Gray, L., & Brazer, S. R. (1992). Aspiration after stroke: Lesion analysis by brain MRI. *Dysphagia, 7*(3), 170–173.

Alberty, J., Oelerich, M., Ludwig, K., Hartmann, S., & Stoll, W. (2000). Efficacy of Botulinum toxin A for treatment of upper esophageal sphincter dysfunction. *Laryngoscope, 110*(7), 1151–1156.

Aviv, J. E., Kaplan, S. T., Thomson, J. E., Spitzer, J., Diamond, B., & Close, L. G. (2000). The safety of flexible endoscopic evaluation of swallowing with sensory testing (FEEST): An analysis of 500 consecutive evaluations. *Dysphagia, 15*(1), 39–44.

Aviv, J. E., Martin, J. H., Sacco, R. L., Zagar, D., Diamond, B., Keen, M. S., & Blitzer, A. (1996). Supraglottic and pharyngeal sensory abnormalities in stroke patients with dysphagia. *Annals of Otology, Rhinology, and Laryngology, 105*, 92–97.

Bartolome, G., & Neumann, S. (1993). Swallowing therapy in patients with neurological disorders causing cricopharyngeal dysfunction. *Dysphagia, 8*(2), 146–149.

Bhattacharyya, N., Kotz, T., & Shapiro, J. (2003). The effect of bolus consistency on dysphagia in unilateral vocal cord paralysis. *Otolaryngology— Head and Neck Surgery, 129*(6), 632–636.

Blitzer, A., & Sulica, L. (2001). Botulinum toxin: Basic science and clinical uses in otolaryngology. *Laryngoscope, 111*(2), 218–226.

Brin, M. F., & Younger, D. (1988). Neurologic disorders and aspiration. *Otolaryngologic Clinics of North America, 21*(4), 691–699.

Brodtkorb, E., Wyzocka-Bakowska, M. M., Lillevold, P. E., Sandvik, L., Saunte, C., & Hestnes, A. (1988). Transdermal scopolamine in drooling. *Journal of Mental Deficiency Research, 32*, 233–237.

Bushmann, M., Dobmeyer, S. M., Leeker, L., & Perlmutter, J. S. (1989). Swallowing abnormalities and their response to treatment in Parkinson's disease. *Neurology, 39*, 1309–1314.

Bulow, M., Olsson, R., & Ekberg, O. (2001). Videomanometric analysis of supraglottic swallow, effortful swallow, and chin tuck in patients with pharyngeal dysfunction. *Dysphagia, 16*(3), 190–195.

Bulow, M., Olsson, R., & Ekberg, O. (2003). Videoradiographic analysis of how carbonated thin liquids and thickened liquids affect the physiology of swallowing in subjects with aspiration on thin liquids. *Acta Radiology, 44*(4), 366–372.

Camelo, A. L., Awad, R. A., Madrazso, A., & Aguilar, F. (1997). Esophageal motility disorders in Mexican patients with Duchenne's muscular dystrophy. *Acta Gastroenterology Latinoamerica, 27*, 119–122.

Castell, J. A., Castell, D. O., Schultz, A. R., & Georgeson, S. (1993). Effect of head position on the dynamics of the upper esophageal sphincter and pharynx. *Dysphagia, 8*(1),1–6.

Chaudhuri, G., Hildner C. D., Brady, S., Hutchins, B., Aliga, N., & Abadilla, E. (2002) Cardiovascular effects of the supraglottic and super-supraglottic swallowing maneuvers in stroke patients with dysphagia. *Dysphagia, 17*(1), 19–23.

Chen, M. Y., Donofrio, P. D., Frederick, M. G., Ott, D. J., & Pikna, L. A. (1996). Videofluoroscopic evaluation of patients with Guillain-Barre syndrome. *Dysphagia, 11*(1), 11–13.

Costantini, M., Zaninotto, G., Anselmino, M., Marcon, M., Iurilli, V., Boccu, C., Feltrin, G. P., Angelini, C., & Ancona, E. (1996). Esophageal motor function in patients with myotonic dystrophy. *Digestive Diseases and Sciences, 41,* 2032–2038.

Crary, M. A. (1995). A direct intervention program for chronic neurogenic dysphagia secondary to brainstem stroke. *Dysphagia, 10*(1), 6–18.

Crary, M. A., & Groher, M.E. (2000). Basic concepts of surface electromyographic biofeedback in the treatment of dysphagia: A tutorial. *American Journal of Speech-Language Pathology, 9,* 116–25.

Dalakas, M. C. (1998). Controlled studies with high-dose intravenous immunoglobin in the treatment of dermatomyositis, inclusion body myositis, and polymyositis. *Neurology, 51,* S37–S45.

Daniels, S. K., Brailey, K., & Foundas, A. L. (1999). Lingual discoordination and dysfunction following acute stroke: Analyses of lesion localization. *Dysphagia, 14,* 85–92.

Daniels, S. K., & Foundas, A. L. (1999). Lesion localization in acute stroke patients with risk of aspiration. *Journal of Neuroimaging, 9*(2), 91–98.

De Swart, B. J. M., Verheij, J. C. G. E., & Beurskens, C. H. G. (2003). Problems with eating and drinking in patients with unilateral facial paralysis. *Dysphagia, 18*(4), 267–273.

Ding, R., & Logemann, J. A. (2000). Pneumonia and stroke patients: A retrospective study. *Dysphagia, 15*(2), 51–57.

D'Onofrio, V., Annese, V., Miletto, P., Leandro, G., Marasco, A., Sodano, P., & Iaquinto, G. (2000). Long-term follow-up of achalasic patients treated with botulinum toxin. *Diseases of the Esophagus, 13*(2), 96–101.

Drake, W., O'Donoghue, S., Bartram, C., Lindsay, J., & Greenwood, R. (1997). Eating in side-lying facilitates rehabilitation in neurogenic dysphagia. *Brain Injury, 11*(2), 137–142.

Dunn, K. W., Cunningham, C. E. & Backman, J. E. (1987). Self-control and reinforcement in the management of a cerebral-palsied adolescent's drooling. *Developmental Medicine and Child Neurology, 29*(3), 305–310.

Dworkin, J. P., & Nadal, J. C. (1991). Nonsurgical treatment of drooling in a patient with closed head injury and severe dysarthria. *Dysphagia, 6*(1), 40–49.

Fradet, G., Pouliot, D., Robichaud, R., St. Pierre, S., & Bouchard, J. P. (1997). Upper esophageal sphincter myotomy in oculopharyngeal muscular dystrophy: Long-term clinical results. *Neuromuscular Disorders, 7,* Supplement 1, S90–S95.

Freed, M. L., Freed, L., Chatburn, R. L., & Christian, M. (2001). Electrical stimulation for swallowing disorders caused by stroke. *Respiratory Care*, *46*(5), 466–474.

Goyal, R. K. (2001). Esophagus in *Harrison's Principles of Internal Medicine*, *15th ed.* (Eds. Braunwald, E., Fauci, D. L., Kasper, S. L., Hauser, D. L., Longo, & J. L. Jameson). 1642–1649. New York: McGraw-Hill.

Hamdy, S., Aziz, Q., Rothwell, J. C., Crone, R., Hughes, D., Tallis, R. C., & Thompson, D. G. (1997). Explaining oropharyngeal dysphagia after unilateral stroke. *Lancet*, *350*(9079), 686–692.

Hamdy, S., Aziz, Q., Rothwell, J. C., Power, M., Singh, K. D., Nicholson, D. A., Tallis, R.C., & Thompson, D. G. (1998). Recovery of swallowing after dysphagic stroke relates to functional reorganization in the intact motor cortex. *Gastroenterology*, *115*(5), 1104–1112.

Hamdy, S., Jilani, S., Price, V., Parker, C., Hall, N., & Power, M. (2003). Modulation of human swallowing behaviour by thermal and chemical stimulation in health and after brain injury. *Neurogastroenterological Motility*, *15*(1), 69–77.

Hillel, A., Dray, T., Miller, R., Yorkston, K., Konikow, N., Strande, E., & Browne, J. (1999). Presentation of ALS to the otolaryngologist/head and neck surgeon: Getting to the neurologist. *Neurology*, *53*(8 Suppl), S22–S25.

Horner, J., Buoyer, F. G., Alberts, M. J., & Helms, M. J. (1991). Dysphagia following brainstem stroke: Clinical correlates and outcome. *Archives of Neurology*, *48*(11), 1170–1173.

Horner, J., & Massey, E. W. (1988). Silent aspiration following stroke. *Neurology*, *38*(2), 317–319.

Horner, J., Massey, E. W., & Brazer, S. R. (1990). Aspiration in bilateral stroke patients. *Neurology*, *40*(11), 1686–1688.

Horner, J., Massey, E. W., Riski, J. E., Lathrop, D. L., & Chase, K. N. (1988). Aspiration following stroke: Clinical correlates and outcome. *Neurology*, *38*(9), 1359–1362.

Huckabee, M. L., & Cannito, M. P. (1999). Outcomes of swallowing rehabilitation in chronic brainstem dysphagia: A retrospective evaluation. *Dysphagia*, *14*(2), 93–109.

Johnson, E. R., McKenzie, S. W., Rosenquist, C. J., Lieberman, J. S., & Sievers, A. E. (1992). Dysphagia following stroke: Quantitative evaluation of pharyngeal transit times. *Archives of Physical Medicine and Rehabilitation*, *73*(5), 419–423.

Kagel, M. C., & Leopold, N. A. (1992). Dysphagia in Huntington's disease: A 16-year retrospective. *Dysphagia*, *7*(2), 106–114.

Kahrilas, P. J., Logemann, J. A., Krugler, C., & Flanagan, E. (1991). Volitional augmentation of upper esophageal sphincter opening during swallowing. *American Journal of Physiology*, *260*(3 Pt 1), 450–456.

Kawai, S., Tsukuda, M., Mochimatsu, I., Enomoto, H., Kagesato, Y., Hirose, H., Kuroiwa, Y., & Suzuki, Y. (2003). A study of the early stage of dysphagia in amytrophic lateral sclerosis. *Dysphagia*, *18*(1), 1–8.

Kern, M. K., Jaradeh, S., Arndorfer, R. C., & Shaker, R. (2001). Cerebral cortical representation of reflexive & volitional swallowing in humans. *AJP-Gastrointestinal and Liver Physiology*, *28* (3), G-354–360.

Kirshner, H. S. (1989). Causes of neurogenic dysphagia. *Dysphagia, 3*(4), 184–188.

Kluin, K. J., Bromberg, M. B., Feldman, E. L., & Simmons, Z. (1996). Dysphagia in elderly men with myasthenia gravis. *Journal of the Neurological Sciences, 138*(2), 49–52.

Kobayashi, H., Hoshino, M., Okayama, K., Sekizawa, K., & Sasaki, H. (1994). Swallowing and cough reflexes after onset of stroke. *Chest, 105*(5), 1623.

Koheil, R., Sochaniwskyj, A. E., Bablich, K., Kenny, D. J., & Milner, M. (1987). Biofeedback techniques and behavior modification in the conservative remediation of drooling by children with cerebral palsy. *Developmental Medicine and Child Neurology, 29*(1), 19–26.

Lacau Saint-Guily, J., Perie, S., Willig, T. N., Chaussade, S., Eymard, B., & Angelard, B. (1994). Swallowing disorders in muscular diseases: Functional assessment and indications of cricopharyngeal myotomy. *Ear, Nose, and Throat Journal, 73*(1), 34–40.

Langmore, S. E., Terpenning, M. S., Schork, A., Chen, Y., Murray, J. T., Lopatin, D., & Lowsche, W. J. (1998). Predictors of aspiration pneumonia: How important is dysphagia? *Dysphagia, 13*(2), 69–81.

Larsen, G. L. (1973). Conservative management for incomplete dysphagia paralytica. *Archives of Physical Medicine and Rehabilitation, 54*(4), 180–185.

Lazarus, C., & Logemann, J. A. (1987). Swallowing disorders in closed head trauma patients. *Archives of Physical Medicine and Rehabilitation, 68*(2), 79–84.

Lazarus, C., Logemann, J. A., & Gibbons, P. (1993). Effects of maneuvers on swallowing function in a dysphagic oral cancer patient. *Head & Neck, 15*(5), 419–424.

Lazarus, C., Logemann, J. A., Huang, C. F., & Rademaker, A. W. (2003). Effects of two types of tongue strengthening exercises in young normals. *Folia Phoniatrica et Logopaedica, 55*(4), 199–205.

Lazzara, G., Lazarus, C., & Logemann, J. A. (1986). Impact of thermal stimulation on the triggering of the swallowing reflex. *Dysphagia, 1*, 73–77.

Leelamanit, V., Limsakul, C., & Geater, A. (2002). Synchronized electrical stimulation in treating pharyngeal dysphagia. *Laryngoscope, 112*(12), 2204–2210.

Leopold, N. A., & Kagel, M. C. (1985). Dysphagia in Huntington's disease. *Archives of Neurology, 42*(2), 57–60.

Leopold, N. A., & Kagel, M. C. (1996). Prepharyngeal dysphagia in Parkinson's disease. *Dysphagia, 11*(1), 14–22.

Leopold, N. A., & Kagel, M. C. (1997). Pharyngo-esophageal dysphagia in Parkinson's disease. *Dysphagia, 12*(1), 11–18.

Lewin, J. S., Hebert, T. M., Putnam, J. B., & DuBrow, R. A. (2001). Experience with the chin tuck maneuver in postesophagectomy aspirators. *Dysphagia, 16*(3), 216–219.

Linke, R., Witt, T. N., & Tatsch, K. (2003). Assessemnt of esophageal function in patients with myasthenia gravis. *Journal of Neurology, 250*(5), 601–606.

Logemann, J. A. (1993). The dysphagia diagnostic procedure as a treatment efficacy trial. *Clinics in Communication Disorders, 3*(4), 1–10.

Logemann, J. A. (1983). *Evaluation and treatment of swallowing disorders.* San Diego, CA: College-Hill Press.

Logemann, J. A. (1998). *Evaluation and treatment of swallowing disorders* (2nd ed.). Austin: Pro-Ed.

Logemann, J. A., Kahrilas, P. J., Kobara, M., & Vakil, N. B. (1989). The benefit of head rotation on pharyngoesophageal dysphagia. *Archives of Physical Medicine and Rehabilitation, 70*(110), 767–771.

Logemann, J. A., Pauloski, B. R., Colangelo, L., Lazarus, C., Fujiu, M., & Kahrilas, P. J. (1995). Effects of a sour bolus on oropharyngeal swallowing measures in patients with neurogenic dysphagia. *Journal of Speech and Hearing Research, 38*(33), 556–563.

Logemann, J. A., Pauloski, B. R., Rademaker, A. W., & Colangelo, L. A. (1997). Super-supraglottic swallow in irradiated head and neck cancer patients. *Head and Neck, 19*(16), 535–540.

Love, R. J., & Webb, W. G. (1992). *Neurology for the speech language pathologist.* (2nd ed.) Boston: Butterworth-Heinemann.

Marcon, M., Briani, C., Ermani, M., Menegazzo, E., Iurilli, V., Feltrin, G. P., Novelli, G., Gennarelli, M., & Angelini, C. (1998). Positive correlation of CTG expansion and pharyngoesophageal alterations in myotonic dystrophy patients. *Italian Journal of Neurological Sciences, 19*(2), 75–80.

Marie, I., Hachulla, E., Levesque, H., Reumont, G., Ducrotte, P., Cailleux, N., Hatron, P. Y., Devulder, B., & Courtois, H. (1999). Intravenous immunoglobins as treatment of life threatening esophageal involvement in polymyositis and dermatomyositis. *Journal of Rheumatology, 26*(12), 2706–2709.

Martin, B. J. W., Logemann, J. A., Shaker, R., & Dodds, W. J. (1993). Normal laryngeal valving patterns during three breath hold maneuvers: A pilot investigation. *Dysphagia, 8*(1), 11–20.

Martin, R. E., Goodyear, B. G., Gati, J. S., & Menon, R. S. (2001). Cerebral cortical representation of automatic and volitional swallowing in humans. *Journal of Neurophysiology, 85,* 938–950.

Meng, N. H., Wang, T. G., & Lien, I. N. (2000). Dysphagia in patients with brainstem stroke: Incidence and outcome. *American Journal of Physical Medicine and Rehabilitation, 79*(2), 170–175.

Mosier, K., & Bereznaya, I. 2001. Parallel cortical networks for volitional control of swallowing in humans. *Experimental Brain Research, 140*(3), 280–289.

Mosier, K. M., Liu, W. C., Maldjian, J. A., Shah, R., & Modi, B. (1999). Lateralization of cortical function in swallowing: A functional MR imaging study. *American Journal of Neuroradiology, 20*(8), 1520–1526.

Nagaya, M., Kachi, T., & Yamada, T. (2000). Effect of swallowing training on swallowing disorders in Parkinson's disease. *Scandinavian Journal of Rehabilitation Medicine, 32*(1), 11–15.

Neubrand, M., Scheurlen, C., Schepke, M., & Sauerbruch, T. (2002). Long-term results and prognostic factors in the treatment of achalasia with botulinum toxin. *Endoscopy, 34*(7), 519–523.

Neverlien, P. O., Sorumshagen, L., Eriksen, T., Grinna, T., Kvalshaugen, H., & Lind, A. B. (2000). Glycopyrrolate treatment of drooling in an adult male patient with cerebral palsy. *Clinical Experiments in Pharmacological Physiology*, *27*(4), 320–322.

Nilsson, H., Ekberg, O., Olsson, R., & Hindfelt, B. (1998). Dysphagia in stroke: A prospective study of quantitative aspects of swallowing in dysphagic patients. *Dysphagia*, *13*(1), 32–38.

Nishino, T. (1993). Swallowing as a protective reflex for the upper respiratory tract. *Anesthesiology*, *79*(3), 588–601.

Ohmae, Y., Ogura, M., Kitahara, S., Karaho, T., & Inouye, T. (1998). Effects of head rotation on pharyngeal function during normal swallow. *Annals of Otology, Rhinology, and Laryngology*, *107*, 344–348.

Pelletier, C. A., & Lawless, H. T. (2003). Effect of citric acid and citric acid-sucrose mixtures on swallowing in neurogenic oropharyngeal dysphagia. *Dysphagia*, *18*(4), 231–241.

Perie, S., Eymard, B., Laccourreye, L., Chaussade, S., Fardeau, M., & Lacau-St. Guily, J. (1997). Dysphagia in oculopharyngeal muscular dystrophy: A series of 22 French cases. *Neuromuscular Disorders*, *7*, Supplement 1, S96-S99.

Perlman, A. L. (1991). The neurology of swallowing. *Seminars in Speech and Language*, *12*, 171–184.

Rasley, A., Logemann, J. A., Kahrils, P. J., Rademaker, A. W., Pauloski, B. R., & Dodds, W. J. (1993). Prevention of barium aspiration during videofluoroscopic swallowing studies: Value of change in posture. *American Journal of Roentology*, *160*(5), 1005–1009.

Richter, J. E. (1995). Motility disorders of the esophagus. In T. Yamada (Ed.), *Textbook of gastroenterology*. Philadelphia: J. B. Lippincott.

Robbins, J. A., Levine, R. L., Maser, A., Rosenbek, J. C., & Kempster, G. B. (1993). Swallowing after unilateral stroke of the cerebral cortex. *Archives of Physical Medicine and Rehabilitation*, *74*(12), 1295–1300.

Robbins, J. A., Logemann, J. A., & Kirshner, H. S. (1986). Swallowing and speech production in Parkinson's disease. *Annals of Neurology*, *19*(3), 283–287.

Rosenbek, J. C., Roecker, E. B., Wood, J. L., & Robbins, J. (1996). Thermal application reduces the duration of stage transition after stroke. *Dysphagia*, *11*(4), 225–233.

Sciortino, K., Liss, J. M., Case, J. L., Gerritsen, K. G., & Katz, R. C. (2003). Effects of mechanical, cold, gustatory, and combined stimulation of the human anterior faucial pillars. *Dysphagia*, *18*(1), 16–26.

Secil, Y., Aydogdu, I., & Ertekin, C. (2002). Peripheral facial palsy and dysfunction of the oropharynx. *Journal of Neurology, Neurosurgery, and Psychiatry*, *72*(3), 391–393.

Seikel, J. A., King, D. W., & Drumright, D. G. (1997). *Anatomy and physiology for speech, language, and hearing*. San Diego, CA: Singular Publishing Group.

Setzen, M., Cohen, M. A., Perlman, P. W., Belafsky, P. C., Guss, J., Mattucci, K. F., & Ditkoff, M. (2003). The association between laryngopharyngeal sensory deficits, pharyngeal motor function, and the prevalence of aspiration with thin liquids. *Otolaryngology Head and Neck Surgery*, *128*(1), 99–102.

Shaker, R., Easterling, C., Kern, M., Nitschke, T., Massey, B., Daniels, S., Grande, B., Kazandjian, M., & Dikeman, K. (2002). Rehabilitation of swallowing by exercise in tube-fed patients with pharyngeal dysphagia secondary to abnormal UES opening. *Gastroenterology, 122*(5), 1314–1321.

Shaker, R., Kern, M., Bardan, E., Taylor, A., Stewart, E. T., Hoffmann, R. G., Arndorfer, R. C., Hofmann, C., & Bonnevier, J. (1997). Augmentation of deglutive upper esophageal sphincter opening in the elderly by exercise. *American Journal of Physiology, 272*, G1518–G1522.

Shapira, J., Becker, A., & Moskovitz, M. (1999). The management of drooling in children with neurological dysfunction: A review and case report. *Specialty Care in Dentistry, 19*(4), 181–185.

Sharkawi, A. E., Ramig, L., Logemann, J. A., Pauloski, B. R., Rademaker, A. W., Smith, C. H., Pawlas, A., Baum, S., & Werner, C. (2002). Swallowing and voice effects of Lee Silverman Voice Treatment (LSVT): A pilot study. *Journal of Neurology, Neurosurgery, and Psychiatry, 72*(1), 31–36.

Shaw, G. Y., & Searl, J. P. (2001). Botulinum toxin treatment for cricopharyngeal dysfunction. *Dysphagia, 16*(3), 161–167.

Shott, S. R., Myer, C. M., & Cotton, R. T. (1989). Surgical management of sialorrhea. *Otolaryngology, Head, and Neck Surgery, 101*(1), 47–50.

Smithard, D. G., O'Neill, P. A., England, R. E., Park, C. L., Wyatt, R., Martin, D. F., & Morris, J. (1997). The natural history of dysphagia following stroke. *Dysphagia, 12*(4), 188–193.

Stephens, R. E., Addington, W. R., & Widdicombe, J. G. (2003). Effect of acute unilateral middle cerebral artery infarcts on voluntary cough and the laryngeal cough reflex. *American Journal of Physical Medicine and Rehabilitation, 82*(5), 379–383.

St. Guily, J. L., Perie, S., Willig, T. N., Chaussade, S., Eymard, B., & Angelard, B. (1994). Swallowing disorders in muscular diseases: Functional assessment and indications of cricopharyngeal myotomy. *Ear, Nose, and Throat Journal, 73*(1), 34–40.

Thomas, F. J., & Wiles, C. M. (1999). Dysphagia and nutritional status in multiple sclerosis. *Journal of Neurology, 246*(8), 677–682.

Veis, S. L., & Logemann, J. A. (1985). Swallowing disorders in persons with cerebrovascular accident. *Archives of Physical Medicine and Rehabilitation, 66*(6), 372–375.

Vigderman, A. M., Chavin, J. M., Kososky, C., & Tahmoush, A. J. (1998). Aphagia due to pharyngeal constrictor paresis from acute lateral medullary infarction. *Journal of the Neurological Sciences, 155*(2), 208–210.

Welch, M. V., Logemann, J. A., Rademaker, A. W., & Kahrilas, P. J. (1993). Changes in pharyngeal dimensions effected by chin tuck. *Archives of Physical Medicine and Rehabilitation, 74*(2), 178–181.

Willig, T. N., Paulus, J., Lacau-St. Guily, J., Beon, C., & Navarro, J. (1994). Swallowing problems in neuromuscular disorders. *Archives of Physical Medicine and Rehabilitation, 75*(11), 1175–1181.

CHAPTER 7

Physiological Bases of Structural Etiologies of Dysphagia and Treatment Strategies

LEARNING OBJECTIVES

After completing the chapter and reviewing the study questions, you should be able to:

- Describe and discuss structural etiologies of dysphagia

- Understand how anatomical alterations modify swallowing physiology

- Describe and discuss a variety of structural etiologies of dysphagia due to acute changes and progressive transformations

- Understand the anatomic/physiologic rationale for treatment strategies

- Apply your understanding of anatomy and physiology to management decisions when selecting therapeutic strategies.

INTRODUCTION

It is easy to imagine that any change or defect in the structures involved in deglutition can disrupt a safe and efficient swallow. Anatomical defects or variations in the bony structures, cartilages, muscles, and recesses can cause changes in the mechanical and aerodynamic forces that are necessary to guide the bolus along its intended path. Such anatomical variations or defects may be due to congenital malformations (e.g., cleft palate), acute changes (e.g., trauma, infections, tracheotomy), or progressive transformations (e.g., osteophytes, diverticula, neoplasms). Because this book is dedicated to mature deglutition, congenital malformations will not be discussed here as their sequelae are most pertinent to developmental or pediatric dysphagia. The purpose of this chapter is to discuss acute and progressive structural etiologies of dysphagia and to present physiologically-based treatment options for these mechanical defects.

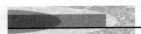

ACUTE STRUCTURAL CHANGES

Acute changes to the structures of deglutition may result from an accidental trauma, or they may occur as negative side effects of medical treatments or surgeries designed to save a person's life or to treat other serious problems. Acute structural changes may also result from exposure to infections, toxins, or chemical agents. Signs and symptoms of dysphagia that arise from these acute structural changes are determined by the location and nature of the changes. Symptoms can range from mild discomfort to florid aspiration and choking.

Accidental Trauma

Gun shot wounds, motor vehicle accidents, and falls have the potential to interfere with deglutition when damage occurs somewhere along the aerodigestive tract. Oral, pharyngeal, and esophageal dysphagia may result depending on the level of the injury. Management may be medical or behavioral, depending on the extent of the damage.

Medical-Surgical Trauma

The upper alimentary tract is particularly vulnerable to structural insult secondary to attempts to restore or create a breathing passageway in patients who require resuscitation. It is also vulnerable due to its close proximity to the spinal cord, vertebral column, and cardiopulmonary system. Surgeries in any of these areas, for any reason, can impinge on its structure as well as innervation.

Endotracheal Intubation

Dysphagia related to endotracheal intubation (when a breathing tube is placed through the mouth or nose into the trachea to allow ventilation during surgery or during respiratory distress) can occur acutely or secondary to prolonged intubation. Arytenoid dislocation can occur during intubation if the endotracheal tube hits the arytenoid cartilage on the way to the trachea, resulting in vocal fold paralysis (MacArthur & Healy, 1995). When the vocal folds are unable to close, the risk for aspiration increases. Prolonged endotracheal intubation (i.e., longer than eight hours) has been shown to increase risk of aspiration after extubation (Leder, Cohn, & Moller, 1998). An endotracheal tube alters the sensory abilities of the larynx (Leder, et al., 1998). As the length of intubation time increases, edema, irritation, and granulation tissue may occur in the larynx. Over an extended time, subglottic stenosis (narrowing) may occur. Leder and colleagues (1998) studied deglutition in 20 trauma patients who had orotracheal intubation for 48 hours or more and found that 45 percent demonstrated aspiration 24 hours following extubation. Many patients who have had prolonged orotracheal aspiration aspirate silently, without any overt signs of dysphagia such as coughing or choking (Leder, et al., 1998). Aspiration following extubation is often transient—often no longer observed after 48 hours. It is therefore recommended that patients who have had prolonged endotracheal intubation be objectively assessed for aspiration and/or be restricted from oral intake for at least 24–48 hours following extubation (Leder, et al., 1998).

Tracheotomy

A tracheotomy is a surgical procedure that places a tube below the cricoid cartilage in order to bypass the upper airway in patients with chronic or acute upper airway obstruction (Nash, 1988), respiratory failure (Bach & Alba, 1990), chronic obstructive sleep apnea (Heffner, Miller, & Sahn, 1986), or pulmonary toilet (a condition in which patients are unable to clear their secretions adequately). The tracheostomy tube is placed below the cricoid cartilage, through the trachea, between the third and fourth tracheal rings, bypassing the upper airway (laryngeal area), thus allowing a greater volume of inspired air available for oxygenation. The surgical operation, itself, is referred to as a tracheotomy. After there is a permanent or temporary opening into the trachea with a tube, it is referred to as a tracheostomy.

Although a commonly used procedure, the presence of a tracheostomy tube is not without complications. Deglutitive aspiration is a major problem for patients with a tracheostomy (Betts, 1965; Cameron, Reynolds, & Zuidema, 1973; Elpern, Jacobs, & Bone, 1987; Tolep, Getch, & Criner, 1996). Many times a tracheostomy is used as a solution to long-term aspiration, but in reality may lead to more aspiration. The cause of aspiration is unknown; however, it is likely due to multiple factors. Mechanical changes that affect swallowing following tracheostomy placement include decreased laryngeal elevation, obstruction by the cuff, and decreased subglottic pressure. Table 7-1 summarizes the symptoms associated with tracheostomy-related dysphagia.

Two neurophysiologic factors, desensitization of the protective cough reflex and loss of coordination of laryngeal closure, are interrelated and have also been cited as the cause for aspiration in tracheostomy patients (Buckwalter & Sasaki, 1984; Nash, 1988). Desensitization of the larynx and loss of the protective reflexes occur in tracheostomy patients due to chronic air diversion through the tracheostomy tube. Diversion of normal airflow over time elevates the stimulation threshold necessary

Table 7-1. Symptoms associated with tracheotomy-induced dysphagia.

Decreased laryngeal elevation	The tracheostomy tube is in a relatively fixed position in regard to the strap muscles and skin of the neck, therefore limiting the rostrocaudal excursion of the laryngotracheal framework. Limited laryngeal elevation and anterior rotation causes the duration of the vocal cord closure to be significantly shorter when compared to normal controls (Buckwalter & Sasaki, 1984; Shaker, Dodds, Dantas, Hogan, & Anrndorfer, 1990; Shaker, Milbrath, Ren, Campbell, Toohill, & Hogan, 1995).
Obstruction by the cuff	External pressure of the cuff on the esophagus can cause material to pool above the cuff level and then spill into the airway when the cuff is deflated or when the patient inhales in a forceful manner (Betts, 1965; Cameron, et al., 1973; Feldman, Deal, & Urquhart, 1966; Weber, 1974).
Decreased subglottic pressure	When respiratory airflow is routed out of the neck via the tracheostomy tube, the airflow through the vocal folds and oral cavity is greatly reduced or entirely absent, depending on how tightly the tracheostomy tube fits against the tracheal wall. Reduction of normal laryngeal airflow or subglottic pressure leads to a buildup or stasis in the supraglottic region that may be aspirated after the swallow (Dettelbach, Gross, Mahlmann, & Eibling, 1995; Siebens, Tippett, Kirby, & French, 1993).
Reduction of the adductor vocal fold reflex	Diversion of the normal airflow over time elevates the stimulation threshold necessary for laryngeal adduction, leading to delayed and uncoordinated laryngeal closure (Buckwalter & Sasaki, 1984).

for laryngeal adduction, leading to delayed laryngeal closure (Buckwalter & Sasaki, 1984). Uncoordinated laryngeal closure (adduction) occurs due to chronic airway bypass leading to desensitization and atrophy of the muscles. Disuse atrophy of the swallowing musculature may occur with prolonged placement of a tracheostomy tube (DeVita & Spierer-Rundback, 1990).

Tracheostomy Cuffs

Tracheostomy tubes are either cuffed or uncuffed (Figures 7-1a and 7-1b). A cuff is a soft balloon at the end of the tube that can be inflated to hold the tube snuggly against the tracheal wall (Figure 7-2a). A cuff is inflated (Figure 7-2b) when the patient requires mechanical ventilation. Deflation of the cuff (Figure 7-2c) prior to swallowing trials is recommended. If the cuff is inflated tightly against the tracheal wall it may interfere with laryngeal elevation or may rub against the tracheal wall. Prolonged irritation of the tracheal tissue can lead to formation of granulation tissue, scarring, and sometimes the development of a tracheoesophageal fistula (abnormal opening between the trachea and esophagus) (Tippett & Siebens, 1995). Cuff status (inflated vs. deflated) has not been found to affect the incidence of penetration or aspiration (Suiter, McCullough, & Powell, 2003).

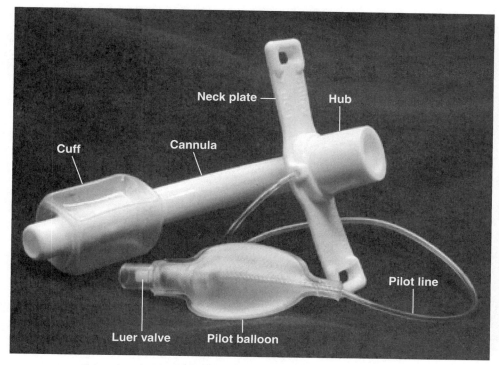

Figure 7-1a. Photo of a cuffed tracheostomy tube.

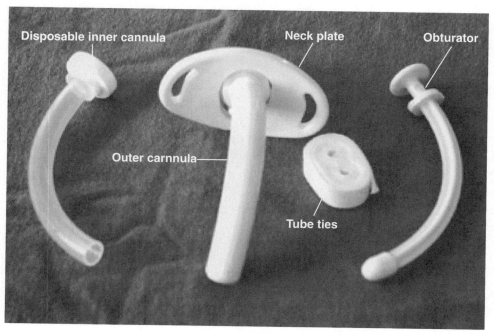

Figure 7-1b. Photo of a cuffless tracheostomy tube.

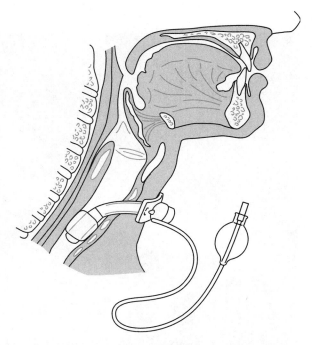

Figure 7-2a. Photo of an inflated, cuffed tracheostomy tube in place.

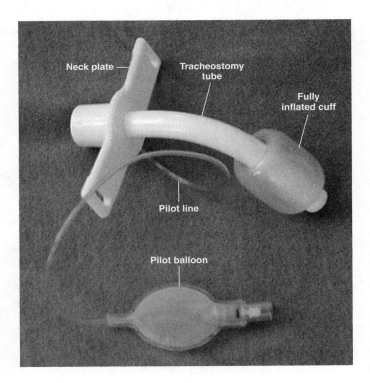

Figure 7-2b. Photo of an inflated, cuffed tracheostomy tube.

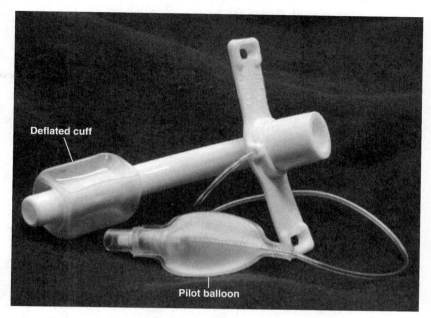

Figure 7-2c. Photo of a deflated, cuffed tracheostomy tube.

Inflatable Cuffs *Do Not* Prevent Aspiration

It is important to note that an inflated cuff does not prevent aspiration. The cuff will be examined from an anatomical perspective. The tracheostomy tube is placed below the cricoid cartilage. Therefore, the tracheostomy tube is below the larynx and below the vocal folds that are housed in the larynx. Aspiration occurs when material being swallowed enters the airway below the true vocal folds. Therefore, it is easy to see that if food or liquid is sitting on top of the inflated cuff, that material has *already* been aspirated. It has also been shown that an inflated cuff does not prevent all material from entering the lungs (Bone, Davis, Zuidema, & Cameron, 1974; Dettelbach, et al., 1995). Material sitting on the inflated cuff can seep around the cuff into the trachea and lungs. If the doctor has given permission to deflate the cuff for swallowing trials, it is important to thoroughly suction above the cuff prior to deflation in order to remove all accumulated food and secretions.

Tracheostomy Fenestrations

A tracheostomy tube can be **fenestrated** or **non-fenestrated** (see Figure 7-3). A fenestrated tube has a hole or window cut into the tube to allow greater airflow through the upper airway. A fenestrated tube may be used to allow for better airflow for speech production or to prepare the

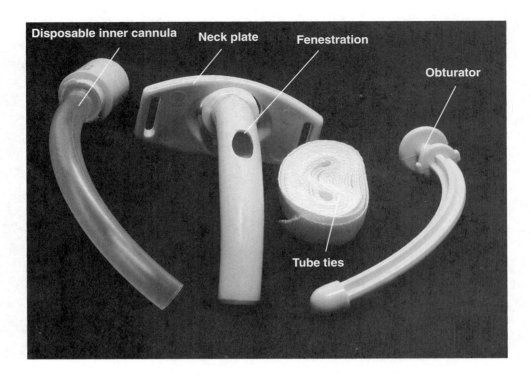

Figure 7-3a. Photo of a fenestrated tracheostomy tube.

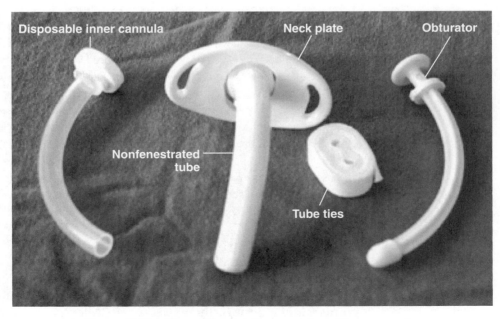

Figure 7-3b. Photo of a non-fenestrated tracheostomy tube.

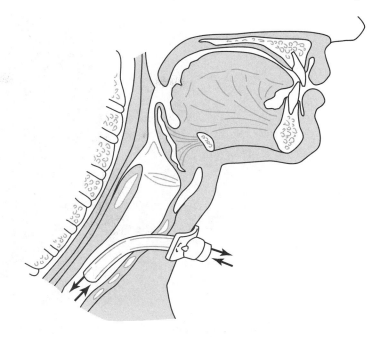

Figure 7-3c. Cuffless, non-fenestrated tracheostomy tube in place.

patient for **decannulation** (removal of the tube). A non-fenestrated tube does not have a hole cut out. This is recommended for patients who require mechanical ventilation, for small children, and for patients who develop granulation tissue due to the open window creating irritation of the tracheal tissue.

Decannulation—removal of the tracheostomy tube—will often permit return to oral feeding and may reduce or eliminate aspiration (Dettelbach, et al., 1995; Eibling & Gross, 1996). Many patients, however, are not ready for decannulation. For these patients, a one-way speaking valve is often recommended (Figure 7-4). A one-way speaking valve attaches to the outside opening of a cuffless or deflated tracheostomy tube. The one-way valve allows air to pass into the tracheostomy, but not out through it. The valve remains open during inhalation, allowing air into the lungs. Upon exhalation, the valve closes and air flows around the tracheostomy tube, up through the vocal folds, allowing the vocal folds to vibrate for speech.

It has been hypothesized that a one-way speaking valve can decrease aspiration and improve swallow function by restoring more

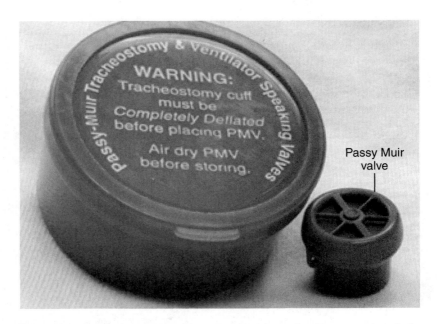

Passy Muir
valve

Figure 7-4a. Photo of a speaking tracheotomy valve (Passy-Muir valve).

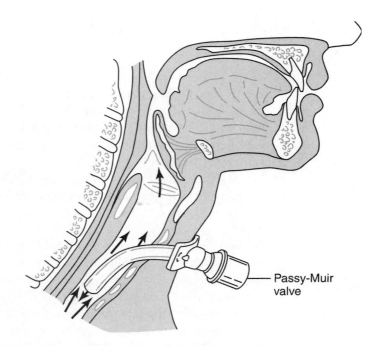

Passy-Muir
valve

Figure 7-4b. Passy-Muir speaking valve attached to tracheostomy tube.

normal subglottic and glottic air flow (Suiter, et al., 2003; Dettelbach, et al., 1995; Stachler, Hamlet, Choi, & Fleming, 1996). Return of airflow through the larynx should, therefore, restore protective laryngeal reflexes and reduce or prevent aspiration. Research has indicated that use of a one-way valve does reduce the severity of aspiration, however, controversy over whether the incidence of aspiration is reduced remains.

Dettelbach, et al. (1995) found that patients wearing a one-way speaking valve were better able to sense and clear supraglottic penetration. Suiter and colleagues (2003) found that the one-way valve significantly reduced the incidence and severity of aspiration of thin liquids; however, the study also indicated that use of the one-way valve resulted in an increase in oral residue, posterior pharyngeal wall residue, and cricopharyngeal residue. This exacerbation of oral and pharyngeal residue with use of the one-way valve, therefore, also needs to be assessed in this population during clinical examination. Stachler and colleagues (1996) used scintigraphy to quantify aspiration in head and neck cancer patients with tracheostomy and found that all subjects aspirated both with and without valve use; however, the amount of aspiration was significantly smaller with the one-way valve in place. Another study using scintigraphy to measure aspiration found that occlusion of the tracheostomy tube reduced or eliminated aspiration in some head and neck cancer patients (Muz, Hamlet, Mathog, & Farris, 1994).

Other research, however, has questioned whether occlusion of the tracheostomy tube reduces the incidence of aspiration (Leder, 1999). In the acute care setting, the occlusion status of the tracheostomy tube did not affect the incidence of aspiration for both medical (Leder, Tarro, & Burnell, 1996) and head and neck cancer patients (Leder, Ross, Burrell, & Sasaki, 1998). These results were repeated in a study of 20 consecutive patients who used a one-way speaking valve for the first time without change in incidence of aspiration (Leder, 1999). Leder and colleagues (2001) conducted another study that used manometry to examine the biomechanics of the pharyngeal swallow in tracheostomy patients with and without tracheal tube occlusion. Results indicated that occlusion status had no significant effect on manometric pressure measurements of the upper esophageal sphincter and pharynx (Leder, Joe, Hill, & Traube, 2001). The use of a one-way valve to decrease the *incidence* of aspiration is therefore controversial, however it may decrease the *amount* of aspiration. Given the conflicting reports in the literature regarding the effect of tracheostomy tube occlusion and swallowing physiology, further investigations are warranted.

CLINICAL NOTE

7-2

Use of the Modified Evan's Blue Dye Test in Detecting Aspiration in Tracheostomy Patients

The modified Evan's blue dye test (MEBDT) is a simple, inexpensive, bedside procedure that is frequently used to assess swallowing safety in patients with tracheostomy tubes. Food and liquid are dyed blue and fed to the patient. Suctioned secretions are then monitored for blue dye. Any evidence of blue dye is considered positive for aspiration. Recent investigations, however, have questioned the diagnostic accuracy of the test (Donzelli, Brady, Wesling, & Craney, 2001; Thompson-Henry & Braddock, 1995). Donzelli and colleagues (2001) conducted a FEES examination simultaneously with an MEBDT. The MEBDT showed an overall 50 percent false-negative error rate for the detection of aspiration compared with the FEES. Results of the study indicated that the MEBDT failed to identify aspiration of trace amounts (zero percent) and identified aspiration in 67 percent of patients who aspirated more than trace amounts. Belafsky, Blumenfeld, LePage, and Nahrstedt (2003) conducted a similar study in which the FEES examination was conducted simultaneously with the MEBDT. These authors found the sensitivity of the MEBDT in predicting aspiration to be slightly higher (82 percent). Research has shown, therefore, that the MEBDT is not a completely accurate test for detecting aspiration. Results support the use of the MEBDT as an initial screening test in the detection of aspiration. The FEES or MBS tests could then be used to definitively determine whether or not the patient is aspirating.

Other benefits of a one-way valve include: reinstatement of laryngeal abductor and adductor reflexes (Buckwalter & Sasaki, 1984), improvements in smell (Stachler, et al., 1996), decreased amounts of upper airway secretions (Passy, Baydur, Prentice, & Darnell-Neal, 1993), better clearing of pharyngeal and laryngeal residue after the swallow (Muz, et al., 1994), and ability to produce a productive volitional cough (Leder, et al., 1996).

Cervical Spine Surgery

Dysphagia following anterior cervical spine surgery (Martin, Neary, & Diamant, 1997), thyroid surgery (Kelchner, Stemple, Gerdeman, Le Borgne, & Adam, 1999), and cardiac surgery has been reported (Rosous, et al., 2000). This is not a surprising consequence given the close proximity of the aerodigestive system to these structures. The anterior approach to the cervical spine now serves as the surgical access most often used for cervical spine disease. Anterior surgical spine surgery can result in denervation, esophageal perforation, postoperative hematoma formation, edema, and infection (Daniels, Mahoney, & Lyons, 1998). Baron and colleagues (2003) examined the world literature to determine the occurrence of dysphagia, hoarseness, and unilateral vocal fold motion impairment following anterior cervical diskectomy and fusion and calculated these to be 12.3%, 4.9%, and 1.4% respectively. Older patients may be at higher risk for dysphagia following anterior surgical spine surgery (Baron, Solimen, Gaughan, Simpson, & Young, 2003). Swallowing symptoms vary considerably, perhaps in part due to the level of the surgery (i.e., C2-C7) (Martin, et al., 1997). Vocal fold paralysis is often, but not always, a factor in the dysphagia. Injury to the glossopharyngeal (CN IX), vagus (CN X), and hypoglossal (CN XII) nerves can occur. Post-surgical edema of the posterior pharyngeal wall can prevent full epiglottic deflection, reduced pharyngeal wall contraction, and reduced opening of the upper esophageal sphincter (Martin, et al., 1997). Swallowing symptoms that have been reported include: impaired bolus formation, premature spillage of material into the pharynx, reduced tongue propulsion, reduced hyolaryngeal elevation, reduced epiglottic inversion, reduced pharyngeal wall contraction, reduced upper esophageal sphincter opening, silent aspiration, and absent pharyngeal swallow (Daniels, et al., 1998; Martin, et al., 1997). Some patients require enteral feeding for several weeks to months (Martin, et al., 1997). The majority of patients with persistent dysphagia and dysphonia following anterior cervical spine surgery have complete resolution of the symptoms within 12 months of the procedure (Morpeth & Williams, 2000). Vocal fold medialization surgery and swallowing therapy can assist recovery (Daniels, et al., 1998; Morpeth & Williams, 2000). The speech-language pathologist should choose the therapy techniques appropriate for the presenting dysphagic symptoms. Examples include: bolus control and lingual exercises, thermal stimulation, supersupraglottic swallow, Mendelsohn maneuver, and effortful swallow. Head postures and the Shaker exercises may be contraindicated in this population due to the nature of the cervical spine surgery.

Carotid Endarterectomy

Dysphagia following both carotid endarterectomy (removal of plaques from the carotid artery) and thyroid surgery may result if damage occurs to the recurrent laryngeal nerve (RLN) resulting in a paralyzed vocal fold. The open airway prevents the vocal folds serving as the last line of defense against aspiration. When a nerve is damaged during surgery, it is often recommended that the patient wait six months to a year before permanent treatment of the vocal fold paralysis is undertaken in order to see if the vocal function returns. Approximately 60 percent of patients with vocal fold paralysis spontaneously recover recurrent laryngeal nerve (RLN) function within one year of onset and many of the remaining 40 percent can compensate to satisfactory voice levels (Tucker, 1995). Laryngeal electromyography (EMG) involves placing small hooked wire electrodes into the muscles of the larynx to examine the electrical activity in the muscles. EMG can confirm paralysis and help predict if recovery will occur. Medical-surgical treatment for a paralyzed vocal fold is medialization via thyroplasty or injection of a biomechanical substance to bulk up the paralyzed vocal fold. The patient can be taught compensatory swallowing techniques such as the head turn, head tilt, or super-supraglottic swallow to prevent aspiration. Vocal function exercises may be used in an attempt to enhance glottal closure. Vocal Function Exercises are a series of four exercises developed by Stemple (1993; 2000).

CLINICAL NOTE

7-3

Vocal Function Exercises Can Enhance Glottal Closure

Vocal Function Exercises are a series of four exercises developed by Stemple (1993). The following exercises should each be done as softly as possible twice, two times a day (b.i.d.) with a slightly nasalized tone (Stemple, 1993). While a soft loudness level is to be used, the voice must be fully engaged and not breathy.

1. Sustain the vowel /i/ for as long as possible on the musical note F above middle C for all female patients and boys and F below middle C for mature male patients (goal = 40–45 seconds).

2. Glide from your lowest tone to your highest tone on the word *knoll* (goal = no voice breaks). Feel a buzz on the lips.

3. Glide from your highest note to your lowest note on the word *knoll* (goal = no voice breaks). Feel a buzz on the lips.

4. Sustain the musical notes C, D, E, F, and G as long as possible on the *knoll* minus the *kn*.

The patient can push the palms of the hand together while performing these exercises in order to add an isometric push and to increase effort of closure (Stemple, 2000).

Structural Changes Secondary to Infection, Chemical Agents, and Toxins

Dysphagia secondary to infection can result from fungal, bacterial, viral, or chemical agents (Groher, 1997).

Fungal Infections

A fungal infection occurring in the aerodigestive tract can cause dysphagia. **Candidiasis** or **thrush** is a fungal infection caused by an overgrowth of a yeast (fungus). In the mouth, candidiasis looks like creamy white patches or small red spots on the tongue, hard palate, gums, or pharynx. Crusting on the corners of the mouth may be a symptom of thrush. Candida causes dysphagia when there is a fungus overgrowth in the mouth, pharynx, or esophagus. Thrush is a common early sign of acquired immunodeficiency syndrome (AIDS) and can lead to dysphagia characterized by difficulty swallowing, alteration in taste, and odynophagia (pain when swallowing). Thrush is also common in patients with xerostomia (dryness of the mouth) or from long-term use of antibiotics. Lack of saliva increases the risk of oral infections in these patients. Xerostomia can result from radiation therapy, Sjögren's syndrome (an autoimmune disease that causes dry mouth and dry eyes; Sjögren's was discussed in Chapter 6), or from the use of medications. Over 400 medications are known to have xerostomia as a side effect. Treatment for thrush may include antimicrobial medications, lozenges, and mouth rinses. Dietary management of thrush includes avoiding alcohol and cigarettes and monitoring sugar and dairy intake.

Infections

Bacterial infections that can cause problems in swallowing include Ludwig's angina and botulism. **Ludwig's angina** is an acute bacterial infection that causes rapid inflammation of the tissues of the submandibular and sublingual spaces. It occurs more often in adults following infection of the roots of the teeth, but can also occur in children (Hartmann, 1999). Symptoms include severe neck pain and swelling, fever, difficulty breathing, drooling, and dysphagia (Hartmann, 1999). Ludwig's angina can be life threatening due to airway compromise; however, patients usually recover without complications. Appropriate therapy includes maintenance of the airway, antibiotics, and surgical drainage when indicated (Moreland, Corey, & McKenzie, 1988).

Botulism is a severe and often fatal intoxication resulting from ingestion of a bacterial toxin in contaminated food. It is characterized clinically by a symmetric, descending paralysis often preceded by gastrointestinal manifestations and cranial nerve involvement (Shapiro, Hatheway, & Swerdlow, 1998). Presenting signs and symptoms include nausea, vomiting, abdominal pain, diarrhea (early) or constipation (late), xerostomia, blurred vision, diplopia, dysarthria, dysphagia, and muscle weakness (Shapiro, et al., 1998). Antitoxin can be beneficial if administered early in the course of illness (Shapiro, et al., 1998).

Herpes simplex is a viral infection that can cause cranial nerve palsies. If the vagus nerve is affected, the patient will present with hoarseness and dysphagia (Bachor, Bonkowsky, & Hacki, 1996; Bachor, Bonkowsky, & Hacki, 1996). Herpes simplex can also cause blisters on the skin, in the mouth, or in the pharynx that can lead to difficulty swallowing due to pain and irritation (Groher, 1997).

In both bacterial and viral infections, inflamation of the oral and pharyngeal structures can significantly impair deglutition because of pain and the impeded pathway. **Epiglottitis** is inflammation of the epiglottis and supraglottic structures commonly associated with a bacterial infection. It characteristically occurs in children ages two to seven years old, but can occur in adults (Stanley & Liang, 1988). Epiglottitis has an abrupt onset of fever, sore throat, dysphagia, drooling, muffled voice, respiratory distress, and lethargy. Airway management is of primary concern in epiglottitis. Diagnosis can be aided through the use of X-ray or fiberoptic visualization of the epiglottis. **Pharyngitis** is swelling of the pharynx that may cause transient dysphagia. Pharyngitis can be caused by either bacterial or viral infections.

Chemical Agents

Ingestion of chemical agents can lead to caustic (burn) injuries to the tissues in the oral cavity, pharynx, and larynx. Children account for the highest incidences of caustic injuries due to accidental ingestion of household chemical agents. Tongue fixation, hypopharyngeal stenosis, epiglottis injuries, incomplete laryngeal closure, and esophageal stenosis can lead to dysphagia characterized by nasopharyngeal regurgitation, pharyngeal stasis, and aspiration (Scott, Jones, Eisele, & Ravich, 1992).

PROGRESSIVE TRANSFORMATIONS

Not all structural changes that cause dysphagia occur acutely or can be linked with a particular event or disease process. Some occur over long periods of time, and some are present at birth but do not cause problems until later in life. Most of these structural changes are related to slow bone growth or slow degradation of muscular and/or mucosal tissue. As such, the dysphagia signs and symptoms in these progressive transformations may appear gradually, over the course of months or even years.

Osteophytes

Osteophytes are bony outgrowths from the spinal cervical vertebrae occurring most often in the elderly. Degenerative joint disease, ankylosing spondylosis, and diffuse idiopathic skeletal hyperostosis (DISH) can all cause cervical osteophyte formation. DISH, also known as Forrestier's disease, is characterized by extensive spinal osteophyte formation that can lead to the formation of a giant cervical osteophyte. The majority of osteophytes are asymptomatic; however, progressive dysphagia sometimes results. If the osteophytes are large, they may narrow the pharyngeal or esophageal spaces leading to mechanical obstruction (Di Vito, 1998). Aspiration may occur if the osteophyte directs the bolus toward the laryngeal vestibule or if the osteophyte interferes with epiglottic deflection. The diagnosis of osteophyte-induced dysphagia should be made by videofluoroscopy. Surgical treatment is sometimes necessary if the dysphagia is not amendable to therapy.

Esophageal Abnormalities

There are a number of structural defects of the upper digestive tract, below the level of the UES, that can result in symptoms of oropharyngeal dysphagia in adults. The speech-language pathologist must be knowledgeable enough to recognize structural defects in the esophagus that require medical follow up by the radiologist or referring physician. While esophageal symptoms of structural disorders are not managed primarily by behavioral treatment provided by speech-language pathol-

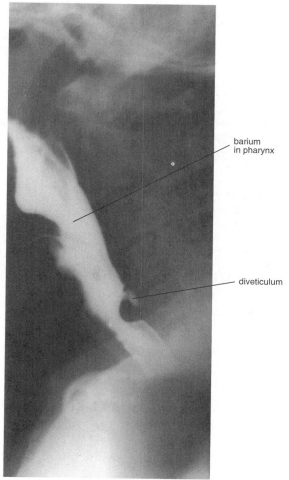

barium
in pharynx

diveticulum

Figure 7-5. Fluoroscopic image of Zenker's diverticulum.

ogists, an understanding and recognition of structural disorders and symptomatology is necessary in order for the speech-language pathologist to effectively communicate with the patient and physician.

Diverticula

Pharyngoesophageal diverticula are outpouchings of mucosa through muscle or membrane in the pharynx or esophagus. One common form is **Zenker's diverticulum** which occurs at the level of the cricopharyngeus, at the UES, in a region that typically has fewer muscle fibers or is congenitally weaker than the surrounding muscle. An example of Zenker's on radiographic study is seen in Figure 7-5. This region handles high pressure peristaltic waves during swallowing so it is no surprise that it can be the location of mucosa herniating through the muscle wall. Interestingly, manometric studies conducted on patients with Zenker's diverticulum have not indicated abnormally high pressures or disturbed peristalsis at the UES (Knuff, Benjamin, & Castell, 1982). This type of structural problem often occurs in the presence of gastroesophageal reflux disease and hiatal hernia (Low & Rubesin, 1993). Recent research indicates that laryngopharyngeal reflux may alter normal function of the UES (Blitzer & Sulica, 2001).

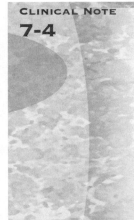

CLINICAL NOTE

7-4

Symptoms Associated with Zenker's Diverticulum

Zenker's diverticula are most common in persons over 60 years of age. Small Zenker's diverticula are usually asymptomatic, but larger ones may collect food and can eventually cause esophageal obstruction. At first a Zenker's diverticulum develops posteriorly, but as it enlarges it protrudes to one side, usually the left. Symptoms of Zenker's diverticulum may include: progressive dysphagia, regurgitation of undigested food, noisy deglutition, sensation of mucus collecting in the throat, bad breath, weight loss, and/or aspiration. Pneumonia is a potentially serious complication. A Zenker's divertuculum may cause swelling in the lateral part of the neck. Patients may learn to empty the diverticulum by applying gentle manual pressure to the side of the neck. Symptomatic diverticula are often treated surgically by doing a diverticulectomy (removal of the diverticulum) with concurrent cricopharyngeal myotomy. Other forms of treatment include endoscopic stapling and carbon dioxide laser surgery (Veenker & Cohen, 2003).

Other types of herniations can also occur in the pharynx. **Lateral pharyngeal pouches** occur when mucosa herniates through the thyrohyoid membrane forming a pouch with a relatively large opening. Most often, material will fill the pouch during the swallow and empty. A **lateral pharyngeal diverticulum**, on the other hand, has a narrow neck that increases the chances of material remaining after the swallow has been completed. While this type of diverticulum, or pouch, is usually asymptomatic, dysphagia may result if material caught is cleared during non-swallow periods. Unexpected material in the pharynx when the airway is not protected, as during a swallow, can be aspirated. Symptomatic diverticula are often surgically repaired. Diverticula may be found within 10 cm of the LES and are referred to as epiphrenic diverticula. Whether patients with epiphrenic diverticula are symptomatic or not appears to be related to the structure of the diverticula, as in the pharyngeal diverticula discussed above. Esophageal motility abnormalities may play a role in the development of the diverticula and in the symptomatology, though the relationship between dysmotility and diverticula is not fully agreed upon in the current literature (Fasano, Levine, Rubesin, Redfern, & Laufer, 2003).

Gastroesophageal Reflux Disease

Gastroesophageal reflux disease (GERD) may be considered an example of a structural problem resulting, in part, from a neuromuscular problem. Mucosal changes are brought about by frequent or chronic exposure to acidic stomach contents as a result of an LES that allows material to reflux into the esophagus, or a UES that allows reflux into the pharynx or larynx. Episodes of reflux are common in all individuals, often on a daily basis. Difficulties arise when the problem occurs too often or chronically over a long period. The most common symptom is heartburn or substernal pain (discomfort behind the sternum). Other signs of reflux problems may include dysphagia, odynophagia, vocal hoarseness, nocturnal coughing, nausea, a globus sensation (lump in the throat), and a bad taste in the mouth upon awakening. These symptoms considered all together are often referred to as **dyspepsia**. While many people with reflux will have these overt symptoms, asymptomatic individuals are also encountered. The muscosal changes, which can include erythema (redness from engorged capillaries) and edema, are usually evident in areas that have been exposed to the reflux material such as the esophagus proper, the posterior portion of the laryngeal vestibule, and the vocal folds. When the reflux escapes the esophagus through the UES it is frequently termed **laryngopharyngeal reflux**. Reflux esophagitis is graded on a zero to six scale with zero indicating a normal esophagus and six indicative of ulcerations and the presence of strictures (Tytgat, 1995). GERD is not a minor problem to be ignored. Long-term exposure of esophageal mucosa to reflux may result in pre-cancerous changes. This metaplasia, or change in tissue, is called **esophageal columnar metaplasia** or **Barrett's esophagus**. This disorder represents the change of stratified squamous mucosa to columnar mucosa and can be seen in Figure 7-6. The risk of developing esophageal cancer (adenocarcinoma) is approximately 30 times higher in people with Barrett's esophagus. While considered an atypical presentation of GERD, laryngospasm may result and when protracted lead to **syncope** (loss of consciousness). Recent or concurrent viral or bacterial upper respiratory infection with

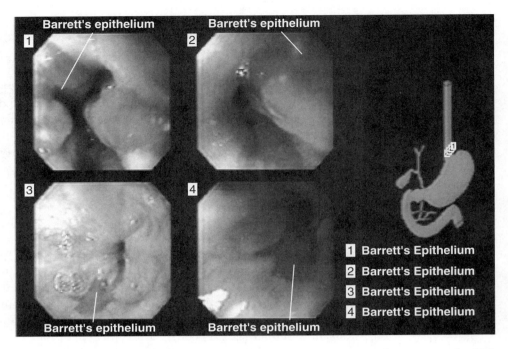

Figure 7-6. Endoscopic image of Barrett's esophagus. (*Courtesy of V. Duane Bohman.*)

significant and possibly violent cough is hypothesized to increase the amount of reflux resulting in the laryngospasm. The laryngospasm is thought to be elicited by sensory information carried by the superior laryngeal nerve (SLN) and motor control through the recurrent laryngeal nerve (RLN) (Maceri & Zim, 2001).

Treatment for GERD progresses from behavioral strategies, to medical-pharmalcological management, to surgical treatment or may be a combination of strategies. Behavioral strategies include raising the head of the bed slightly to assist gravity in keeping stomach contents where they belong, avoiding large meals that cause high intragastric pressure on the LES, avoiding foods known to lessen LES pressure (such as fried, fatty foods, peppermint and spearmint flavored foods, caffeine, and alcohol), and allowing at least three hours between eating a meal and laying down. Pharmacological options include a number of drugs, specifically proton pump inhibitors or histamine-2 receptor antagonists, designed to reduce acid production. A recent meta-analysis of 13 studies found that while both types of medications reduced reflux symptoms as compared to a placebo, proton pump inhibitors worked the best (van Pinxteren, Numans, Lau, de Wit, Hungin, & Bonis, 2003). When all options have failed to control the reflux disorder current surgical options include Hill's posterior gastropexy and Belsey's and Nissen's fundoplication. These three procedures are designed to improve

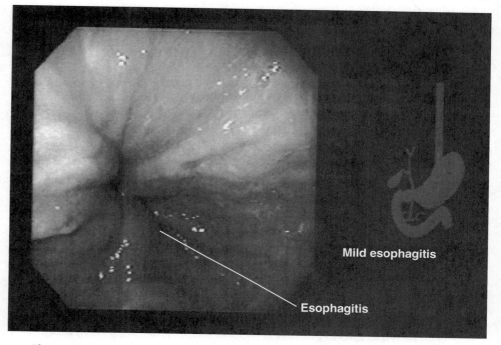

Mild esophagitis

Esophagitis

Figure 7-7. Endoscopic image of esophagitis. (*Courtesy of V. Duane Bohman.*)

LES function by either anchoring the gastroesophageal junction or wrapping it with stomach tissue and suturing the wrap in place thereby creating a mechanical barrier to reflux (Orlando, 1995).

Esophagitis

Esophagitis is a general term that means there are inflammatory changes present in the esophagus as can be seen in Figure 7-7. A number of factors can result in esophagitis, some of which have been described earlier in the chapter as having an effect on the oral and pharyngeal regions. Infection by candida, herpes virus, HIV, and cytomegalovirus results in esophagitis. The type of lesions found in the esophagus will differ based on the type of infection. Candida results in plaquelike lesions along the length of the esophagus while herpes lesions may appear as multiple small ulcerations. HIV and cytomegalovirus cause large ulcerations. Medications that may become stuck to the mucosa of the esophagus can result in drug-induced esophagitis. The medication causes an ulceration of the tissue as the pill dissolves. This can happen with vitamins, aspirin, antibiotics, or anti-inflammatory medications. There are many different grading scales for esophagitis in clinical use but most share common characteristics. Often a grade of zero or one is normal and five or six is severe, indicating Barrett's esophagus (Kahrilas & Ergun, 1994). Treatment targets the cause of the esophagitis and includes medication

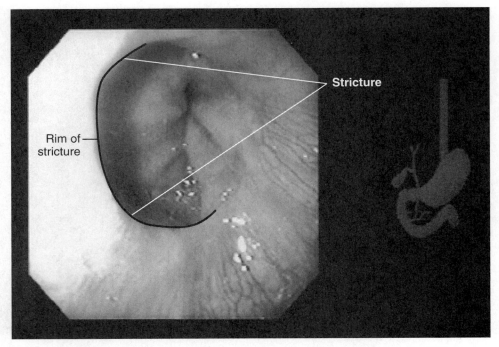

Figure 7-8. Endoscopic image of an esophageal stricture. (*Courtesy of V. Duane Bohman.*)

to reduce reflux, to clear up bacterial or yeast infections, or to reduce severity of viral infections with antiviral drugs.

Strictures and Webs

Strictures are narrowings of a tube caused by inflammation, external compression, or scarring following chemical or mechanical trauma as illustrated in Figure 7-8. A web, in comparison, is the formation of a tissue band or ridge. Webs are often congenital but may be acquired in later life. A specific syndrome, called the Plummer-Vinson syndrome, is most often diagnosed in middle-aged women. The syndrome consists of symptomatic hypopharyngeal (region between the hyoid bone and the cricoid cartilage) webs and iron-deficiency anemia. Dysphagia, when present, is often to solid food. Webs are treated medically by dilating the region to stretch or break the fibers of the web.

Within the esophagus, the chronic exposure to reflux may lead to a reflux stricture. These are often located in the esophagus body. Another result of reflux may be the development of a **Schatzki's ring**, a thin ridge of tissue located in the lower espohagus just above the LES (Figure 7-9). Often this allows a hiatal hernia to slide through the ring. Again, as with webs, dysphagia occurs often with solid foods. Sympto-

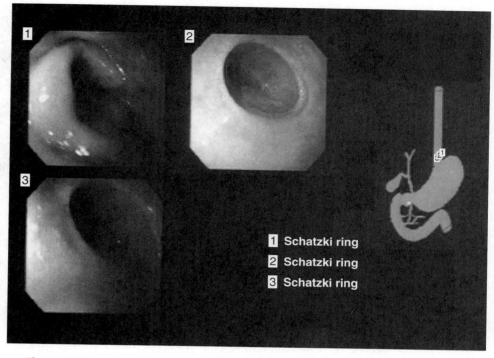

Figure 7-9. Endoscopic image of Schatzki ring. (*Courtesy of V. Duane Bohman.*)

matic rings are often treated by dilation. The purpose of any dilation procedure is to stretch or break the fibrous tissue without causing significant trauma that would lead to a reoccurrence.

Hiatal Hernia

The main body of the esophagus is housed in the thoracic cavity. At the inferiormost end, slightly above the LES, the esophagus pierces through the diaphragm (at the **hiatus**) and into the abdominal cavity. The pressure gradients are different in the abdominal and thoracic cavities. A herniation of stomach tissue through the hiatus of the diaphragm may result from increased intra-abdominal pressure pushing the stomach up through the opening or from the esophagus shortening in reaction to reflux, thereby pulling the stomach tissue up through the hiatus (Boyce & Boyce, 1995). A hiatal **hernia** is the intrusion of stomach tissue up through the esophageal opening (hiatus) in the diaphragm into the thoracic cavity. On endoscopic examination the tissue differences between gastric and esophageal mucosa are evident, as shown in Figure 7-10. It often co-occurs with LES dysfunction and GERD.

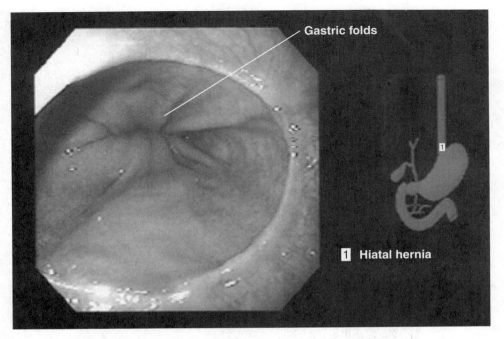

Figure 7-10. Endoscopic image of a hiatal hernia. (*Courtesy of V. Duane Bohman.*)

 HEAD AND NECK CANCER

Head and neck cancer is the most frequent cause of structural dysphagia. Cancer of the head and neck may be treated with surgery, radiation, or both. Chemotherapy may also be used in conjunction with the above. All treatments have the potential to lead to dysphagia.

Surgical Treatment for Cancer

Surgical resection for cancer located in the head and neck region results in specific deficits that are consistent with the anatomical and/or neurological alteration. Although specific patterns of dysphagia can be ascertained according to the type of surgery, it is important to note that every patient is different and may not present with the same type and degree of dysphagia following similar surgeries. The extent of surgery is dictated by the type, location, and severity of the cancer. Reconstruction following surgical removal of structures attempts to restore the anatomy and physiology as close to normal as possible (Logemann, 1985). Prognosis for return to oral feeding is dependent on the extent of surgery, the presence of pre- or post-operative radiation therapy, the development of post-operative complications, the presence of concomitant diseases (e.g., pulmonary disease, stroke), and the patient's capability to learn and follow directions (Denk, Swoboda, Schima, & Eibenberger, 1997; Groher, 1997; Logemann, 1998; Rademaker, et al., 1993). The following sections review surgical resection and reconstruction for head and neck cancer, specifically addressing varying degrees of cancer of the lips, mandible, tongue, anterior tongue/floor of mouth, tonsil/base of tongue, palate, pharynx, and larynx. (Note: More than one of these structures is often involved.)

Lip Resection

Lip resection can result in the inability to contain the bolus in the mouth due to motor and sensory deficits resulting in drooling and loss of bolus control. Bolus control problems occur if over three-fourths of the upper lip is resected (McConnel & O'Conner, 1994). If the anterior mandible is resected along with the labial muscles, there will be sensory deficit in the skin and mucous membranes of the lower lip and skin of the chin due to loss of the inferior alveolar nerve, a sensory branch of the trigeminal nerve (CN V) (Kronenberger & Meyers, 1994).

Mandibulectomy

Surgical removal of the anterior portion of the mandible (**mandibulectomy**) will greatly affect deglutition by disrupting multiple muscle attachments integral to swallow function. Recall the muscular attachments that are located at the anterior portion of the mandible include genioglossus, geniohyoid, mylohyoid, anterior digastric. These patients may present with drooling, impairment in oral manipulation of the bolus, reduced hyolaryngeal elevation, and aspiration (Kronenberger & Meyers, 1994; McConnel & Logemann, 1990). Mandibulectomy involves removal of a portion of the mandible and is often accompanied by radical changes in the tongue and floor of the mouth (Kronenberger & Meyers, 1994). The most important factor in determining the postoperative dysphagia is the amount of mandible that has been removed (Kronenberger & Meyers, 1994). The jaw is often reconstructed with metal plates or with bone and soft tissue (Kronenberger & Meyer, 1994). Chewing can be affected if the occlusal relationships of the teeth are disrupted or if teeth have been extracted (see radiation therapy). Prosthetic appliances will be more successful in patients with more bone and dentition present postoperatively (Kronenberger & Meyer, 1994).

Glossectomy

Occasionally, a tumor will involve only the tongue. The tumor can be treated by removal of the affected region within the tongue (**glossectomy**). If part of the tongue is removed and the tongue is sutured together, there will be a reduction in tongue mass and range of motion (Logemann, 1985). Patients with a **partial glossectomy** will have oral stage dysphagia characterized by difficulties with bolus formation and propulsion, increased oral transit time, and increased difficulty with thicker consistencies (Furia, Carrarra de Angelis, Martins, Barros, Carneiro, & Kowalski, 2000). If one longitudinal half of the tongue is intact following resection, the patient will be able to make palatal contact with the tongue to initiate the swallow; however, bolus control will be impaired (Logemann, 1985). Removal of half of the *mobile* tongue (**hemiglossectomy**) without reconstruction will generally not result in serious swallowing problems and the patients can resume oral eating within a week postoperatively without aspiration (Hirano, Kuroiwa, Tanaka, Mausuoka, Sato, & Yoshida, 1992).

Surgical resection of the anterior portion of the tongue and the floor of the mouth with distal flap reconstruction (without altering mandibular alignment) has been shown to result in oral stage dysphagia characterized by oral residue on the anterior floor of the mouth, tongue blade, and hard palate (Pauloski, et al., 1993). Due to the anterior location of the surgical resection, the pharyngeal stage is not significantly changed, with laryngeal closure and cricopharyngeal opening remaining within normal limits (Pauloski, et al., 1993). Paste and cookie consistencies are the most difficult for this population to handle efficiently (Pauloski, et al., 1993).

Surgical resection of the base of tongue, faucial arch, and hemimandibulectomy (removal of one-half of the mandible) has been shown to result in oral and pharyngeal dysfunction characterized by increased oral and pharyngeal residue and increased oral transit times (Logemann, et al., 1993). The patient may have delayed triggering of the pharyngeal swallow and reduced pharyngeal wall contraction leading to residue in the valleculae (Logemann, 1998). Paste and cookie consistencies are the most difficult for this population to handle efficiently (Logemann, et al., 1993). Similar to the patients with anterior tongue surgery, the laryngeal valving and cricopharyngeal opening is not significantly affected following tonsil/tongue base resection (Logemann, et al., 1993).

Generally, if 50 percent or more of the tongue is resected, greater severity of swallowing impairment is expected (Logemann, 1998). Prognosis for **total glossectomy**, removal of all of the tongue, depends on whether mandible resection accompanies the glossectomy, the size of the tumor, and/or whether surrounding muscles are also removed. Resection of the anterior portion of the mandible will affect hyolaryngeal elevation, increasing the chances of aspiration. In a study of 20 patients who had undergone various degrees of surgical resection for oral cancer, it was found that a diagnosis of a large tumor, extensive removal of the tongue base, removal of the geniohyoid and mylohyoid muscles, and removal of the lateral pharyngeal wall resulted in poorer outcome (Hirano, Kuroiwa, Tanaka, Matsuoka, Sato, & Yoshida, 1992). Some patients who have undergone a total glossectomy can never eat by mouth due to severe and chronic aspiration (Furia, et al., 2000; Hirano, et al., 1992). If surgery for total glossectomy involves only the intrinsic musculature of the tongue, the prognosis for swallowing is good (Frazell & Lucas, 1962). The patient will need to use gravity to transfer the bolus from the oral cavity into the pharynx; the intact suprahyoid musculature will ensure adequate laryngeal elevation and protection; the intact pharyngeal musculature will lead to normal bolus propulsion.

Surgery of the Palate

Resection of the hard and soft palates may be necessary due to cancer of the palates themselves, involvement from tumors located in the tonsillar area, or for tumors involving the sinuses (Kronenberger & Meyers, 1994). Surgical resection of the hard palate can result in abnormal communication of the oral and nasal cavities. This is typically handled prosthetically with good results. If all or part of the soft palate or velum is resected, the patient will be unable to get normal velopharyngeal closure resulting in nasal regurgitation and loss of normal aerodynamic pressures. Surgical, behavioral, or prosthetic management can help reduce nasal regurgitation.

Treatment for Oral Cancer

Following medical oral cancer management behavioral treatments to improve swallow function, compensating for structural and functional defects and maximizing use of the remaining structures becomes the focus for the speech-language pathologist.

ORAL-MOTOR EXERCISES

The use of oral-motor exercises for treatment of dysphagia is sometimes questioned. Perlman, Luschei, and Du Mond (1989) found that swallowing generates more activity in the superior constrictor muscle than in any non-swallowing task. This provides some evidence that employment of aerodigestive musculature is strongest during swallowing when compared to other aerodigestive functions such as talking and gagging. It is, therefore, important to focus on functional swallowing exercises as much as possible. In patients with head and neck cancer, however, the efficacy of oral-motor exercises is warranted (Logemann, Pauloski, Rademaker, & Colangelo, 1997; Sonies, 1993). Exercise programs can improve muscle strength, coordination, and mobility. Resistive exercises are used to build muscle strength, while range-of-motion exercises increase structural mobility. Head and neck cancer patients often experience reduced strength and mobility of the swallowing structures due to reconstruction and possible **fibrosis** (change of muscle fibers into connective tissue) following radiation treatment. Oral-motor exercises should begin with physician permission after sufficient healing time has occurred. Oral-motor exercises should be performed in front of a mirror in order to present feedback to the patient. Another form of biofeedback is surface electromyography (sEMG), which records muscle activity through electrodes applied to the skin surface. Biofeedback with sEMG can enhance learning of muscle movements by displaying muscle activity to the patient via auditory and/or visual display (Crary & Groher, 2000). The patient can perform oral-motor exercises with infrequent supervision in most cases if the patient is cognitively able to follow directions. Frequent video recordings of the exercises can help monitor progress. Protocols for exercises for weak labial, mandibular, and tongue musculature are presented in Figures 7–11, 7–12, and 7–13.

SENSORY STIMULATION

Stimulation of the areas affected by surgical resection following cancer, such as the face, lips, and oral cavity, may be necessary to create sensory awareness. Decreased sensation may affect the patient's ability to hold, manipulate, and propel the bolus. If facial areas lack sensation, the fingertips or a washcloth can be used to apply a light, circular massage to the impaired areas (Sonies, 1993). Areas within the oral cavity can be stroked and/or pressure from a frozen lemon glycerin swab can be applied. Having the patient identify distinct points in the mouth that the clinician touches can monitor progress. Thermal tactile application can be used to enhance the swallowing response in patients with a delayed pharyngeal swallow. Once the patient is safely able to attempt trials of food and liquid by mouth, the bolus can be manipulated to increase the sensation by presenting a sour bolus, a cold bolus, a bolus requiring chewing, and/or a larger bolus (Logemann, 1998; Logemann, Pauloski, Colangelo, Lazarus, Fujiu, & Kahrilas, 1995).

INTRAORAL PROSTHETICS

Intraoral prosthetics may also be used to augment swallowing function in patients following treatment for oral cancer. Oral cancer patients with significant loss of tongue tissue or with surgical removal of the hard and/or soft palate may benefit from intraoral prosthetics (Logemann, Kahrilas, Hurst, Davis, & Krugler, 1989). Intraoral prosthetics are constructed by a maxillofacial prosthodontist. Patients may experience initial aversion to the prosthesis and may need to desensitize to the presence of the prosthesis over time. Patients experiencing difficulty with velopharyngeal closure may present with the complaint of nasal regurgitation. These patients can benefit from a **palatal lift prosthesis**, which mechanically maintains closure of the soft palate. A palatal lift prosthesis attaches anteriorly to the teeth and has an extended, posterior tailpiece that lifts the velum into an elevated position. Patients who are edentulous (toothless) can be fitted with a combination denture-plus-speech bulb or palatal obturator. Patients with significant resection of the hard and soft palates may benefit from a large **palatal obturator**. A palatal obturator appliance can be developed to functionally close a large palatal defect and restore speech and

Figure 7-11. Weak labial musculature can be exercised by instructing the patient to perform the following exercises several times each.

Pucker your lips and hold them for several seconds.
Spread your lips into a big smile for several seconds.
Open your mouth widely and try to close your lips together without closing your jaw.
Close your lips tightly, press them together, and hold for several seconds.
Close your lips tightly against a tongue blade (or a stack of tongue blades) and hold the blade(s) with your lips while it is gently pulled away (clinician or client holds tongue blade[s] and gently pulls away providing resistance).
Say *pa-pa-pa-pa* as quickly and as accurately as you can.
Say *ba-ba-ba-ba* as quickly and as accurately as you can.
Say *ma-ma-ma-ma* as quickly and as accurately as you can.

Figure 7-12. Reduced mandible movement can be exercised by instructing the patient to perform the following exercises several times each.

Open your mouth as wide as possible and hold it for several seconds.
Close your jaws together as tightly as possible and hold it for several seconds.
Move your jaw to the left side as far as possible and hold it for several seconds.
Move your jaw to the right side as far as possible and hold it for several seconds.
Move your jaw in a circular fashion several times.
Open your jaw from a closed position while firm resistance is provided from under the chin (clinician or client presses firmly up against the chin while the patient attempts to open the jaw).
Bite down with your teeth on a tongue blade (or a stack of tongue blades) and hold the blade(s) with your teeth as it is gently pulled away (clinician or client holds tongue blade[s] and gently pulls away providing resistance).
Move your jaw to the left side as far as possible while firm resistance is provided from the left side (clinician or client firmly presses against the left side of the jaw while the client attempts to lateralize).
Move your jaw to the right side as far as possible while firm resistance is provided from the right side (clinician or client firmly presses against the right side of the jaw while the client attempts to lateralize).

Figure 7-13. Weak tongue musculature can be exercised by instructing the paient to perform the following exercises several times each.

Open your mouth and stick out your tongue. Hold your tongue steadily out in front without resting it on your lower lip. Hold it for several seconds.
Stick out your tongue and elevate it to your nose and hold it for several seconds.
Stick out your tongue and depress it toward your chin and hold it for several seconds.
Move your tongue to the left corner of your mouth and hold it for several seconds.
Move your tongue to the right corner of your mouth and hold it for several seconds.
Move your tongue in a circular fashion around your lips several times.
Move your tongue from the left to the right corner as quickly as possible.
Open your mouth and move your tongue along the hard palate from the front to the back several times.
Stick your tongue straight out against a tongue blade and push against resistance for several seconds (clinician or client holds tongue blade providing firm resistance).
Stick your tongue out and move your tongue to the left corner against resistance from a tongue blade (clinician or client holds tongue blade against the left side of the tongue providing firm resistance).
Stick your tongue out and move your tongue to the right corner against resistance from a tongue blade (clinician or client holds tongue blade against the right side of the tongue providing firm resistance).
Inside your mouth, press your tongue against the left cheek and push against resistance from a hand placed on the outside of the cheek (clinician or client holds hand flat against left cheek providing firm resistance).
Inside your mouth, press your tongue against the right cheek and push against resistance from a hand placed on the outside of the cheek (clinician or client holds hand flat against right cheek providing firm resistance).
Move the gauze to the right side of your mouth with your tongue (clinician forms a bolus out of a gauze pad and holds on to one end while the client manipulates it in her mouth) (Logemann, 1998).
Move the gauze to the left side of your mouth with your tongue.
Move the gauze to the back of your mouth with your tongue.
While the tongue tip is held with gauze, pull your tongue back as hard as possible for several seconds (clinician or client holds the tongue tip and provides resistance).

swallowing. A **palatal reshaping prosthesis** can be used to recontour the dimensions of the hard palate to fit the tongue following partial glossectomy. The acrylic appliance is shaped to fill in the areas of the hard palate where the patient's tongue cannot make sufficient contact. Use of the prosthesis can significantly improve the patient's ability to use the tongue to propel the bolus through the pharynx (Logemann, et al., 1989).

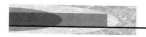

PHARYNGEAL CANCER

Pharyngeal wall tumors may warrant resection. Following resection, a reduction in pharyngeal elevation and contraction will lead to stasis in the valleculae, pyriform sinuses, and pharyngeal wall. As always, it is important to determine where the resection occurred in order to target the more functional side (if there is one) in therapy. A head turn or head tilt should be attempted during dynamic assessment of the swallow.

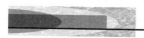

LARYNGEAL CANCER

Laryngeal cancer is classified as supraglottic, glottic, or subglottic based on the epicenter of the lesion. The **supraglottic** (above the glottis) region includes the epiglottis, false vocal folds, ventricles, aryepiglottic folds, and arytenoids. The **glottis** includes the true vocal folds. The **subglottic** (below the glottis) region begins about one centimeter below the true vocal folds and extends to the lower border of the cricoid cartilage. The surgical removal of the larynx is called a **laryngectomy**. When possible, laryngeal cancer is treated by removing parts of the larynx (partial laryngectomy) rather than the entire structure (total laryngectomy). The goal of treatment is complete cancer excision while maintaining function. All major laryngeal procedures have the risk of dysphagia. A majority of patients experience some aspiration after partial laryngectomy (Kronenberger & Meyers, 1994). The extent of the resection and type of closure affects swallow recovery. Forms of laryngeal surgery for cancer include: supraglottic laryngectomy, hemilaryngectomy, near-total laryngectomy, and total laryngectomy.

Supraglottic Laryngectomy

Supraglottic laryngectomy (sometimes referred to as a horizontal laryngectomy) involves the removal of the hyoid bone and the top of the larynx. The structures that are removed differ in each individual, but may involve removal of the epiglottis, aryepiglottic folds, false vocal folds, and sometimes base of the tongue, with preservation of the true vocal folds. The suprahyoid musculature, which elevates the larynx during swallowing, is severed or resected (Kronenberger & Meyers, 1994). The remaining larynx, therefore, is often suspended under the tongue base in order to improve airway protection and to facilitate opening of the upper esophageal sphincter. The patient has a functional voice postoperatively, but the patient has lost the top two tiers of airway protection important for safe swallowing. If the superior laryngeal nerve is damaged on one or both sides, supraglottic sensation will be reduced or absent, increasing the risk for silent aspiration. If the resection includes more structures such as one arytenoid cartilage and pyriform sinus, then the recovery of the swallowing function will become more complicated with the risk of aspiration greatly increased. Three main factors predispose the supraglottic laryngectomy patient to aspiration: (1) reduced hyolaryngeal elevation due to resection of suprahyoid musculature; (2) removal of the top two tiers of laryngeal airway protection; (3) delay in triggering of laryngeal elevation (McConnel, Mendelsohn, & Logemann, 1987). A nasogastric tube is routinely placed at surgery to provide nutritional supplementation until the tissues have healed sufficiently to allow swallowing trials (generally 10 to 14 days). Supraglottic laryngectomy patients with tongue base resection have a longer rehabilitation period than those without tongue resection (Denk, et al., 1997; Rademaker, et al., 1993). A supraglottic swallow or super-supraglottic swallow can be used to protect the laryngeal airway from penetrated material by focusing on timing and effort of true vocal fold closure. Patients often use supraglottic and super-supraglottic swallows for the first two to three months post-operatively, but often these maneuvers are not continued over time (Logemann, 1985; Logemann, et al., 1992). Range-of-motion exercises to improve tongue movement and arytenoid movement can also be implemented if necessary. A modified barium swallow should be conducted to determine if the swallow maneuver is effective in preventing aspiration.

Hemilaryngectomy

Hemilaryngectomy (sometimes referred to as a vertical laryngectomy) involves removal of one false vocal cord, one true vocal fold, and a portion of the thyroid cartilage on one side. The epiglottis and arytenoid cartilages are generally left intact. The surgical half of the larynx is then reconstructed to midline so that the intact vocal fold has tissue to make contact with for voicing and swallowing. Tight closure of the remaining vocal fold against the rebuilt tissue is often impaired post-operatively, thus reducing the ability to protect against aspiration (Logemann, 1985).

If an arytenoid cartilage is also resected, there is an increased risk of aspiration due to reduced glottic closure, reduced arytenoid-to-epiglottis contact, and impaired cricopharyngeal opening (McConnel & O'Connor, 1994). Laryngeal elevation during the swallow may be asymmetrical, with the intact side of the larynx elevating higher with better arytenoid-to-epiglottis contact (Schoenrock, King, Everts, Schneider, & Shumrick, 1972). Following hemilaryngectomy, the patient may need to use the chin-tuck, head-turn, or combined-swallow technique to eliminate aspiration. Hemilaryngectomy patients generally have a shorter rehabilitation time than supraglottic laryngectomy patients (Denk, et al., 1997). Most hemilaryngectomy patients do not have major problems with aspiration; however, if the arytenoid cartilage is involved, the rehabilitation period will be much longer (McConnel & O'Connor, 1994). These patients may need to use the supraglottic swallow maneuver and/or laryngeal adduction exercises to improve swallowing (Logemann, 1998).

Near-Total Laryngectomy

Near-total laryngectomy involves removal of the larynx while leaving a large part of the supraglottic area, such as the epiglottis. A fistula is constructed in the supraglottic area so that when the person occludes the permanent stoma, airflow can pass through the fistula to vibrate the walls of the pharynx. There is not a lot of information about the effects of this procedure on swallowing. Severe aspiration can result in some cases resulting in the need for total laryngectomy (Suits, Cohen, & Everts, 1996).

Total Laryngectomy

Total laryngectomy involves removal of the entire cricoid cartilage, thyroid cartilage, epiglottis, hyoid bone, arytenoids, true vocal folds, and false vocal folds. The trachea is sectioned between the second and third tracheal rings in order to create a permanent stoma in the neck for breathing. This results in permanent separation of the gastrointestinal tract from the respiratory tract as seen in Figures 7-14a and 7-14b. Patients need to be counseled pre-operatively on the permanent changes that they will experience in breathing, swallowing, and speaking. Changes that occur secondary to total laryngectomy that are important to eating and swallowing are reviewed in the following paragraphs.

Changes in the pathways for breathing will alter the taste of food for some laryngectomy patients. Why does this happen? When the patient breathes in and out through the stoma in the neck, the nasal passages are

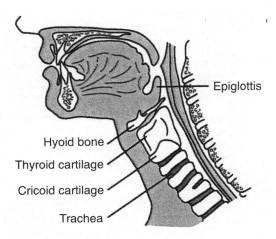

Figure 7-14a. Lateral view of normal oropharyngeal and laryngeal region.

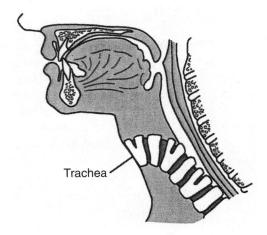

Figure 7-14b. Lateral view of oropharyngeal region following laryngectomy.

no longer used for the transport of air. By bypassing the nose, the patient will experience significant disability in the sense of smell leading to a decrease in the sense of taste. Patients who have a reduced sense of taste often have a decrease in appetite. Patients with laryngectomy can learn to induce nasal airflow by doing a nasal airflow-inducing technique simply described to patients as a *polite yawn* (yawning with lips closed) (Hilgers, van Dam, Keyzers, Koster, van As, & Muller, 2000). This technique involves lowering the jaw, floor of mouth, tongue, and soft palate while keeping the lips closed. The maneuver induces negative pressure in the oral cavity and oropharynx, generating nasal airflow and permitting odorous substances to reach the olfactory epithelium (Hilgers, et al.,

2000). Hilgers and colleagues (2000) successfully taught 15 of 33 (46%) total laryngectomy patients who had no sense of smell to learn to smell by using the *polite yawn* technique in one 30-minute session.

Swallowing changes also take place following total laryngectomy. Intuitively, it would seem that separating the pathway for breathing from the pathway for swallowing would solve many of the difficulties that can occur during swallowing. The pathway is now much simpler; the bolus now travels from the oral cavity to the esophagus without risk of material entering the larynx (penetration and aspiration). The complex interactions between laryngeal closure and bolus propulsion are no longer necessary. What then can possibly go wrong during this simplified passage? Post-surgical changes to the anatomy following total laryngectomy have the potential to affect swallowing motility. Alteration in pharyngeal musculature can lead to difficulty in bolus propulsion, post-operative fistula development can lead to aspiration, strictures can lead to difficult bolus passage, muscle spasms can lead to difficult bolus passage, and diverticula can lead to pocketing of food.

The pharyngeal muscles will not function normally following surgery because they have been surgically cut and then put back together, often with large portions being removed, thus affecting the ability of the pharyngeal muscles to segmentally constrict and move the bolus through the pharynx. Bolus transport will, therefore, rely more on tongue propulsion and gravity. The patient will complain of inability to clear the pharynx in one swallow.

Pharyngocutaneous **fistula**, an opening that occurs in the pharynx at the surgical site during healing, is the most common complication following total laryngectomy (Redaelli-de-Zinis, Ferrari, Tomenzoli, Premoli, Parrinello, & Nicolai, 1999). Factors that may lead to the development of a fistula include pre-operative radiation therapy, faulty surgical technique, advanced tumor size, poor nutritional status, and underlying medical disorders (Boyce & Meyers, 1989). A fistula can lead to aspiration of material from the pharynx into the trachea. A videofluoroscopic examination of swallowing will detect the presence of a post-operative fistula. In the majority of cases a fistula will close with proper wound care; however, it is sometimes necessary to surgically suture the pharyngeal mucosa or to close it with a flap of tissue from pharyngeal musculature or from tissue from another site such as part of the jejunum, a segment of the small intestine (Redaeilli-de-Zinis, et al., 1999). If it is determined with the use of manometry that the fistula developed due to excessive tension at the pharyngeal suture line, a cricopharyngeal myotomy can diminish peak pharyngeal pressures during swallowing, thereby reducing resistance at the pharygo-esophageal junction (Horowitz & Sasaki, 1993).

A stricture is a narrowing or stenosis that can occur in the pharynx or upper esophagus due to extensive resection or due to scar tissue formation. A stricture impedes the flow of the bolus creating more difficulty with thicker viscosities and solid foods. A stricture may be treated by the use of dilation or by surgery. In order to dilate the stricture, the patient is taught to swallow rubber catheters, called bougies, that are gradually increased in size in order to open up the stricture (Logemann, 1998). This treatment often has to be repeated at regular intervals when the symptoms return. A surgical treatment for a stricture is a cricopharyngeal myotomy, where the cricopharyngeus muscle is cut vertically in order to relax the muscle. Horowitz and Sasaki (1993) found that a cricopharyngeal myotomy reduces sphincteric pressure thus allowing easier bolus flow into the esophagus.

Following total laryngectomy, some patients present with a **spasm** in the pharyngoesophageal segment (PES), which leads to difficulty swallowing. A videofluoroscopic examination can be used to determine if the difficulty swallowing is due to a stricture or if it is due to a spasm (Crary & Glowasky, 1996). If it is determined that it is a spasm, injection of botulinum has been demonstrated to improve swallowing function (Crary & Glowasky, 1996). **Botulinum Toxin Type A (Botox)** is produced from the *Clostridium botulinum* bacteria. Botox works by inhibiting the presynaptic release of acetylcholine at the neuromuscular junction reducing the hypercontraction of the muscles. Injection of small amounts of Botox into the muscle decreases spasticity by reducing hyperactive muscle contraction. Botox affects only the muscles where it is injected. The reduction in strength and spasticity is temporary and most patients need to be re-injected every three to six months. A second treatment for PES spasm is a cricopharyngeal myotomy (Horowitz & Sasaki, 1993).

While less common than stricture, recurrent neoplasm, and neuromuscular dysfunction, a pharyngeal **diverticulum** (out-pouching of the wall) can also be the cause of post-laryngectomy dysphagia (Sobol, Prince, & Cronin, 1990). In post-laryngectomy patients, the diverticulum develops in the anterior pharyngeal wall. The patient will complain of difficulty clearing pharyngeal residue and regurgitating undigested material. Videofluoroscopy should be used in identifying a diverticulum. Treatment of a diverticulum depends on the severity of symptoms. Behavioral treatment includes neck postures, digital manipulation, and alteration of food consistencies (Sobol, et al., 1990). Surgical removal of a diverticulum can be accomplished with endoscopic laser surgery (Lippert, Folz, Rudert, & Werner, 1999) or with open pharyngoplasty (Sobol, et al., 1990).

Some total laryngectomy patients will have a fold of tissue at the base of the tongue, which appears to be an epiglottis when viewed on lateral videofluoroscopy. This fold of tissue is often referred to as a **pseudoepiglottis** and occurs more often in laryngectomy patients with vertical surgical closures (100%) than in patients with a "T"-shaped closure (67%) (Davis, Vincent, Shapshay, & Strong, 1982). When the patient swallows, the fold of tissue widens and collects food and liquid (Logemann, 1998). This pocket may be so large that it can obstruct the bolus from passing through the pharynx. The effects of the pseudoepiglottis should be examined during videofluoroscopy in order to visualize how the dimensions of the pocket change when filled with food and liquid. Treatment includes surgical removal of the tissue fold or diets restricted to liquids and thin pastes (Logemann, 1998). During videofluoroscopy the treatment strategy of a head turn can be attempted to see if it is successful in channeling the food out of the pathway of the pseudoepiglottis (Logemann, 1998).

Pharyngolaryngoesophagectomy

A **pharyngolaryngoesophagectomy** involves removal of the pharynx, larynx, and esophagus and is used to treat extensive head and neck tumors. After removal of the structures, the stomach is pulled up and attached to the pharynx (**gastric pull-up procedure**). The patient can swallow following the procedure but may experience the aforementioned difficulties associated with total laryngectomy. Backflow of material into the mouth and nose may also be a postoperative complication of this surgery (Johansson, Johnsson, Groshen, & Walther, 1999; Logemann, 1998). Postural techniques such as extending the neck or rotating the head should be attempted to determine if they eliminate the backflow (Logemann, 1998). The long-term survival rates for patients following pharyngolaryngoesophagectomy is smaller due to the fact that the tumors are more extensive, often extending into bone, cartilage, or soft tissues (Hartley, Bottrill, & Howard, 1999).

ESOPHAGEAL NEOPLASMS

Very few tumors of the esophagus are benign. It is estimated that less than 10 percent of all tumors diagnosed are non-malignant (Goyal, 2001). Of malignant tumors, nearly 90 percent are squamous cell carcinomas and the majority of the remaining 10 percent are adenocarcinoma (the kind resulting from metaplastic changes associated with Barrett's esophagus). Esophageal squamous cell cancer has a relatively high incidence and is the fifth most common cancer in adult males (Goyal, 2001). Symptom onset includes solid food dysphagia leading to difficulties with semisolids and liquids. Progression is relatively rapid and also includes weight loss and possibly voice problems if the recurrent laryngeal nerve is involved in the thoracic cavity. On average, diagnosis is made in advanced stages of the disease. Treatment is often surgical with resection of the area and may be **palliative** in nature. Radiation treatment generally follows surgery. Prognosis is often poor with a five-year survival rate ranging from less than 5 percent to 8 percent (Goyal, 2001; Reid & Thomas, 1995).

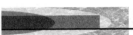

RADIATION TREATMENT FOR HEAD AND NECK CANCER

Radiation therapy uses high-energy radiation directed to the area of the tumor and to the adjacent lymph nodes to damage cancer cells and stop them from growing. Radiation therapy is usually given five days a week for five to six weeks. Radiation therapy may be used alone, combined with chemotherapy, or combined with surgery. There are a variety of protocols that vary according to tumor location, stage, and whether the cancer has spread. A medical team working with the patient determines appropriate course of treatment. Whenever possible, the use of radiation with or without chemotherapy is advocated over surgery as a treatment for patients with advanced laryngeal cancer in order to preserve the larynx and voice. Quality of life measures in patients who have received radiotherapy plus chemotherapy have been found to be higher than in patients who have received surgery plus radiotherapy (Terrell, Fisher, & Wolf, 1998). Terrell and colleagues (1998) found that the radiation-plus-chemotherapy group reported significantly less bodily pain, better scores on mental health, lower levels of depression, and better emotional well-being than compared to the surgery-plus-radiation group.

Radiation therapy and surgery are often used together in a variety of combinations to treat laryngeal cancer. Radiation can be used to shrink a large tumor before surgery or to destroy cancer cells that may remain in the area after surgery, with the latter scenario occurring more often. Tissue that has been irradiated is more difficult to heal and is more at risk for post-surgical complications such as fistula development. Surgery can also be used to successfully remove a recurrent tumor after radiation therapy used alone fails (Quer, Leon, Orus, Venegas, Lopez, & Burgues, 2000).

Radiation therapy to the head and neck region can lead to immediate and long-term dysphagia due to xerostomia, tissue necrosis, edema, sensory changes, tissue fibrosis, and/or trismus. Xerostomia, dryness of the mouth, can result when the mucus-producing glands fall within the focus of the radiation beam. The dryness increases with higher levels of radiation exposure. Saliva is important because it acts as a lubricant and promotes wound healing in the oral cavity. Saliva protects dentition by neutralizing alkaline and acidic foods. A dental exam should precede radiation therapy in order to prepare the oral cavity for radiation by extracting infected teeth. Daily use of fluoride gel is also prescribed for patients before, during, and after radiation therapy in order to reduce the risk of dental caries. Reduction in saliva can lead to difficulty transporting the bolus, discomfort in chewing and swallowing, and an increase in oral infections and dental caries. When salivary flow is decreased, it increases the concentration of bacteria within the saliva (Langmore, et al., 1998). If the person aspirates food and liquid that is mixed with saliva with an overgrowth of bacteria, or if the person aspirates the bacteria-laden saliva alone, the chances for developing pneumonia are increased (Langmore, et al., 1998). A patient with xerostomia will have more difficulty manipulating a dry, absorbent food material resulting in longer mastication time and increased oral and pharyngeal residue (Hamlet, et al., 1997). Patients will complain of a sticky, more viscous saliva that is difficult to expectorate. Xerostomia in radiation patients is irreversible and must be treated in a palliative manner through the use of diet modification, artificial saliva, oral moisturizer, humidification, or salivary stimulation through the use of tart sugarless candies, chewing gum, medication (pilocarpine, salagen, biotene), or electrical stimulation (Papas, Fernandez, Castano, Gallagher, Trivedi, & Shrotriya, 1998). Patients need to be taught good oral hygiene and instructed to schedule regular dental examinations.

Radionecrosis, damage and breakdown of soft tissue and bone due to radiation, is a potential, although uncommon, complication of radiation to the head and neck. Radionecrosis of the temporal bone, midface, mandible, and larynx has been reported following radiation treatment for head and neck cancer (Fitzgerald & Koch, 1999). The majority of patients with radionecrosis present with these symptoms within one year of treatment; however, delayed presentations up to several decades after radiotherapy for cancer of the larynx have been reported (Fitzgerald & Koch, 1999). Laryngeal radionecrosis can lead to aspiration, odynophagia (pain when swallowing), respiratory obstruction, and hoarseness. Surgical treatment, such as a tracheostomy or total laryngectomy, is often necessary. Hyperbaric oxygen therapy, a means of providing additional oxygen to the tissues of the body to promote healing, has also proven to be beneficial in some patients with advanced laryngeal radionecrosis (Filntisis, Moon, Kraft, Farmer, Scher, & Piantadosi, 2000). Filntisis and colleagues (2000) studied 18 patients with severe radionecrosis of the larynx and found that 13 (72.2%) had major improvement following hyperbaric oxygen therapy thus avoiding the need for a total laryngectomy.

Post-radiation **edema** (swelling) of the laryngeal tissues can lead to dysphagia and dysphonia. **Mucositis** (inflammatory changes to the mucosa) can cause pain and tenderness when swallowing. Edema and mucositis will generally resolve within three to six months following the completion of therapy. Treatment involves hydration, humidification, acid suppression, and occasionally the use of steroids and antibiotics.

Tissue fibrosis occurs as a result of damage to small blood vessels in the radiated area (Logemann, 1998). Fibrosis can continue for many years following treatment. Fibrosis of tissue following radiation can lead to reduced posterior tongue base motion, reduced laryngeal elevation, and restricted epiglottis base to arytenoid contact (Lazarus, 1993). This can lead to stasis and aspiration before and after the swallow, sometimes necessitating non-oral feeding. These patients often benefit from the super-supraglottic swallow and the Mendelsohn maneuver (Lazarus, 1993; Logemann, 1998). Patients receiving radiation should begin range of motion exercises for the tongue, jaw, and larynx before radiation begins and continue to use these exercises forever to maintain function and prevent fibrosis (Logemann, 1998).

Trismus historically has been defined as tonic contraction of the muscles of mastication and describes the early symptom of tetanus also called *lock-jaw*. More recently, the term trismus has been used to describe any restriction to mouth opening including restrictions caused by trauma, disease, surgery, or radiation. When trismus occurs secondary to radiation of the head and neck, dysphagia often accompanies it. Cancers treated with radiation that occur in the nasopharyngeal region, including the base of the tongue, salivary glands, maxilla, and mandible, are most likely to result in trismus. Trismus can lead to problems with communication, nutrition, and oral hygiene. Limited mouth opening may result in compromised mastication, poor bolus formation, and increased oral and pharyngeal residue. These factors increase the incidence of aspiration. Treatments of trismus include stretching of the muscles along with passive motion and injection of Botox into the bilateral masseter, temporalis, lateral, and medial pterygoid muscles (Spillane, Shelton, & Hasty, 2003) and surgery (Dimitroulis, 2002).

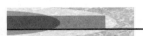

Alteration, big or small, of the anatomy of the aerodigestive tract can lead to dysphagia. Dysphagia is not only due to the structural anomalies but also to the altered peripheral neurological system that typically accompanies anatomical change. Mechanical and aerodynamic forces in swallowing are highly coordinated and vulnerable to transformation. This chapter presented structural etiologies of dysphagia due to acute changes (e.g., trauma, infections, tracheotomy) and progressive transformations (e.g., osteophytes, diverticula, neoplasms). The underlying physiological principles for treatment strategies were discussed and speech-language pathologists were encouraged to apply their understanding of physiology to the selection of remedial or compensatory strategies in clinical practice.

STUDY QUESTIONS

1. What is endotracheal intubation and how does it increase the risk of aspiration?

2. Describe xerostomia and its possible causes.

3. What are the mechanical and neurophysiologic factors that may cause aspiration following tracheostomy placement?

4. What are osteophytes and how can they result in dysphagia?

5. Describe Zenker's diverticulum and its implications for swallowing.

6. What is a glossectomy and how may it affect swallowing?

7. What is a supraglottic laryngectomy and why may it lead to aspiration?

8. What is a stricture and how may it affect swallowing?

9. Describe the impact of radiation therapy on deglutition.

REFERENCES

Bach, J., & Alba, A. (1990). Tracheostomy ventilation: A study of efficacy with deflated cuffs and cuffless tubes. *Chest, 97*(3), 679–683.

Bachor, E., Bonkowsky, V., & Hacki, T. (1996). Herpes simplex virus type I reactivation as a cause of a unilateral temporary paralysis of the vagus nerve. *European Archives of Otorhinolaryngology, 253,* 297–300.

Baron, E. M., Solimen, A. M., Gaughan, J. P., Simpson, L., & Young, W. F. (2003). Dysphagia, hoarseness, and unilateral true vocal fold motion impairment following anterior cervical diskectomy and fusion. *Annals of Otology, Rhinology, and Laryngology, 112*(11), 921–926.

Betts, R. H. (1965). Post-tracheostomy aspiration. *New England Journal of Medicine, 273,* 155.

Blitzer, A., & Sulica, L. (2001). Botulinum toxin: Basic science and clinical uses in otolaryngology. *Laryngoscope, 111*(2), 218–226.

Bone, D. K., Davis, J. L., Zuidema, G. D., & Cameron, J. L. (1974). Aspiration pneumonia: Prevention of aspiration in patients with tracheostomies. *Annals of Thoracic Surgery, 18*(1), 30–37.

Boyce, S. E., & Meyers, A. D. (1989). Oral feeding after total laryngectomy. *Head and Neck Surgery, 11*(3), 269–273.

Boyce, G. A., & Boyce Jr., H. W. (1995). Esophagus: Anatomy and structural anomolies. In T. Yamada (Ed.), *Textbook of gastroenterology* (2nd ed.). Philadelphia: J. B. Lippincott.

Buckwalter, J. A., & Sasaki, C. (T.) (1984). Effect of tracheostomy on laryngeal function. *Otolaryngologic Clinics of North America, 17*(1), 41–48.

Cameron, J. L., Reynolds, J., & Zuidema, G. D. (1973). Aspiration in patients with tracheostomies. *Surgery, Gynecology & Obstetrics, 136*(1), 68–70.

Crary, M. A., & Glowasky, A. L. (1996). Using Botulinum Toxin A to improve speech and swallowing function following total laryngectomy. *Archives of Otolaryngology, Head, and Neck Surgery, 122*(7), 760–763.

Crary, M. A., & Groher, M. E. (2000). Basic concepts of surface electromyographic biofeedback in the treatment of dysphagia: A tutorial. *American Journal of Speech-Language Pathology, 9*, 116–125.

Daniels, S. K., Mahoney, M. C., & Lyons, G. D. (1998). Persistent dysphagia and dysphonia following cervical spine surgery. *Ear, Nose and Throat Journal, 77*(6), 472–475.

Davis, R. K., Vincent, M. E., Shapshay, S. M., & Strong, M. S. (1982). The anatomy and complications of "T" versus vertical closure of the hypopharynx after laryngectomy. *Laryngoscope, 92*(1), 16–22.

Denk, D. M., Swoboda, H., Schima, W., & Eibenberger, K. (1997). Prognostic factors for swallowing rehabilitation following head and neck cancer surgery. *Acta Otolaryngology (Stockholm), 117*(15), 769–74.

DeVita, M. A., & Spierer-Rundback, L. (1990). Swallowing disorders in patients with prolonged orotracheal intubation or tracheostomy tubes. *Critical Care Medicine, 18*(12), 1328–1330.

Dimitroulis, G. (2002). A review of 56 cases of chronic closed lock treated with temporomandibular joint arthroscopy. *Journal of Oral and Maxillofacial Surgery, 60*(5), 519–524.

DiVito, J. (1998). Cervical osteophytic dysphagia: Single and combined mechanisms. *Dysphagia, 13*(1), 58–61.

Dettelbach, M., Gross, R., Mahlmann, J., & Eibling, D. (1995). Effect of the Passy-Muir Valve on aspiration in patients with tracheostomy. *Head & Neck, 17*(4), 297–302.

Dixon-Wood, V. L. (1997). Counseling and early management of feeding and language skill development for infants and toddlers with cleft palate. In K. R. Bzoch (Ed.), *Communicative disorders related to cleft lip and palate* (4th ed.). Austin, TX: Pro-Ed.

Donzelli, J., Brady, S., Wesling, M., & Craney, M. (2001). Simultaneous modified Evan's blue dye procedure and video nasal endoscopic evaluation of the swallow. *Laryngoscope, 111*(10), 1746–1750.

Eibling, D. E., & Gross, R. D. (1996). Subglottic air pressure: A key component of swallowing efficiency. *Annals of Otology, Rhinology, & Laryngology, 105*(4), 253–258.

Elpern, E., Jacobs, E., & Bone, R. (1987). Incidence of aspiration in tracheally intubated adults. *Heart & Lung, 16*(5), 527–531.

Fasano, N. C., Levine, M. S., Rubesin, S. E., Redfern, R. O., & Laufer, I. (2003). Epiphrenic diverticulum: Clinical and radiographic findings in 27 patients. *Dysphagia, 18*(1), 9–15.

Feldman, S., Deal, C., & Urquhart, W. (1966). Disturbance of swallowing after tracheostomy. *The Lancet, 1*(7444), 954–955.

Filntisis, G. A., Moon, R. E., Kraft, K. L., Farmer, J. C., Scher, R. L., & Piantadosi, C. A. (2000). Laryngeal radionecrosis and hyperbaric oxygen therapy: Report of 18 cases and review of the literature. *Annals of Otology, Rhinology, and Laryngology, 109*(6), 554–562.

Fitzgerald, P. J., & Koch, R. J. (1999). Delayed radionecrosis of the larynx. *American Journal of Otolaryngology, 20*(4), 245–249.

Frazell, E. L., & Lucas, J. C. (1962). Cancer of the tongue: Report on the management of 1,554 patients. *Cancer, 15,* 1085–1099.

Furia, C. L., Carrarra de Angelis, E., Martins, N. M., Barros, A. P., Carneiro, B., & Kowalski, L. P. (2000). Videofluoroscopic evaluation after glossectomy. *Archives of Otolaryngology, Head, and Neck Surgery, 126*(3), 378–383.

Goyal, R. K. (2001). Esophagus. In *Harrison's principles of internal medicine* (15th ed.). (Eds. Braunwald, E., Fauci, D. L., Kasper, S. L., Hauser, D. L., Longo, & Jameson, J. L.). New York: McGraw-Hill.

Groher, M. E. (1997). *Dysphagia: Diagnosis and treatment.* Boston: Butterworth-Heinemann.

Hamlet, S., Faull, J., Klein, B., Aref, A., Fontanesi, J., Stachler, R., Shamsa, F., Jones, L., & Simpson, M. (1997). Mastication and swallowing in patients with postirradiation xerostomia. *International Journal of Radiation Oncology Biology Physics, 37*(4), 789–796.

Hartley, B. E., Bottrill, I. D., & Howard, D. J. (1999). A third decade's experience with the gastric pull-up operation for hypopharyngeal carcinoma: Changing patterns of use. *Journal of Laryngology and Otology, 113*(3), 241–243.

Hartmann, R. W. (1999). Ludwig's angina in children. *American Family Physician, 60*(1), 109–112.

Heffner, J. E., Miller, K. S., & Sahn, S. A. (1986). Tracheostomy in the intensive care unit: Part 1: Indications, techniques, and management. *Chest, 90*(2), 269–274.

Hilgers, F. J., van Dam, F. S., Keyzers, S., Koster, M. N., van As, C. J., & Muller, M. J. (2000). Rehabilitation of olfaction after laryngectomy by means of a nasal airflow-inducing maneuver: The "polite yawning" technique. *Archives of Otolaryngology, Head, and Neck Surgery, 126*(6), 726–732.

Hirano, M., Kuroiwa, Y., Tanaka, S., Mausuoka, H., Sato, K., & Yoshida, T. (1992). Dysphagia following various degrees of surgical resection for oral cancer. *Annals of Otology, Rhinology, and Laryngology, 101,* 138–141.

Horowitz, J. B., & Sasaki, C. T. (1993). Effect of cricopharyngeus myotomy on postlaryngectomy pharyngeal contraction pressures. *Laryngoscope, 103*(2), 138–140.

Johansson, J., Johnsson, F., Groshen, S., & Walther, B. (1999). Pharyngeal reflux after gastric pull-up esophagectomy with neck and chest anastomoses. *Journal of Thoracic and Cardiovascular Surgery, 118*(6), 1078–1083.

Kahrilas, P. J., & Ergus, G. A. (1994). Esophageal dysphagia. *Acta Oto-Rhino-Laringologica Belgique, 48*(2), 171–190.

Kelchner, L. N., Stemple, J. C., Gerdeman, E., Le Borgne, W., & Adam, S. (1999). Etiology, pathophysiology, treatment choices, and voice results for unilateral adductor vocal fold paralysis: A 3-year retrospective. *Journal of Voice, 13*(4), 592–601.

Knuff, T. E., Benjamin, S. B., & Castell, D. O. (1982). Pharyngoesophageal (Zenker's) diverticulum: A reappraisal. *Gastroenterology, 82*(4), 734–736.

Kronenberger, M. B., & Meyers, A. D. (1994). Dysphagia following head and neck cancer surgery. *Dysphagia, 9*(4), 236–244.

Langmore, S. E., Terpenning, M. S., Schork, A., Chen, Y., Murray, J. T., Lopatin, D., & Loesche, W. J. (1998). Predictors of aspiration pneumonia: How important is dysphagia? *Dysphagia, 13*(2), 69–81.

Lazarus, C. L. (1993). Effects of radiation therapy and voluntary maneuvers on swallowing functioning in head and neck cancer patients. *Clinics in Communication Disorders, 3*(4), 11–20.

Leder, S. B. (1999). Effect of a one-way tracheostomy speaking valve on the incidence of aspiration in previously aspirating patients with tracheostomy. *Dysphagia, 14*(1), 73–77.

Leder, S. B., Joe, J. K., Hill, S. E., & Traube, M. (2001). Effect of tube occlusion on upper esophageal sphincter and pharyngeal pressures in aspirating and nonaspirating patients. *Dysphagia, 16*(2), 79–82.

Leder, S. B., Cohn, S. M., & Moller, B. A. (1998). Fiberoptic endoscopic documentation of the high incidence of aspiration following extubation in critically ill trauma patients. *Dysphagia, 13*(4), 208–212.

Leder, S. B., Ross, D. A., Burrell, M. I., & Sasaki, C. T. (1998). Tracheostomy tube occlusion status and aspiration in early postsurgical head and neck cancer patients. *Dysphagia, 13*(3), 167–171.

Leder, S. B., Tarro, J. M., & Burrell, M. I. (1996). Effect of occlusion of a tracheostomy tube on aspiration. *Dysphagia, 11*(4), 254–258.

Lippert, B. M., Folz, B. J., Rudert, H. H., & Werner, J. A. (1999). Management of Zenker's diverticulum and postlaryngectomy pseudodiverticulum with the CO_2 laser. *Otolaryngology, Head and Neck Surgery, 121*(6), 809–814.

Logemann, J. A. (1998). *Evaluation and treatment of swallowing disorders* (2nd ed.). Austin: Pro-Ed.

Logemann, J. A. (1985). The relationship of speech and swallowing in head and neck surgical patients. *Seminars in speech and language, 6*, 351–359.

Logemann, J. A., Kahrilas, P. J., Hurst, P., Davis, J., & Krugler, C. (1989). Effects of intraoral prosthetics on swallowing in patients with oral cancer. *Dysphagia, 4*(2), 118–120.

Logemann, J. A., Pauloski, B. R., Colangelo, L., Lazarus, C., Fujiu, M., & Kahrilas, P. J. (1995). Effects of a sour bolus on oropharyngeal swallowing measures in patients with neurogenic dysphagia. *Journal of Speech and Hearing Research, 38*(3), 556–563.

Logemann, J. A., Pauloski, B. R., Rademaker, A. W., & Colangelo, L. (1997). Speech and swallowing rehabilitation in head and neck cancer patients. *Oncology, 11*(5), 651–659.

Logemann, J. A., Pauloski, B. R., Rademaker, A. W., Cook, M. A., Graner, D., Milianti, F., Beery, Q., Stein, D., Bowman, J., Lazarus, C., Heiser, M. A., & Baker, T. (1992). Impact of the diagnostic procedure on outcome measures of swallowing rehabilitation in head and neck cancer patients, *Dysphagia, 7*(4), 179–186.

Logemann, J. A., Pauloski, B. R., Rademaker, A. W., McConnel, F. M. S., Heiser, M. A., Cardinale, S., Shedd, D., Stein, D., Beery, Q., Johnson, J., & Baker, T. (1993). Speech and swallow function after tonsil/base of tongue resection with primary closure. *Journal of Speech and Hearing Research, 36*(5), 918–926.

Low, V. H. S., & Rubesin, S. E. (1993). Contrast evaluation of the pharynx and esophagus. *Radiologic Clinics of North America, 31*(6), 1265–1291.

MacArthur, C. J., & Healy, G. B. (1995). Acquired voice disorders in the pediatric population. In J. A. Rubin, R. T. Sataloff, G. S. Korovin, & W. J. Gould (Eds.), *Diagnosis and treatment of voice disorders.* New York: Igaku-Shoin.

Maceri, D. R., & Zim, S. (2001). Laryngospasm: An atypical manifestation of severe gastroesophageal reflux disease (GERD). *Laryngoscope, 111*(11 Pt 1), 1976–1979.

Martin, R. E., Neary, M. A., & Diamant, N. E. (1997). Dysphagia following anterior cervical spine surgery. *Dysphagia, 12*(1), 2–8.

McConnel, F. M. S., & O'Conner, A. (1994). Dysphagia secondary to head and neck surgery. *Acta Oto-rhino-laryngologica Belgium, 48*(2), 165–170.

McConnel, F. M. S., & Logemann, J. A. (1990). Diagnosis and treatment of swallowing disorders. In C. W. Cummings (Ed.), *Otolaryngology, Head, and Neck Surgery.* (Update II). St. Louis, MO: Mosby.

McConnel, F. M. S., Mendelsohn, M. S., & Logemann, J. A. (1987). Manofluorography of deglutition after supraglottic laryngectomy. *Head & Neck Surgery, 9*(3), 142–150.

Moreland, L. W., Corey, J., & McKenzie, R. (1988). Ludwig's angina: Report of a case and review of the literature. *Archives of Internal Medicine, 148*(2), 461–466.

Morpeth, J. F., & Williams, M. F. (2000). Vocal fold paralysis after anterior cervical diskectomy and fusion. *Laryngoscope, 110*(1), 43–46.

Muz, J. M., Hamlet, S., Mathog, R. H., & Farris, R. (1994). Scinitigraphic assessment of aspiration in head and neck cancer patients with tracheostomy. *Head & Neck, 16*(1), 17–20.

Nash, M. (1988). Swallowing problems in the tracheostomized patient. *Otolaryngologic Clinics of North America, 21*(4), 701–709.

Papas, A. S., Fernandez, M. M., Castano, R. A., Gallagher, S. C., Trivedi, M., & Shrotriya, R. C. (1998). Oral prilocarpine for symptomatic relief of dry mouth and dry eyes in patients with Sjögren's syndrome. *Advances in Experimental Medicine and Biology, 438,* 973–978.

Pauloski, B. R., Logemann, J. A., Rademaker, A. W. McConnel, F. M. S., Heiser, M. A., Cardinale, S., Shedd, D., Lewin, J., Baker, S. R., Graner, D., Cook, B., Milianti, F., Collins, S., & Baker, T. (1993). Speech and swallowing function after anterior tongue and floor of mouth resection with distal flap reconstruction. *Journal of Speech and Hearing Research, 36*(2), 267–227.

Perlmann, A. J., Luschei, E. S., & Du Mond, C. E. (1989). Electrical activity from the superior pharyngeal constrictor during reflexive and nonreflexive tasks. *Journal of Speech and Hearing Research, 32*(4), 749–754.

Quer, M., Leon, X., Orus, C., Venegas, P., Lopez, M., & Burgues, J. (2000). Endoscopic laser surgery in the treatment of radiation failure of early laryngeal carcinoma. *Head & Neck, 22*(5), 520–523.

Rademaker, A. W., Logemann, J. A., Pauloski, B. R., Bowman, J., Lazarus, C., Sisson, G., Milianti, F., Graner, D., Cook, B., Collins, S., Stein, D., Beery, Q., Johnson, J., & Baker, T. (1993). Recovery of postoperative swallowing in patients undergoing partial laryngectomy. *Head & Neck, 15*(4), 325–334.

Redaelli-de-Zinis, L. O., Ferrari, L., Tomenzoli, D., Premoli, G., Parrinello, G. & Nicolai, P. (1999). Postlaryngectomy pharyngocutaneous fistula: Incidence, predisposing factors, and therapy. *Head & Neck, 21*(2), 131–138.

Reid, B. J., & Thomas, C. R. (1995) Esophageal neoplasms. In T. Yamada (Ed.), *Textbook of gastroenterology.* (2nd ed.). Philadelphia: J. B. Lippincott

Rousou, J. A., Tighe, D. A., Garb, J. L, Krasner, H., Engelman, R. M., Flack, J. E., & Deaton, D. W. (2000). Risk of dysphagia after transesophageal echocardiography during cardiac operations. *Annals of Thoracic Surgery, 69*(2), 486–489.

Schoenrock, L. D., King, A. Y., Everts, E. C., Schneider, H. J., & Shumrick, D. (1972). Hemilaryngectomy: Deglutition evaluation and rehabilitation. *Transcripts of the American Academy of Opthalmology and Otology, 76*(3), 752–757.

Scott, J. C., Jones, B., Eisele, D. W., & Ravich, W. J. (1992). Caustic ingestion of the upper aerodigestive tract. *Laryngoscope, 102*(1), 1–8.

Shaker, R., Dodds, W., Dantas, R., Hogan, W., & Arndorfer, R. (1990). Coordination of deglutitive glottic closure with oropharyngeal swallowing. *Gastoenterology, 98*(6), 1478–1484.

Shaker, R., Milbrath, M., Ren, J., Campbell, B., Toohill, R., & Hogan, W. (1995). Deglutitive aspiration in patients with tracheostomy: Effect of tracheostomy on the duration of vocal cord closure. *Gastroenterology, 108*(5), 1357–1360.

Shapiro, R. L., Hatheway, C., & Swerdlow, D. L. (1998). Botulism in the United States: A clinical and epidemiological review. *Annals of Internal Medicine, 129*, 221–228.

Siebens, A. A., Tippett, D. C., Kirby, N., & French, J. (1993). Dysphagia and expiratory air flow. *Dysphagia, 8*(3), 266–269.

Sobol, S. M., Prince, K., & Cronin, D. (1990). Anterior neopharyngeal diverticulum following laryngectomy. *Head & Neck, 12*(6), 520–523.

Sonies, B. C. (1993). Remediation challenges in treating dysphagia post head/neck cancer: A problem oriented approach. *Clinics in Communication Disorders, 3*(4), 21–26.

Spillane, K. S., Shelton, J. E., & Hasty, M. F. (2003). Stroke-induced trismus in a pediatric patient: Long-term resolution with Botulinum Toxin A. *American Journal of Physical Medicine and Rehabilitation, 82*(6), 485–488.

Stachler, R. J., Hamlet, S. L., Choi, J., & Fleming, S. (1996). Scintigraphic quantification of aspiration reduction with the Passy-Muir valve. *Laryngoscope, 106*(2 Pt. 1), 231–234.

Stanley, R. E., & Liang, T. S. (1988). Acute epiglottitis in adults: The Singapore experience. *Journal of Laryngology and Otology, 102*(11), 1017–1021.

Stemple, J. C. (Ed.). (1993) *Voice therapy: clinical studies.* St Louis, MO: Mosby Yearbook.

Stemple, J., (Ed.). (2000) *Voice therapy: clinical studies* (2nd ed.). San Diego, CA: Singular Publishing Group.

Suiter, D. M., McCullough, G. H., & Powell, P. W. (2003). Effects of cuff deflation and one-way tracheostomy speaking valve placement on swallow physiology. *Dysphagia, 18*(4), 284–292.

Suits, G. W., Cohen, J. I., & Everts, E. C. (1996). Near total laryngectomy: Patient selection and technical considerations. *Archives of Otolaryngology, Head, and Neck Surgery, 122*(5), 473–475.

Terrell, J. E., Fisher, S. G., & Wolf, G. T. (1998). Long-term quality of life after treatment of laryngeal cancer: The Veterans Affairs Laryngeal Cancer Study Group. *Archives of Otolaryngology, Head and Neck Surgery, 124,* 964–971.

Thompson-Henry, S., & Braddock, B. (1995). The modified Evan's blue dye procedure fails to detect aspiration in the trachestomized patient: Five case reports. *Dysphagia, 10*(3), 172–174.

Tippett, D. C., & Siebens, A.A. (1995). Preserving oral communication in individuals with tracheostomy and ventilator dependency. *American Journal of Speech Language Pathology, 4*(2), 55–61.

Tolep, K., Getch, C., & Criner, G. (1996). Swallowing dysfunction in patients receiving prolonged mechanical ventilation. *Chest, 109*(1), 167–172.

Tucker, H. M. (1995). Laryngeal reinnervation. In J. S. Rubin, R. T. Sataloff, G. S. Korovin, & W. J. Gould. *Diagnosis and treatment of voice disorders.* New York: Igaku-Shoin.

Tytgat, G. N. (1995). Upper gastrointestinal endoscopy. In T. Yamada (Ed.), *Textbook of gastroenterology* (2nd ed.) Philadelphia: J. B. Lippincott.

Van Pinxteren, B., Numans, M. E., Lau, J., de Wit, N. J., Hungin, A. P., & Bonis, P. A. (2003). Short-term treatment of gastroesophageal reflux disease. *Journal of General Internal Medicine, 18*(9), 755–763.

Veenker, E., & Cohen, J. I. (2003). Current trends in management of Zenker's diverticulum. *Current Opinions in Otolaryngology, Head and Neck Surgery, 11*(3), 160–165.

Weber, B. (1974). Eating with a Trach. *American Journal of Nursing, 74*(8), 1439.

EPILOGUE

Future Directions

Our understanding of the anatomical and physiological basis of deglutition will continue to evolve past the rudimentary level that currently exists. What do we currently know? Scientific study has identified the basic morphological structures involved in deglutition. We have moved away from a conceptualization of rigid sequential involvement of structures to a soft assembly of structures. We have begun to appreciate the immense variability within and between individuals to swallow safely and efficiently. We have begun to appreciate an increased number of variables that affect deglutition including bolus characteristics and differences attributable to sex, age, and physical robustness. The flexibility of swallow motor activity is being expanded exponentially in current research findings. Early results suggest that cortical regions of activation may differ in the relative distribution of activity depending on the specific eating task such as volitional dry vs. wet swallows (Mosier, Liu, Maldjian, Shah, & Modi, 1999). As well, different activation patterns have been observed depending on subject attentional states (Binonfski, Buccino, & Taylor, 1998). Individuals with intact neuromuscular systems have been shown to produce highly variable activation patterns to the left or right cortical hemispheres during various swallow maneuvers (Hamdy, Aziz, & Rothwell; Singh, Barlow, Hughes, Tallis, & Thompson, 1996). Preliminary data on normal adult subjects suggest that the historic view of the swallow being controlled by a complex, but relatively fixed, reflex system may be simplistic or inaccurate. What has historically been considered a rigid pattern, centrally controlled, is being observed dynamically to change with a high level of flexibility. Non-invasive means to assess neural metabolic function promises to rapidly advance our understanding of brain plasticity in stereotypic behaviors such as deglutition.

Where do we need to go from here? Improved imaging techniques from a cellular-to-organ system level will provide critical missing elements in our current understanding of this complex biological function. Functional imaging techniques (such as functional MRI) used while the action of interest, such as deglutition, is produced by a person is moving to the forefront of research diagnostic imaging techniques in this field. Exact neural structures that register metabolic activity during swallow currently are being identified and the patterns of activation and pattern variability are being explored. Through interdisciplinary study, motor theories underlying human volitional behaviors are being explored for their ability to explain swallow function (Mosier & Bereznaya, 2001). Just as motor theories for central pattern generators were extended from research on simple organisms and stereotypic human behavior to swallow in the 1980s, more complex models are being explored today.

We need to better understand the neurophsyiologcal mechanisms underlying many of the disease states that lead to dysphagia—from GERD to Alzheimer's and MS. A more thorough foundation in normal function and its inherent variability is needed to provide a solid point of comparison for disordered function. As the number of studies (and as a result, sample size) increases, our understanding of normal variation within and between individuals should increase as well. Peer-reviewed research will be critical to establishing a solid foundation for both normal and disordered deglutition.

Speech-language pathologists must remain in both the clinical and research arenas as this field matures. As professionals dealing with patients on a daily basis we are poised to ask the questions that research needs to explore under carefully controlled conditions without bias or threats to validity. Speech-language pathologists will be best served and challenged within their careers if they do not become mere technicians. Within our training programs we need to emphasize that clinical practice and research are not dichotomous entities. As anatomy and physiology of a mechanism should be integral to treatment and management strategy development for that mechanism, so too should research be a critical component of clinical practice. We look to the practitioners to drive and inform the research questions of interest. A current example of this synergistic relationship between clinical practice and research is the attention being given to poor interrater reliability in interpreting results from videofluoroscopic examinations. Clinicians who practice are the key people to solve this obstacle. Standardization of the rheological qualities of contrast materials for modified barium swallow studies and therapeutic foods for patients with dysphagia are significant challenges for practicing clinicians. They are well positioned to ask the pertinent questions, design the studies, and carry the results into mainstream practice.

As a profession we must also be critical thinkers and reviewers of methods and materials that are on the market. We must look to peer-reviewed publications to lead the way in establishing a strong theoretical base to our clinical work. The peer review process is essential to maintaining an objective approach with high standards within the field of deglutition and dysphagia management. Our methods and procedures must stand up to rigorous and thorough testing before being adopted into general clinical practice. A current example is our limited understanding of what pulse oximetry is able or unable to tell us about physiological function during the act of mealtime swallow function. While quickly brought into clinical use because of ease and the noninvasive nature of monitoring, it appears that saturation levels are not a direct signal of aspiration. With further research, this methodology may, or may not, be able to provide us with less direct, but clinically useful, information. Incorporation into clinical use should only occur after the underlying hypothesis has shown some positive results in controlled trials. **Deep pharyngeal stimulation** is another clinical method that currently has little more than anecdotal support yet has been disseminated widely in training workshops to speech-language pathologists eager to help dysphagic patients. Dr. Logemann has addressed this issue eloquently in the *Dysphagia Audio Digest* (2002) review of *A Framework for Managing Controversial Practices* (Duchan, Calculator, Sonnenmeier, Diejl, & Cumley, 2001). Dr. Logemann applies the principles found in this article to the practice of dysphagia treatment with methodologies lacking published efficacy data. She outlines six main areas that clinicians and researchers should address in the decision making process when considering adoption of a controversial practice. These areas include:

1. Knowing the source of the controversy and carefully consider the underlying rationale for the procedure/technique; review outcome data; understand the risks and benefits possibly offered; be clear on what the perceived effectiveness of the treatment is

2. Appreciating how the controversial techniques fit into the realm of accepted methods

3. Establishing and using formal informed consent procedures with controversial practices

4. Providing patient-specific criteria for implementation, including incusion/exclusion criteria and careful monitoring of progress

5. Seeking out specialized training in the use of the practice

6. Keeping careful documentation records and having a non-biased professional evaluate effectiveness.

If these areas are carefully addressed, clinicians will honor their code of ethics as well as advance the state-of-the-art in dysphagia management.

As members of the health care team, speech-language pathologists need to take an active role in disseminating findings from outcome-based measures. We need to provide administrators, who make service-delivery decisions, with hard data showing the efficacy and efficiency of dysphagia management. Cost effectiveness remains a powerful tool in receiving institutional support in these days of managed care and escalating medical costs. Backing statements up with carefully conducted research findings adds credibility to the field of speech-language pathology and earns the respect and trust needed in a clinical environment. A strong research base will also enable speech-language pathology to remain in a prominent position in the broader medical community that shapes government health care policy. Speech-language pathologists are *front-row observers* to the effect of governmental healthcare decisions such as caps being placed on Part B Medicare. Member advocacy has assisted in service provision with the development of new CPT codes for diagnosis and treatment of dysphagia.

Speech-language pathologists are also well positioned to share current literature findings with interdisciplinary team members in their work settings. Despite literature dating back to the late 1980s demonstrating that the gag reflex is not predictive of pharyngeal phase dysphagia severity or aspiration risk, most (if not every) speech-language pathologist in clinical practice has had to refute the findings of an intact gag and the implication that oral feeding is safe. A nine-year-old article in *Lancet* (Davies, Kidd, Stone, & MacMahon, 1995) showed that 20 to 40 percent of normal, healthy, swallowing adults do *not* have a gag response. This information has not filtered down to all practicing clinicians and continues to have significant clinical implications.

The field of dysphagia will continue to challenge professionals and gains in our understanding of the anatomy, physiology, and pathophysiology of disorders will have a positive impact on people worldwide. It is our hope that speech-language pathologists continue to lead the advancement of knowledge and quality of care.

REFERENCES

Binkofski, F., Buccino, G., & Taylor, J. G. (1998). Attention modulates motor cortex activation: A fMRI study. *Neuroimage, 7,* S84.

Davies, A. E., Kidd, D., Stone, S. P., & MacMahon, J. (1995). Pharyngeal sensation and gag reflex in healthy subjects. *Lancet, 345*(8948), 487–488.

Duchan, J. F., Calculator, S., Sonnenmeier, R., Diehl, S., & Cumley, G. D. (2001). A framework for managing controversial practices. *Language, Speech, and Hearing Services in the Schools, 32*(3), 133–141.

Hamdy, S., Aziz, Q., Rothwell, J. C., Singh, K. D., Barlow, J., Hughes, D. G., Tallis, R. C., & Thompson, D. G. (1996). The cortical topography of human swallowing musculature in health and disease. *Nat Med., 2*(11), 1217–1224.

Logemann, J. A. (2002). *Dysphagia Audio Digest Volume 9*, Tape 1. Illinois: Northern Speech Services.

Mosier, K., & Bereznaya, I. (2001). Parallel cortical networks for volitional control of swallowing in humans. *Experimental Brain Research, 140*(3), 280–289.

Mosier, K. M., Liu, W. C., Maldjian, J. A., Shah, R., & Modi, B. (1999). Lateralization of cortical function in swallowing: A functional MR imaging study. *American Journal of Neuroradiology, 20*(8), 1520–1526.

Cranial Nerve Examination

(adapted from information in Love & Webb, 1992; Perlman, 1991; Seikel, King, & Drumright, 1997)

CRANIAL NERVE	MOTOR TEST	SENSORY TEST	UPPER MOTOR NEURON INTERPRETATION	LOWER MOTOR NEURON INTERPRETATION
V	Patient: clench teeth Clinician: palpate masseter and temporalis muscles Observation: note symmetry and muscle mass Patient: raise, lower, and lateralize mandible Clinician: offer manual resistance to movements Observation: note strength, symmetry, smoothness, and range of motion of movements Patient: swallow	Patient: close eyes Clinician: light touch, cold and warm, to facial quadrants, anterior 2/3 of tongue, teeth, inner cheek, hard and soft palates Observation: report of tingling, accuracy in localization of touch	**Unilateral UMN:** typically, no motor or sensory findings, sometimes mild and transient deficits **Bilateral UMN:** difficulty chewing; hypertonia in muscles of mastication; sensory deficits; reduced hyolaryngeal elevation with submandibular muscle involvement; significant oral phase deficits with impact on pharyngeal phase	**Unilateral LMN:** mandible deviates *toward* the side of paralysis or paresis upon lowering; muscle hypotonia, and atrophy apparent; impaired hyolaryngeal elevation; ipsilateral sensory dysfunction; likely mild to moderate oral phase deficits **Bilateral LMN:** significantly impaired chewing abilities; muscle hypotonia bilaterally; bilateral sensory deficits; significantly impaired hyolaryngeal elevation; significant oral phase deficits with negative impact on pharyngeal phase

CRANIAL NERVE	MOTOR TEST	SENSORY TEST	UPPER MOTOR NEURON INTERPRETATION	LOWER MOTOR NEURON INTERPRETATION
	Clinician: locate hyoid Observation: extent and speed of hyolaryngeal elevation			
VII	Patient: wrinkle forehead; close both eyes, left eye, right eye; close mouth; smile, pucker, alternate X 3; frown, pout, puff cheeks with air, /pa/ repetitions as fast as possible Clinician: assess symmetry and tone at rest; assess symmetry and range of movements; assess crispness and speed of /pa/ repetitions	Test a variety of tastes (sweet, salty, sour, vinegar) presented to the anterior 2/3 of the tongue	**Unilateral UMN:** spastic paralysis, weakness of contralateral lower face and neck; weakness apparent during voluntary but not emotional movements; reduced salivary secretion contralaterally, reduced taste sensation from contralateral anterior 2/3 of the tongue **Bilateral UMN:** spastic paralysis of the entire face; severe loss of salivary secretion; loss of sense of taste from the anterior 2/3 of the tongue; significant oral phase deficits	**Unilateral LMN:** flaccid paralysis of entire ipsilateral face; no, or substantially impaired movement of all facial structures for both voluntary and emotional movements; eye tearing; drooling from corner of mouth; loss of salivation ipsilaterally; loss of taste from the ipsilateral anterior 2/3 of the tongue; significant oral phase deficits **Bilateral LMN:** flaccid paralysis of the entire face; hypotonia and atrophy; severe loss of salivary secretion and sense of taste from the anterior 2/3 of the tongue; severe oral phase deficits
IX	Motor to stylopharyngeus—cannot be tested alone	Patient: close eyes Clinician: lightly touches, warm and cold, the right and left sides of posterior 1/3 of the tongue, faucial pillars, palatine tonsils, posterior pharyngeal wall Observation: evidence of accurate sensation Patient: open mouth Clinician: applies variety of tastes to posterior 1/3 of tongue Obervation: evidence of acuity and distinction of tastes	**Unilateral UMN:** little evidence of contralateral weakness or sensory loss **Bilateral UMN:** complete loss of sensation and taste from the posterior 1/3 of the tongue; complete loss of sensation from the faucial pillars and posterior pharyngeal wall; impaired salivation from parotid gland; impaired or absent gag; significant pharyngeal phase deficits, particularly with pharyngeal phase initiation	**Unilateral LMN:** loss of touch, pain, thermal, and taste sensation in the ipsilateral posterior 1/3 of tongue; ipsilateral loss of sensation to faucial pillars and posterior pharyngeal wall; loss of salivary secretion from ipsilateral parotid gland **Bilateral LMN:** complete loss of sensation and taste from the posterior 1/3 of the tongue; complete loss of sensation from faucial pillars and posterior pharyngeal wall; difficulty in initiation of pharyngeal phase

CRANIAL NERVE	MOTOR TEST	SENSORY TEST	UPPER MOTOR NEURON INTERPRETATION	LOWER MOTOR NEURON INTERPRETATION
IX, X, XI	Patient: sustain "ah" Clinician: observe (supplement with visualization techniques if feasible or necessary) Observations: velar movement symmetry; movement of lateral pharyngeal wall; quality of phonation and resonance		**Unilateral UMN:** little or mild effect on velar movement **Bilateral UMN: (pseudobulbar palsy)** may show velopharyngeal closure deficits for speech that are more severe than for swallowing; hypernasal, nasal air emission; strained, strangled voice quality; less likely to have nasal regurgitation during swallowing; difficulty swallowing on command; less difficulty with nonvolitional swallow intiation; pharyngeal swallow response may be delayed or absent; significant pharyngeal phase deficits	**Unilateral LMN:** ipsilateral paralysis of the velar and pharyngeal musculature; velum deviates away from lesion; pharyngeal stasis and pyriform pooling ipsilaterally **Bilateral LMN:** no or extremely impaired velopharyngeal closure; nasal regurgitation; pharyngeal stasis pyriform pooling; severe pharyngeal phase deficits
X	Patient: phonation, talking Clinician: perceptual and/or instrumental assessment Observations: vocal quality; pitch and loudness levels and control Observe opening of cricopharyngeal muscle during videofluoroscopy examination	Fiberoptic Endoscopic Evaluation of Swallowing with Sensory Testing (FEESST): air pulses are delivered to right and left sides of the valleculae, epiglottis, anterior wall of the pyriform sinuses, and aryepiglottic folds (Aviv, Kaplan, Thomson, Spitzer, Diamond, & Close, 2000)	**Unilateral UMN:** mild contralateral vocal fold weakness possible; paralysis is unlikely; contralateral laryngopharyngeal sensory deficit probable (Aviv, et al., 1996) **Bilateral UMN: (pseudobulbar palsy)** strain/struggle characteristics, monopitch due to hypertonicity; hypertonic cricopharyngeal muscle; pyriform pooling; bilateral laryngopharyngeal sensory deficits; increased jaw and gag reflexes and emotional lability (Kirshner, 1989); significant pharyngeal phase deficits	**Unilateral LMN:** deficits vary by lesion location; possible ipsilateral deficit in velar elevation; possible ipsilateral defect in pitch modulation; possible ipsilateral loss of sensation from the laryngopharynx, valleculae, and epiglottis; possible ipsilateral vocal fold paralysis in paramedian position; possible ipsilateral vocal fold paralysis in the intermediate position; decreased opening of the UES. **Bilateral LMN:** deficit pattern depends on level of lesions; possible velar immobility; vocal fold impairment or immobility due to bilateral cricothyroid paralysis, or paralysis of all other intrinsic laryngeal muscles bilaterally; possible loss of sensation from the pharynx, laryngopharynx, valleculae, and epiglottis; decreased opening of the UES; pyriform pooling; severe pharyngeal phase dysphagia with risk of aspiration and choking

CRANIAL NERVE	MOTOR TEST	SENSORY TEST	UPPER MOTOR NEURON INTERPRETATION	LOWER MOTOR NEURON INTERPRETATION
XII	Patient: connected speech, /ka/ and /ta/ repetitions Clinician: perceptual and/or instrumental assessment; examination of tongue appearance and movement in non-speech tasks Observations: articulatory precision, speaking rate, observe tongue for atrophy or fasciculations, reduced or asymmetrical range of movement of the tongue; reduced strength		**Unilateral UMN:** spastic paralysis of contralateral genioglossus muscle; deviation of tongue toward weak side on protrusion (the side **opposite** the lesion when it is UMN) **Bilateral UMN:** weakness on both sides. Unable to protrude the tongue beyond the lips. Increased tone or spasticity, consonant imprecision, and difficulty manipulating the bolus	**Unilateral LMN:** the entire ipsilateral side of the tongue will appear shrunken or atrophied; may see fasciculations or fibrillations, seen as tiny ripplings under the surface of the tongue; the tongue will deviate toward the weak side (the **same** side of the lesion if it is an LMN lesion); reduced range of tongue movement, consonant imprecision **Bilateral LMN:** paralysis of both sides of the tongue characterized by atrophy and fasciculations; movements of the tongue for speech and swallowing will be significantly impaired

Answers to Study Questions

CHAPTER ONE ANSWERS

1. The only true joint on the skull is the temporo-mandibular joint. Its translational and rotational movements are important in mastication.

2. Teeth are responsible for breaking down food and integrating saliva into the bolus through chewing. People who lack a full complement of teeth typically restrict their diets to soft, moist foods that can be manipulated through gumming and tongue movements.

3. **a.** The lips are closed by activation of the perioral muscles of facial expression and innervated by the facial nerve (CN VII). These muscles include the inferior and superior orbicularis oris muscles, the inferior and superior incisivus labii, and for strong closure, the levator and depressor anguli oris muscles.

   b. Activation of the buccinator and risorius muscles provides tone or tenseness to the cheeks. These muscles are innervated by the facial nerve (CN VII).

   c. Activation of the intrinsic tongue muscles that insert laterally into the tongue (particularly transverse fibers) creates a channel in the midline of the tongue. This is important for holding a bolus, particularly a liquid one. All intrinsic tongue muscles are innervated by the hypoglossal nerve (CN XII).

   d. Chewing is accomplished by synergistic activation of the muscles of mastication. These include the masseter, medial pterygoid, and temporalis mus-

cles for jaw elevation, and the lateral pterygoid and anterior belly of the digastric muscles for jaw lowering and translational movement. These muscles are innervated by the mandibular branch of the trigeminal nerve (CN V).

4. The velum does not play an active role during oral preparation or oral transport. Instead, it rests in a low position in the oropharynx where it discourages food or liquid from entering the pharynx prematurely.

5. The bulk of the parotid gland is located over the ramus of the jaw. It is innervated by the glossopharyngeal nerve (CN IX). The sublingual glands are located on the floor of the mouth along the internal surface of the jaw. These glands are innervated by facial nerve fibers (CN VII). The submandibular glands are located beneath the mandible and they also are innervated by the facial nerve (CN VII).

6. Sensory information is critical to oral preparation and oral transport of the bolus. It contributes to an adequate amount of chewing and saliva production in oral preparation, and efficient manipulation of the bolus during oral transport.

CHAPTER TWO ANSWERS

1. The following structural events are associated with the pharyngeal swallow response: velopharyngeal port closure; hyolaryngeal elevation; epiglottic inversion;

true and false vocal fold closure; progressive pharyngeal contraction; and dilation of the UES.

2. The pharyngeal swallow response has been shown to be triggered most efficiently at the anterior faucial pillars, the posterior tongue at the level of the lower edge of the mandible, the valleculae, the pyriform sinuses, and the laryngeal aditus.

3. Pressure differentials are created by adjacent areas of constriction and dilation along the length of the pharynx. These differentials assist in propelling the bolus to the UES. Structures that contribute to the pressure differentials include the posterior tongue and contractions of the superior, middle, and inferior pharyngeal constrictor muscles.

4. Superficial and deep sensory receptors that project to the nucleus tractus solitarius in the medulla instigate the pharyngeal swallow response when the sensory input is of an appropriate pattern and intensity.

5. The majority of swallows commence after a short exhalation and are followed by an exhalation (EXHALE-SWALLOW-EXHALE). Only rarely are normal swallows followed by an inhalation. Patients who are weak or who have difficulty breathing may be inclined to inhale after the apneic period during swallowing. This could put them at risk for aspiration.

CHAPTER THREE ANSWERS

1. The physiology of UES opening is a combination of neurological inhibition to tonic closure of the 2 to 6 cm region and mechanical traction placed on the UES by hyolaryngeal elevation and anterior movement. It is currently believed that the superior and anterior movement of the hyolaryngeal complex is the most significant component of timely UES opening, allowing efficient bolus passage.

2. Blood supply to the esophagus is mainly segmental with specific arteries supplying the three regions—cervical, thoracic, and abdominal portions. The cervical esophagus receives its blood supply from branches of the inferior thyroid artery. The thoracic esophagus receives blood from branches of the aorta, right intercostal, and bronchial arteries. Branches of the left gastric,

short gastric, and left inferior phrenic arteries supply the abdominal esophagus.

3. Both primary and secondary espohageal peristaltic waves are normal sequential stripping waves. The difference is that primary waves are initiated by a swallow, whereas secondary waves are not associated with swallow initiation.

4. The similarities between the UES and LES include the identical role as a valve-like structure designed to keep material from moving in a retrograde direction. Both sphincters receive central and local neural regulation and both are under non-volitional control. Both the UES and LES are tonically closed at rest. UES morphology differs substantially from the LES. The UES has contributions from striated muscle fibers while the LES is solely smooth muscle. The LES is formed by increased thickness of the circular muscle fibers of the esophagus with a histological change in the circular muscle fibers located here. These complete rings of muscle do not insert onto cartilage as in the UES. While the UES relaxes at swallow initiation, the LES relaxes when the peristaltic wave is in the midportion of the esophagus. Unlike the UES, the LES does not appear to be significantly influenced by bolus characteristics.

5. Thank you, Dr. Thomas, for keeping me in the loop. I am assuming that the pooling in the pyriform sinuses is occurring after a swallow that demonstrated normal hyolaryngeal elevation. If not, the problem may be less one of neurological opening of the UES and the result of a myotomy may be disappointing. If hyolaryngeal elevation, as observed by the SLP during the modified barium swallow, was considered abnormal I would like the chance to try some behavioral treatment strategies with Mr. Smith. Would that be a possibility? I have some primary research supporting a series of exercises designed to increase laryngeal elevation—I'll have my office send a copy of the article to you.

CHAPTER FOUR ANSWERS

1. During non-discrete bolus ingestion, food enters and remains in the pharynx before the pharyngeal swallow response is triggered. This is associated with a partial adduction of the vocal folds, preceding even the *leading complex* of submental muscle activity.

2. Motor equivalence refers to a system's ability to accomplish the same motor goal in a number of ways. With regard to swallowing, one example is the many ways a mouthful of food can be manipulated during mastication to obtain a manageable bolus.

3. Bolus size, consistency, and viscosity are the characteristics that have been associated with changes in swallowing parameters.

4. Increased age is associated with mild to moderate reductions in swallow efficiency, including slowing and generally increased transit times.

5. Bolus size, or volume, is one of the primary factors that must be taken into consideration when assessing swallow function. A large bolus will most likely result in structures moving faster and farther than when ingesting a lower volume bolus. OTT and PTT decrease, anterior tongue base movement and elevation of the hyolaryngeal complex begin earlier, the UES opens earlier and has a larger diameter for a longer duration, swallowing apnea increases, and higher lingual and pharyngeal propulsive pressures are created in order to complete the swallow in the same time as that of a smaller bolus.

CHAPTER FIVE ANSWERS

1. The A-P view is the view of choice when examining the symmetry between the right and left sides of the oropharyngeal region during bolus ingestion under fluorography. In this position, the speech-language pathologist can evaluate primary side of bolus transit and pooling or residue following the swallow by seeing the right and left sides independently. This position is also helpful in evaluating the efficacy of treatment strategies such as turning the head to the affected side. Following the swallow, the patient brings the head back into an A-P view for evaluation of residue.

2. The most frequently used test for diagnosis of laryngopharyngeal reflux continues to be 24 hour pH-probe testing. This exam allows frequent sampling over a continuous period rather than a very brief sample at a finite time of day. It is a more sensitive measure to events that may occur during sleep.

3. Barium swallow and modified barium swallow studies have different purposes. The barium swallow study is looking for anatomical defects and motility disorders, primarily in the esophageal phase. A pharyngoesophagram will cover the structures between the oropharynx to the gastric cardia (the part of the stomach where the esophagus connects). An upper gastrointestinal series includes all the structures viewed in a barium swallow with the addition of the stomach and duodenum (the top part of the small intestine). The purpose of a modified barium swallow is to examine anatomy and physiology of the swallow mechanism. It remains the pre-eminent method to view the oral, pharyngeal, and early esophageal phase and to diagnose the underlying cause(s) for the symptoms of aspiration and penetration. As well, it allows visualization of the pharyngeal phase while compensatory strategies are tested for their ability to increase swallow safety and efficiency. This test uses graded bolus sizes enabling the visualization of structures without obliteration by large quantities of barium.

4. Thin barium is not the same as mealtime thin liquids. It differs from, say a cup of coffee, across the characteristics of bolus density (weight), viscosity (thickness), and yield stress (difficulty to propel fluid). As well, it has a much different mouthfeel. (Take a sip and experience the difference!)

5. There is no *one* best method to evaluate swallow function. The method chosen by the physician is determined by the patient's symptoms, the location of the suspected problem, and the information needed to rule out, confirm, or grade specific diseases. A number of methods provide complementary information. One particular imaging method is no better than another—it all depends on the purpose of the study and the information sought. Often, weaknesses inherent in one method can be improved upon by combining techniques, such as adding a fluoroscopic image to a manometric study to provide a maximum amount of diagnostic information.

CHAPTER SIX ANSWERS

1. One symptom of a swallowing disorder that occurs in the oral stage is the pocketing of food in the lateral sulci. This may result from disordered cheek and/or tongue musculature or from disordered sensation between the periodontal structures and mucosa of the cheek. A second

symptom of oral stage dysphagia is drooling. This may result from a dysfunction of the obicularis oris muscle or disordered sensation in the anterior oral cavity and/or lower face. A third symptom of a swallowing disorder that affects the oral stage is prolonged oral transit time. This may result from a dysfunction in tongue musculature, facial musculature, or the muscles of mastication. It could also be the result of decreased oral sensation.

2. Delay in triggering the pharyngeal swallow is a sign of a pharyngeal stage dysphagia. This may result from a dysfunction in the oral, pharyngeal, and/or esophageal musculature or from a sensory dysfunction in the oropharynx and/or laryngopharynx. Aspiration is another sign of a pharyngeal stage disorder. This may result from reduced hyolaryngeal elevation and/or laryngeal closure or from reduced sensation in the mucosa of the larynx. Vallecular stasis is a third sign of a pharyngeal stage swallowing disorder. This may result from reduced tongue base retraction and/or hyolaryngeal elevation or from reduced valleculae and epiglottis sensation.

3. Cerebrovascular accident (CVA) is the number one neurologic cause of dysphagia. Approximately 160,000 to 573,000 (or 42 to 75 percent) stroke patients are affected by dysphagia each year. Many patients who suffer CVA have swallowing difficulty, initially, and then gradually improve with time, with the majority experiencing no major dysfunction after six months.

4. Some common neurological diseases associated with dysphagia include: cerebrovascular disease, traumatic brain injury, brainstem tumor or stroke, ALS, Parkinson's disease, Huntington's disease, multiple sclerosis, and myasthenia gravis.

5. Treatment strategies should be introduced in the following order: postural techniques, techniques to enhance oral sensation, swallowing maneuvers, and diet changes.

6. If the patient presents with unilateral pharyngeal weakness or paresis, unilateral vocal fold paresis, and/or reduced cricopharyngeal relaxation, the head posture of a head-turn to the weaker side may be attempted in an effort to improve swallowing physiology. The physiological rationale for this posture is that it directs the bolus down the stronger side closing the pyriform sinus on the damaged side, increases vocal fold closure by placing extrinsic pressure on the thyroid cartilage, and increases the length of cricopharyngeal sphincter opening and decreases cricopharyngeal resting pressure, thereby reducing pyriform sinus stasis.

CHAPTER SEVEN ANSWERS

1. Endotracheal intubation occurs when a breathing tube is placed through the mouth or nose into the trachea to allow ventilation during surgery or during respiratory distress. It may increase the risk of aspiration because arytenoid dislocation can occur if the endotracheal tube hits the arytenoid cartilage, thus resulting in vocal fold paralysis. Prolonged endotracheal intubation has been shown to increase the risk of aspiration following extubation because the endotracheal tube alters the sensory abilities of the larynx. As the length of intubation increases, edema, irritation, and granulation tissue may occur in the larynx. Subglottic stenosis may also occur over time.

2. Xerostomia, or dryness of the mouth, can result from radiation therapy, Sjögren's syndrome, or the use of medications. Reduction in saliva can lead to difficulty transporting the bolus, discomfort in chewing and swallowing, and an increase in oral infections and dental caries. A person with xerostomia will have difficulty manipulating dry, flaky foods, resulting in longer mastication time and increased oral and pharyngeal stasis.

3. Mechanical changes that may cause aspiration following tracheostomy placement include decreased laryngeal elevation, obstruction by the cuff, and decreased subglottic pressure. Neurophysiologic changes that may result in swallowing problems following tracheostomy placement include desensitization of the larynx resulting in the loss of protective reflexes and uncoordinated laryngeal closure.

4. Osteophytes are bony outgrowths from the spinal cervical vertebrae that occur most often as a result of normal aging. Progressive dysphagia may sometimes result if the osteophytes are large because they may narrow the pharyngeal or esophageal spaces. Aspiration may occur if the osteophyte directs the bolus toward the laryngeal vestibule or if it interferes with epiglottic deflection.

5. Zenker's diverticulum (out-pouching of the wall) is a protrusion of mucosa and submucosa through the posterior muscle layers of the pharynx, typically at the level of the cricopharyngeus muscle. It may develop when there is a discoordination between pharyngeal contraction and cricopharyngeal relaxation or as a result of gastroesophageal reflux. The diverticulum may adversely affect swallowing if food particles gather in the space. Individuals with Zenker's diverticulum will complain of bad breath, regurgitation, sensation of obstruction, and aspiration after the swallow.

6. A glossectomy refers to surgical removal of the tongue as a result of a tumor. Patients with a partial glossectomy will have difficulty with bolus formation and propulsion, oral and pharyngeal residue, increased oral transit time, and increased difficulty with thicker consistencies. Patients with a hemiglossectomy will not experience any serious swallowing problems. Patients with a total glossectomy, on the other hand, experience a more severe swallowing impairment, including decreased lingual control, decreased tongue base retraction, and a delayed pharyngeal swallow.

7. A supraglottic laryngectomy involves the removal of the hyoid bone and the top of the larynx. Structures that may be removed include the epiglottis, aryepiglottic folds, false vocal folds, and the base of the tongue. The three factors that may lead to aspiration in supraglottic laryngectomy patients include reduced hyolaryngeal elevation, removal of the top two tiers of laryngeal airway protection, and delayed triggering of laryngeal elevation.

8. A stricture is a narrowing or stenosis that can occur in the pharynx or upper esophagus as a result of extensive resection or scar tissue formation. A stricture will impede the flow of the bolus creating more difficulty with thicker viscosities and solid foods.

9. Radiation therapy to the head and neck region may result in dysphagia due to xerostomia, tissue necrosis, edema (swelling), sensory changes, and/or tissue fibrosis. Xerostomia, or reduction in saliva, can lead to difficulty transporting the bolus, discomfort in chewing and swallowing, and an increase in oral infections and dental caries. Tissue necrosis, or breakdown of soft tissue and bone, can lead to aspiration, odynophagia, respiratory obstruction, and hoarseness. Tissue fibrosis (change of muscle fibers into connective tissue) can lead to reduced posterior tongue base motion, reduced laryngeal elevation, and restricted epiglottis base to arytenoids contact, all of which may result in aspiration before and after the swallow.

GLOSSARY

achalasia a primary esophageal motor disorder of unknown etiology characterized by insufficient lower esophageal sphincter (LES) relaxation and loss of esophageal peristalsis, esophageal dilation, minimal LES opening with a "bird-beak" appearance, and poor esophageal emptying of barium.

abdominal esophagus short, 0.5 to 2.5cm portion of the esophagus below the diaphragm to the cardiac opening of the stomach.

adrenergic ganglia group of nerve cell bodies of the autonomic nervous system that use norepinephrine as their neurotransmitter; part of thoracic sympathetic chain by which the enteric nervous system sends information to the CNS.

adventitial lymph nodes round or oval bodies located along lymphatic vessels; located on either side of the esophagus; drain lymph from the esophagus.

adventitial veins vessels that drain blood from the cervical and thoracic esophagus.

alveolar process or ridge the thick, spongy bone part of the maxilla that houses the teeth.

angle of the mandible formed by the inferior border of the ramus of the mandible meeting the inferior border of the corpus of the mandible.

anguli pertaining to oral angles.

ansa cervicalis a motor division of the cervical plexus derived from C1, associated with CN XII, and anteriorly placed, and an inferior root that is derived from C2 and C3 and posteriorly placed; branches arise that innervate the infrahyoid muscles (except thyrohyoid).

anterior belly of the digastric suprahyoid muscle with two bellies (anterior and posterior) that are connected by a central tendon; contraction raises the hyoid bone, or if the hyoid is fixed, may assist in depressing the lower jaw; anterior belly originates from the inner surface of the mandible and inserts in the region of the lesser horn of the hyoid bone.

anterior faucial arches see *anterior faucial pillars.*

anterior faucial pillars anterior folds of mucous membrane that extend from both sides of the soft palate to the lateral tongue and enclose the palatoglossus muscle; also called the *palatoglossal arch.*

anterior gastric branches portion of the vagus nerve (CN X) inferior to the diaphragm; division of left vagal trunk that supplies the stomach.

anterior sulcus space in the oral cavity formed between the lips and adjacent alveolar ridge on the upper and lower jaws; also called **labial sulcus.**

anterior vagal trunk portion of the vagus nerve (CN X) inferior to the esophageal plexus but above the diaphragm; previously the left vagus nerve.

aorta large artery that is the main trunk of the systemic arterial system, originating from the left ventricle; artery that serves the thoracic esophagus.

apneic period absence of breathing used to describe the short period during swallow when breath is held.

areolar tissue loose, irregularly arranged connective tissue (collagen and elastic fibers).

aryepiglottic folds paired, submucous muscle tissue that is often quite sparse, located at the superior aspect of the quadrangular membranes of the larynx; run from the side of the epiglottis to the arytenoid cartilages of the larynx.

aspiration material entering the airway below the level of the true vocal folds.

auditory tube the canal which establishes communication between the middle ear and the nasopharynx; also known as the *eustachian tube.*

Auerbach's plexus also known as *plexus myentericus*; network of esophageal nerves located within the layers of the longitudinal and circular muscle of the esophagus.

autonomic division part of the peripheral nervous system that regulates cardiac, smooth muscle, and glands; during swallow this system interacts with the enteric nervous system supplying the esophagus.

autonomic ganglion also known as *visceral gan-glion*; network of nerves located on the sympatheic trunks, on the peripheral plexuses, and within the walls of organs supplied by the autonomic nervous system; consists of two structurally different groups, the *sympathetic ganglia* and *parasympathetic ganglia.*

away opposite direction from a specified place.

azygous vein vein that ascends through the aortic hiatus of the diaphragm and runs along the right side of the thoracic vertebrae and terminates in the superior vena cava; drains blood from the thoracic esophagus.

Barrett's esophagus columnar metaplasia (change in tissue) of the esophagus seen commonly in GERD; sometimes leads to adenocarcinoma—a type of cancer.

bicuspids teeth with two points; premolars, two in front of each molar for a total of eight in humans.

bifid uvula a palatine uvula cleft or split, divided into two parts.

bolus characteristics properties of a unit of food to be swallowed; includes volume, consistency/viscosity, temperature, and taste.

Botulinum Toxin Type A (Botox) neurotoxin produced from the *Clostridium botulinum* bacteria.

botulism a severe and often fatal intoxication resulting from ingestion of a bacterial toxin in contaminated food.

bronchial arteries thick-walled, muscular blood vessels carrying aerated blood; bronchial arteries serve the thoracic esophagus.

buccal sulci (lateral sulci) pocket or side cavity between the cheek and the maxilla and mandible.

buccinator principal muscle of the cheek; also known as the *Bugler's muscle*; can compress the lips and cheeks against the teeth closing off the lateral sulci.

candidiasis a fungal infection caused by an overgrowth of a yeast.

canines (cuspids) large teeth with a single pointed cusp immediately lateral to the lateral incisors; two each in the upper and lower jaw.

celiac ganglia the largest group of prevertebral sympathetic ganglia that is located on the superior part of the abdominal aorta; contains sympathetic neurons that innervate the stomach.

celiac plexus a very large neural plexus responsible for the abdominal viscera.

central incisors chisel-shaped teeth which bear a single root; two central incisors on both upper and lower jaws in humans.

central pattern generator (CPG) hypothetical construct in the central nervous system responsible for a motor program to take place without any peripheral feedback.

central sulcus depression created by a blending of muscle tissue at midline.

cervical esophagus extends from the cricoid cartilage to the thoracic inlet; composed of striated muscle fibers.

chemoreception process by which organisms respond to chemical stimuli; chemical stimuli come in contact with specialized cells called chemoreceptors in the body that transduce the immediate effects directly or indirectly into nerve impulses.

chemoreceptors specialized receptors which are responsible for taste and smell.

chin tuck technique to improve swallow efficiency. Patient tilts head forward, touching chin firmly to chest before the swallow.

chorea unsustained, random, nonstereotyped movements that flow from one body part to another; reminiscent of dancing.

circumvallate papillae V-shaped row of dermis projections (papillae) on the tongue dorsum just anterior to the foramen cecum and sulcus terminalis.

cold a condition of low temperature.

collumellae two ridges of tissue lateral to the philtrum from the vermillion border of the upper lip to the base of the nose.

combination a result or product of putting together or combining.

computed tomography (CT) a cross-sectional imaging technique that uses computer synthesis of X-rays.

condylar process a rounded surface that articulates at the end of a bone; superior border of the mandibular ramus posterior to the coronoid process.

contrast radiography X-ray study in which a radiopaque material that stands out against anatomical structures is administered to the patient prior to, or during, the study.

coronoid process anterior bony projection of the mandible that serves as the point for muscle attachment.

cricothyroid a fan-shaped muscle which arises from the antero-lateral arch of the cricoid cartilage and inserts into the thyroid cartilage.

cricopharyngeal (CP) sphincter another term for the *upper esophageal sphincter (UES)* that recognizes the cricopharyngeal muscle which forms part of the sphincter (see *UES*).

cricopharyngeus muscle major contributor to upper esophageal sphincter also known as the *cricopharyngeal sphincter*; arises from the cricoid cartilage and courses horizontally; is a component of the inferior pharyngeal constrictor muscle.

cuffed tracheostomy tube with a soft inflatable balloon around it which holds the tube snugly against the tracheal wall.

cuffless tracheostomy tube without a soft inflatable balloon around the tube.

Cupid's bow a notch on the upper lip at the vermilion border which forms the base of two columns.

decannulation removal of the tracheostomy tube.

deciduous temporary; falling off and shedding at maturity.

deep cervical vein a large vein that drains deep muscles in the cervical (neck) region; vessel that carries blood from the cervical esophagus.

deep intrinsic veins vessels in the submucosa of the esophagus that drain into larger veins.

deep pharyngeal stimulation also called thermal

neuromuscular re-education of movement, is a therapeutic program that purports to restore muscle strength and reflexes within the pharynx for improved efficient swallow function; treatment directly stimulates the pharyngeal musculature.

deglutition the process by which a bolus of liquid or masticated food is moved from the mouth to the stomach for digestion.

density the compactness of a substance, often expressed as a ratio of mass per unit volume.

depressor anguli oris a vertical facial muscle that inserts into the orbicularis oris; flat, triangular sheet of muscle superficial and lateral to the fibers of the depressor labii inferioris; when contracted can depress the angle of the lip or pull the upper lip down toward the lower lip.

depressor labii inferioris an angular facial muscle; small, flat, quadrangular muscle, located beneath the lower lip just lateral to the midline, pulls the lower lip down and to the side.

digastric muscle suprahyoid muscle with an anterior and posterior belly that are connected by a central tendon (see **anterior belly of digastric** or **posterior belly of digastric**).

dyspepsia gastric upset or indigestion often characterized by burning, nausea, and burping.

diverticulum a blind tube, sac, or process.

dorsal motor nucleus aggregate of vagus nerve cell bodies located in the medulla oblongata.

double-cannula a tracheostomy tube with an inner and outer tube (cannula).

dystonia sustained muscle contractions resulting in fixed postures, torsional movements, and repetitive movements.

edema abnormal collection of fluid in tissue; swelling.

effortful swallow technique to improve swallow efficiency: swallow hard; push and squeeze all of the muscles of the mouth and throat.

electrocoagulation the clotting of blood using an electrocautery, an instrument that uses high frequency current.

endoscopy examination of the interior of a canal using a special instrument, an endoscope.

endotracheal intubation when a breathing tube is placed through the mouth or nose into the trachea to allow ventilation during surgery or during respiratory distress.

enteric nervous system part of peripheral nervous system that controls the smooth muscle fibers of the thoracic and abdominal esophagus.

enteron Greek word meaning intestine or bowels.

enzyme a catalytic substance usually produced by glands, which has a specific effect of promoting chemical change.

epiglottitis an inflammation of the epiglottis and supraglottic structures that results from a bacterial infection.

esophageal columnar metaplasia see *Barrett's esophagus.*

esophageal manometry technique used to measure esophageal pressures with flexible catheters containing pressure transducers.

esophageal plexus network of nerve fibers formed by the intermingling of the vagus nerve with autonomic system-sympathetic fibers.

esophagitis inflammation of the esophagus.

esophagogastric junction location of the lower esophageal sphincter; end of the esophagus and beginning of the stomach.

external thyroarytenoid synomym for *thyromuscularis* portion of the thyroarytenoid muscle of the larynx; lies lateral to the *vocalis* muscle; see *thyroarytenoid muscle.*

false vocal folds outcroppings of mucosal tissue that lie immediately superior and lateral to the true muscular vocal folds and attach anterolaterally to the arytenoid cartilages; also known as the *ventricular folds.*

fascia(e) sheet(s) of fibrous tissue that separates or encloses muscles or groups of muscles.

fenestrated having a hole or window; in a tracheostomy tube, a hole or window cut into the tube to allow greater airflow through the upper airway.

fibrosis formation of fibrous tissue.

fistula a tubular passageway formed by disease, surgery, injury, or congenital defect, usually connecting two organs or going from an organ to the surface of the body.

frenulum (frenum) a fold or reflection of mucous membrane that limits the range of movement of a structure; the upper and lower lip frenum runs from the gingiva at midline to the upper and lower lips, also at midline.

fungiform papillae mushroom shaped tissue elevations found at the sides and tip of the tongue; epithelium of the papillae have taste buds.

ganglion (ganglia, *pl.***)** cluster or clusters of nerve cell bodies located within the peripheral nervous system.

gastric pull-up procedure surgical procedure where esophageal tissue is removed and the thoracic or abdominal esophagus is pulled up and attached to the pharynx.

gastroesophageal reflux disease (GERD) a syndrome characterized by retrograde movement of stomach contents past the lower esophageal sphincter into the esophagus; symptoms may include retrosternal pain, burning, nausea, cough, or burping.

general visceral afferent (GVA) fibers functional classification system that describes sensory component for general cranial nerve function; nerves that carry sensory information from the pharynx, larynx, chest cavity, and abdomen to the nucleus solitarius in the brain stem.

general visceral efferent (GVE) fibers functional classification system that describes motor component for general cranial nerve function; supplies parasympathetic innervation of smooth muscle; nerve fibers that originate in nuclei of oculomotor (CN III), superior salivary nucleus of facial nerve (CN VII), inferior salivary nucleus of the glossopharyngeal (CN IX) and dorsal motor nucleus of vagus (CN X) in upper brainstem and give motor commands to the esophagus, intestinal tract, respiratory system, and cardiac system and are responsible for constriction of the pupil and gland secretion.

genioglossus muscle extrinsic tongue muscle; originates at the mental symphysis and fans out with the lower fibers inserting into the body of the hyoid bone and the lower fibers inserting into the under surface of the tongue; contraction may result in protrusion of the tongue anteriorly, tongue retraction, or formation of a mid-dorsum trough hyoid elevation and anterior motion.

geniohyoid muscle paired cylindrical muscle located above the superior surface of the mylohyoid muscle; arises from a tendon from the mental symphysis and inserts onto the hyoid bone; with fixed mandible contraction results in depression of the mandible or hyoid elevation and anterior motion if the mandible is fixed.

glossectomy surgical removal of the affected region within the tongue.

glottis the space between the vocal folds.

Golgi tendon organs receptors that are sensitive to tension generated within a tendon due to contraction of a muscle.

greater wings of the sphenoid uppermost bilateral plates extending laterally from the body of the sphenoid bone.

hamulus a hook-like extension descending from the medial pterygoid plate.

hard palate the bony part of the roof of the mouth in front of the soft palate.

head back technique to improve swallow efficiency: patient tilts head back during the swallow.

head rotation technique to improve swallow efficiency: patient turns head fully to the weak side before the swallow.

head tilt technique to improve swallow efficiency: patient tilts head to the stronger side prior to the swallow.

hemiglossectomy surgical removal of half of the mobile tongue.

hemilaryngectomy the surgical removal of one false vocal cord, one true vocal fold, and a portion of the thyroid cartilage on one side.

hemiazygous vein vessel in the thoracic cavity that empties into the azygous vein; the thoracic esophagus empties into the left hemiazygous vein.

hepatic branch portion of the vagus nerve (CN X) inferior to the diaphragm; a branch of the anterior vagal trunk that supplies the liver.

hernia protrusion of tissue through a defect in a structure or wall; as in a hiatal hernia where stomach tissue protrudes through the esophageal hiatus of the diaphragm.

herpes simplex infection caused by a herpes virus types I and II, most commonly resulting in a group of vesicles; herpes virus can cause cranial nerve palsies.

hiatus an opening.

hyoepiglottic ligament ligament which attaches the broadest part of the epiglottis to the hyoid bone.

hyoglossus muscle extrinsic tongue muscle; a quadrilateral sheet of muscle arising from the body and greater horns of the hyoid bone with insertion into submucous tissue of the posterior portion of the tongue; contraction retracts and depresses the tongue and may elevate the hyoid bone.

hyolaryngeal complex structures composing the larynx and hyoid.

incisivus labii muscles facial muscles that run in a parallel direction to the orbicularis oris; contraction results in lip pucker.

inferior longitudinal muscle intrinsic tongue muscle; fibers that originate at the hyoid bone and tongue root and terminate in the tongue tip on the undersurface of the tongue; contraction may either shorten the tongue or depress the tip.

inferior pharyngeal constrictors considered strongest pharyngeal muscle with two primary components, the *thyropharyngeus* which arises from the thyroid cartilage, and the *cricopharyngeus* which arises from the cricoid cartilage; muscle fans out and back to interdigitate forming the midline pharyngeal raphe; contributes to sphincteric action of the upper esophagus.

inferior salivary nucleus a group of preganglionic parasympathetic motor neurons located in the reticular formation of the medulla oblongata dorsal to the nucleus ambiguus.

inferior thyroid artery arises from the thyrocervical trunk; vessel carrying oxygenated blood that serves the cervical esophagus.

inferior thyroid vein drains into the left and right brachiocephalic veins; vessel that carries blood from the cervical esophagus.

interarytenoid muscles a muscle complex located on the posterior surfaces of the arytenoid cartilages; known as *oblique* arytenoids and *transverse* arytenoids based on muscle fiber orientation; contraction adducts and creates medial compression of the vocal folds.

intercostal vein veins that accompany the intercostal arteries; drains blood from the thoracic esophagus.

intermaxillary suture suture that courses anteriorly and terminates at the incisive foramen.

intraepithelial channels grooves located among the cells of the epithelium through which venous blood flows.

keratinized development of formation of a horny layer of keratin, a scleroprotein or albuminoid.

labial frenulum fold or reflection of mucous membrane attaching the upper and lower lips to their respective alveolar ridges.

labial sulcus (*anterior sulcus*) space that exists behind the lips as they rest against the teeth and gums.

labii pertaining to lips.

lamina propria thin plate or flat layer; in the larynx contains extracellular matrix, elastic fibers, and connective tissue.

laryngeal aditus entrance into the laryngeal cavity.

laryngeal vestibule supraglottal region between the ventricular folds and the aditus.

laryngectomy the surgical removal of the larynx.

laryngopharyngeal reflux a variant of gastro-esophageal reflux disease where the retrograde material passes through the upper esophageal sphincter as well as the lower esophageal sphincter causing laryngeal and pharyngeal symptoms which may include hoarseness and sore throat.

laryngopharynx refers to the region posterior to the larynx that extends from the hyoid to the esophagus at the level of the sixth cervical vertebra.

lateral cricoarytenoid muscle slightly fan-shaped muscle located deep to the thyroid cartilage; arises from cricoid cartilage and inserts on muscular process of arytenoids; contraction adducts by rotating vocal process toward midline.

lateral incisors two teeth each on upper and lower jaws, flanking the central incisors; similar in shape to the central incisors, but considerably smaller.

lateral pharyngeal diverticulum outpouching of mucous membrane lining resulting from herniation through the pharyngeal muscular wall.

lateral pharyngeal pouches see *lateral pharyngeal diverticulum*.

lateral (external) pterygoid muscle muscle which originates from two heads, one from the lateral portion of the greater wing of the sphenoid bone and the other from the lateral surface of the lateral pterygoid plate; contraction protrudes mandible and creates grinding motion.

lateral pterygoid plates of the sphenoid bone pterygoid bone process which serves as the origin for the medial and lateral pterygoid muscles.

lateral sulci oral cavity spaces formed between the mucous membranes of the cheeks and lateral alveolar ridges; also called **buccal sulci**.

left gastric artery originates from the celiac artery; supplies the abdominal esophagus and the curvature of the stomach.

left inferior phrenic artery originates from the aorta; blood supply to the diaphragm and abdominal esophagus.

lesser wings of the sphenoid bone lowermost bilateral plates extending laterally from the body of the sphenoid bone.

levator anguli oris muscle flat, triangular muscle located above the angle of the mouth but deep to the levator labii superioris; draws corner of mouth upward.

levator labii superioris muscle bilateral muscle originating at the maxilla and inserting into the orbicularis oris of upper lip; elevates the upper lip.

levator veli palatine muscle originates from the apex of petrous portion of temporal bone and lower part of cartilaginous auditory (eustachian) tube and inserts into aponeurosis of soft palate; contraction raises soft palate.

lingual frenulum fold of mucous membrane that runs from the floor of the mouth to inferior tongue surface at midline.

lower esophageal sphincter (LES) musculature of the gastroesophageal junction that is tonically contracted at rest in order to prevent material from refluxing from the stomach and relaxes during swallow.

lower motor neurons motor neurons below the level of the ventral horn.

Ludwig's angina an acute bacterial infection that causes rapid inflammation of the tissues of the submandibular and sublingual spaces.

lymphatic drainage process by which lymph, a yellow-tinged liquid derived from tissue fluids, drains through tissues in channels known as lymph vessels.

macroglossia enlarged tongue.

magnetic resonance imaging a diagnostic technique that uses a large magnetic field, without radiation, to create three-dimensional images with computer synthesis.

mandibular fossa a deep hollow in the squamous portion of the temporal bone at the root of the zygoma, in which rests the condyle of the mandible.

mandibular sling orientation of muscles or mastication formed by the medial pterygoid and masseter muscles which holds the angle of the mandible and straps the ramus to the skull.

mandibulectomy surgical removal of the anterior portion of the mandible.

manofluorography the combination of pressure measurement within the esophagus, UES, and LES with a radiographic study.

manometry measurement of pressures within some structure; measurement of esophageal pressures using pressure-sensitive transducers.

masseter muscle a thick, flat, quadrilateral muscle that covers the lateral surface of the mandibular ramus, arises from the zygomatic arch and on the ramus and coronoid process of the mandible; contraction closes the jaw.

mastoid process protuberance-like projection of the petrous part of the temporal bone.

mechanoreceptors receptors which respond to mechanical pressure or deformation of the receptor and adjacent tissues.

medial (internal) pterygoid muscle a thick quadrilateral muscle that originates primarily in the vertically directed pterygoid fossa and from the medial surface of the lateral pterygoid plate; contraction protrudes and raises the jaw.

medial pterygoid plates narrow pterygoid bone process; forms the posterior boundary of the lateral wall of the nasal cavity.

median raphe a midline groove; median raphe extends the length of the hard palate.

Meissner's plexus also known as *plexus submucosus*; intermingling group of nerve fibers located in the submucosa of esophagus; allows reflexes to be mediated locally and not by CNS.

Mendelsohn maneuver technique to improve swallow efficiency: during swallow when larynx elevates, hold larynx at the top with muscles for several seconds.

mental foramen small opening in the mandible where the mental nerve and blood vessels exit.

mental symphysis point where the two halves of the mandible are joined.

mentalis muscle a vertical facial muscle that arises from the incisive fossa and inserts on skin of the chin; raises base of lower lip.

metastatic disease spread of cancer from the primary location to other sites, organs, or systems.

middle pharyngeal constrictor middle most pharyngeal muscle whose fibers arise from the greater and lesser horns of the hyoid bone, fan out and back to insert in the medial pharyngeal raphe.

midface central portion of the face from the orbit of the eyes down to and including the structures covering the maxilla, such as the lips.

midline raphe the site of union between two symmetrical structures.

molars teeth with a rounded or flattened surface adapted for grinding.

motility disorders movement disorders; motor disturbances in the esophagus.

motor equivalence refers to a system's ability to accomplish the same motor goal in a number of ways.

mucosa lining of tubular structures in the body; consists of epithelium, lamina propria, and smooth muscle in the digestive tract.

mucosal surface a smooth, moist layer of epithelial tissue.

mucositis inflammatory changes to the mucosa.

mucous viscous secretion of the mucous glands.

muscles of facial expression muscles that are activated to accomplish facial movements.

muscular mucosa layer of tissue between the lamina propria and submucosa of the esophagus.

musculus uvulae a small muscle coursing from the palatine bones to the uvula; when contracted, lifts the soft palate.

mylohyoid muscle a thin, troughlike sheet of muscle originating from the mylohyoid line of the mandible to the mental symphysis; forms the muscular floor of the mouth.

myopathy pathological condition of muscle tissue.

myosin ATPase adenosine triphosphatase; an

enzyme in muscle (myosin); metabolic component of upper striated muscle fibers of the esophagus.

nasal cavity the proximal portion of the respiratory passages on either side of the nasal septum, lined with ciliated mucosa, extending from the nares to the pharynx.

nasopharynx cavity located immediately behind the nasal cavity; potentially separated from the oropharynx by the velum.

near-total laryngectomy the surgical removal of the larynx while leaving a large part of the supraglottic area such as the epiglottis.

neurogenic origins arising from or caused by the nervous system.

neuromuscular spindles muscle fibers.

nociceptor peripheral nerve organ for reception and transmission of painful or injurious stimuli.

non-fenestrated literally *without a window*; a tube without a hole or window cut into the tube.

nuclear medicine the branch of medicine that uses radionuclides in the diagnosis and treatment of disease.

nucleus neuroanatomical classification for an aggregate of cell bodies located within the brain or spinal cord (the CNS).

nucleus ambiguus a nucleus located within the reticular formation of the medulla oblongata that contributes to the vagus, glossopharyngeal, and assessory cranial nerves.

nucleus tractus solitarius (NTS) a region of the medullary reticular formation containing the cell bodies that receive afferent information from cranial nerves VII (facial), IX (glossopharyngeal), and X (vagus).

oblique interarytenoid muscle the more superficial of the two arytenoid muscles which originates from the posterior surface of the muscular process and adjacent posterolateral surface of one arytenoid cartilage and inserts near the apex of the opposite cartilage; adducts and creates medial compression of the vocal folds.

obturator an object that closes an opening; a

device used to close palatal defects; a guide that is used during insertion of a tracheostomy tube.

odynophagia painful swallow.

opposite across from.

oral angles corners of the mouth where superior and inferior muscles come together.

oral-motor exercises strengthening exercises for the muscles of the oral cavity and facial expression.

orbicularis oris muscle lip muscle consisting of an oval ring of muscle fibers located within the lips and encircling the mouth.

orbital cavity the cavity or socket of the skull in which the eye and its appendages are situated.

oropharynx cavity located immediately behind the anterior faucial arches of the oral cavity and extending to the level of the hyoid bone.

osteophytes bony outgrowths from the spinal cervical vertebrae.

palatal aponeurosis a broad, thin sheet of connective tissue that gives rise to the muscles of the soft palate and forms the attachment of muscle to bone at the velum.

palatal lift prosthesis an artificial device that mechanically elevates and maintains closure of the soft palate against the pharyngeal wall.

palatal obturator an appliance that can be developed to functionally close a large palatal defect and improve speech and swallowing function.

palatal reshaping prosthesis an artificial device that can be used to recontour the dimensions of the hard palate to fit the tongue following partial glossectomy.

palatal vault the arch-like shape of the hard palate.

palatine bones form the posterior one-quarter of the hard palate.

palatine processes thick, horizontal, medially directed projection forming three-quarters of the hard palate and, on its superior surface, the floor of the nasal cavity.

palatine tonsils rounded masses of lymphoid tissue between the palatoglossus and palatopharyngeal muscles in the oral cavity.

palatoglossus muscle extrinsic tongue muscle; forms anterior pillar of tonsillar fossa; originates from the oral surface of soft palate and inserts on the side of tongue; contraction raises back of tongue and narrows the fauces.

palatopharyngeus muscle posterior faucial pillar; muscle of the soft palate and a longitudinal muscle of the pharynx with fibers originating from the soft palate, region of the pterygoid hamulus, and eustachian tube and inserting into the lateral wall of the pharynx; contraction lowers soft palate and decreases distance between the faucial arches.

palliative reducing the severity of symptoms without changing the course of disease; type of care provided to cancer patients to improve comfort level.

parasympathetic a division of the autonomic nervous system, part of the peripheral nervous system; visceral efferent peripheral system whose function is to decrease or calm activity to bring organs back to equilibrium.

parotid glands the largest set of salivary glands located in the posterior and inferior cheeks.

partial glossectomy partial removal of the tongue.

Passavant's pad a bulge of muscle tissue formed by the fusion of the fibers of the palatopharyngeal muscle with those of the pterygopharyngeal portion of the superior constrictor.

penetration entry of a bolus into the laryngeal vestibule but above the true vocal folds; material does not go below the true vocal folds.

peristalsis movement characterized by phasic muscle contraction and relaxation; esophageal peristalsis carries the food bolus through the esophagus to the stomach.

peritracheal venous plexus a network of vessels that carries blood from the cervical esophagus.

permanent dentition permanent teeth.

pharyngeal peristalsis term once used to characterize the segmental and sequential contraction of the pharyngeal wall.

pharyngeal plexus a bundle of nerves consisting of fibers primarily from the vagus, with additional fibers from the glossopharyngeal nerves and sympathetic trunks and spinal accessory nerves; supplies motor, sensory, and sympathetic innervation to pharynx and soft palate.

pharyngitis inflammation of the pharynx caused by bacterial or viral infections.

pharyngoesophageal (PES) diverticula outpouching of mucosa through the inferior constrictor muscle and the cricopharyngeus muscle; also known as *Zenker's diverticulum*.

pharyngoesophageal (PE) segment see *upper esophageal sphincter*.

pharyngolaryngoesophagectomy the surgical removal of the pharynx, larynx, and esophagus used to treat extensive head and neck cancers.

pharynogoesophagram a radiographic study to examine upper digestive tract motility where the patient ingests a radiopaque bolus and a fluoroscopic image is taken.

philtrum the groove formed between the collumellae.

plexus a network or interjoining of nerves.

plug to occlude; complete occlusion of the tracheostomy tube.

posterior belly of the digastric muscle suprahyoid muscle with two bellies (anterior and posterior) that are connected by a central tendon; posterior belly origin from the mastoid process with insertion onto the greater horn of the hyoid bone; contraction raises the hyoid bone, or if the hyoid is fixed, may assist in depressing the lower jaw.

posterior faucial arches see *posterior faucial pillars*.

posterior faucial pillars posterior folds of mucous membrane that extend from both sides of the posterior soft palate to the lateral pharyngeal wall and encloses the palatopharyngeus muscle; also called the *palatopharyngeal arches*.

posterior pharyngeal raphe seam located at mid-

line on the posteriorpharyngeal wall created by the merging of the superior, middle, and inferior constrictor muscles.

posterior gastric branches portion of the vagus nerve (CN X) inferior to the diaphragm; division of the posterior vagal trunk.

posterior vagal trunk portion of the vagus nerve (CN X) inferior to the esophageal plexus but above the diaphragm; was previously the right vagus nerve.

postganglionic neuron cell bodies of neurons located in autonomic ganglia; relays impulse beyond the ganglia, axon may go to innervated organ or gland.

preganglionic neuron cell bodies of neurons located in a motor nucleus of the central nervous system with termination of efferent fibers in the autonomic ganglia.

premaxilla a bone on either side of the middle line between the nose and mouth, forming the anterior part of each half of the upper jawbone.

preparatory stage also called *oral preparatory phase*; initial stage of the swallow when the bolus is being masticated and formed.

primary peristaltic waves movement characterized by alternate circular contraction and relaxation in the esophagus that is initiated by pharyngeal swallow.

progressive contraction current term used to characterize the segmental and sequential contraction of pharyngeal wall musculature during swallow.

proprioceptors a specialized type of mechanoreceptors that provide information about body position, balance, and equilibrium, especially during locomotion.

pseudoepiglottis a fold of tissue at the base of the tongue, which appears to be an epiglottis when viewed in the lateral plane.

pterygomandibular ligament a tendinous thickening of the buccopharyngeal fascia, separating and giving origin to the buccinator muscle anteriorly and the superior constrictor of the pharynx posteriorly.

pterygomandibular raphe vertical seam created by blending of buccinator and superior pharyngeal constrictor muscles; extends from the hamulus of the medial pterygoid plate at the pterygomandibular ligament.

pyriform sinuses a pear-shaped depression or fossa in the laryngopharynx.

radiation therapy the use of high-energy radiation directed to the area of the tumor and to the adjacent lymph nodes to damage cancer cells and stop them from growing.

radionecrosis damage and breakdown of soft tissue and bone due to radiation.

ramus a branch.

reticular formation a group of neurons diffusely located in the brainstem associated with arousal, attention, cardiac reflexes, and sensorimotor function.

rheology scientific study of the deformation and flow of substances.

right intercostal arteries arise from the thoracic aorta and have multiple branches; arterial vessels that serve the thoracic esophagus.

risorius muscle muscle originating from a fascia covering the masseter muscle and inserting into skin and mucosa at the angle of the mouth; contraction pulls the angle of the mouth in a lateral direction.

root inferior-most part that firmly attaches to a structure; attachment of the tongue at the hyoid bone.

rotation the turning of a body part about its long axis as if on a pivot.

Ruga (rugae, *pl.*) a wrinkle or fold.

saliva fluid secreted by the parotid, sublingual, submaxillary, and other mucous glands in the mouth.

salivary ducts tiny openings in the salivary gland through which saliva is secreted.

salpingopharyngeus muscle muscle that originates

from the inferior border of the medial aspect of the eustachian tube cartilage and courses vertically, intermingling with palatopharyngeal fibers; contraction thought to depress the soft palate.

same identical position when referring to location.

Schatzki's ring an esophageal ring-shaped stricture in the region of the lower esophageal sphincter.

scleroderma autoimmune disease of the connective tissue characterized by formation of fibrosis of tissues and organs of the body.

sclerotherapy medical treatment involving injections of a solution into vessels or tissues to harden or sclerose.

secondary peristaltic waves normal sequential contraction and relaxation of the esophagus that results from distention and localized pressure of a partial bolus within the esophagus.

septum thin wall dividing two cavities or masses of softer tissue.

serous relating to, containing, or producing serum; a substance having a watery consistency.

Shaker exercise technique to improve swallow efficiency: exercise in which person lays flat on back and raises head high enough to see toes without raising shoulders.

short gastric artery arises from the splenic artery; serves the abdominal esophagus and upper part of the stomach.

side lying patient lies down on side during eating and drinking.

single-cannula a tracheostomy tube with one cannula.

somites mesoderm blocks of cells which form in the region of the hindbrain early in development and go on to become all the connective, muscular, and dermal tissue of the body apart from the head.

sour the primary taste sensation produced by acidic stimuli.

spasm an involuntary and abnormal muscular contraction.

speaking valve a valve that can be placed on the end of a tracheostomy tube to permit voicing.

special visceral afferent (SVA) fibers functional classification system that describes sensory component for special cranial nerve function; responsible for sense of taste and smell through cranial nerves I (olfactory), VII (facial), IX (glossopharyngeal), and X (vagus).

special visceral efferent (SVE) fibers functional classification system that describes motor component(s) for special cranial nerve function; controls muscles of facial expression, mastication, phonation, and deglutition through the trigeminal motor nucleus (CN V), facial motor nucleus (CN VII), and nucleus ambiguous (CN IX, CN X, CN XI).

sphenoid bone bat-shaped bone located deep within the cranium; its various processes serve as attachment sites for several muscles associated with swallowing.

stretch reflex the result of neuromuscular receptors firing, which causes the parent muscle to contract.

stricture an abnormal narrowing of a bodily passage.

stronger having or marked by great physical power.

styloglossus muscle extrinsic tongue muscle; originates at the styloid process fanning out as it courses anteriorly and attaches to the side of the tongue; contraction pulls the tongue superiorly and posteriorly.

styloid process a hook-like projection of bone serving as the site of origin for muscles involved in swallowing.

stylopharyngeus muscle a pharyngeal muscle that arises from the styloid process of the temporal bone and courses downward along the side of the pharynx entering between the superior and middle constrictor; contraction elevates and dilates the pharynx.

subephithelial superficial plexus initial level of the venous drainage system of the esophagus receiving blood from the intraepithelial channels and draining to deep intrinsic veins.

subglottic the space below the true vocal folds.

sublingual glands salivary glands located immediately beneath the mucosal surface of the floor of the mouth, along the internal surface of the jaw.

submandibular glands salivary glands located under the mandible, deep to the mylohyoid muscle.

submucosa layer of connective tissue below the mucosa; in the esophagus, the inner most layer.

superior constrictor see *superior pharyngeal constrictor muscles.*

superior longitudinal fibers intrinsic tongue muscle; fibers that originate near the tongue root, travel primarily in the middle section of the tongue and terminate short of the tongue tip contraction may shorten the tongue and raise the tongue tip, or create a trough on the dorsum.

superior pharyngeal constrictor muscle consists of four muscle bundles that arise from the medial pterygoid plate of the sphenoid bone; the pterygomandibular raphe, the mylohyoid line of the mandible, and the sides of the tongue which course up and back to attach at the midline pharyngeal raphe.

superior salivary nucleus a group of preganglionic parasympathetic motor neurons situated rostral and lateral to the inferior salivatory nucleus; governs secretion of the lacrimal, sublingual, and submaxillary glands by way of the facial nerve and the sphenopalatine and submandibular ganglia.

super-supraglottic swallow technique to improve swallow efficiency: maneuver in which person inhales; holds breath and bears down hard; swallows while holding breath hard; coughs; and swallows again.

supraglottic above the glottis.

supraglottic laryngectomy the surgical removal of the hyoid bone and the top of the larynx.

supraglottic swallow technique to improve swallow efficiency: maneuver in which person inhales and holds breath; swallows while holding breath; coughs; swallows again.

sutures immovable joints.

swallow the act of deglutition.

swallower variables the variables of an individual's age, sex, size, oro-pharyngeal-laryngeal morphology, and idiosyncratic motor control strategies which contribute to swallowing.

sympathetic a division of the autonomic nervous system; visceral efferent peripheral system whose function is to increase activity; *fight or flight.*

symptom something that indicates disease or physical disturbance.

syncope loss of consciousness caused by decreased blood flow in the brain.

tachyphagia rapid eating or bolting of food.

tactile thermal application (TTA) technique to improve swallow efficiency: clinical procedure which involves stroking the anterior faucial pillar with a cooled metal dental mirror to increase the speed at which the pharyngeal response is triggered.

temporal bones irregularly shaped bones that form the lateral sides of the cranium.

temporalis muscle a broad, thin, fan shaped muscle that arises from the entire temporal fossa, fibers converge and pass below the zygomatic arch to insert on the mandibular ramus; contraction raises and lateralizes the mandible.

temporomandibular joint (TMJ) formed by the articulation of the condylar process of the mandible at the mandibular fossa of the temporal bone.

tensor veli palatine muscle muscle that arises from the cartilage of the torus tubaris in the pharynx and adjacent bone and courses to the hamulus of the medial pterygoid plate of the sphenoid bone; thought to be responsible for dilating the eustachian tube.

tertiary peristaltic waves in the esophagus, contraction and relaxation that occur during the primary or secondary waves; most often seen in older individuals; may be considered pathologic in younger symptomatic adults.

textured something composed of closely interwoven elements.

thermal tactile application (TTA) see *tactile thermal application*.

thermoreceptors specialized receptors which respond to changes in temperature.

thoracic esophagus forms the bulk of the esophagus from the thoracic inlet to the diaphragm.

thrush see *candidiasis*.

thyroarytenoid muscle (or **thyrocalis**) intrinsic laryngeal muscle; originates on the inner surface of thyroid cartilage and inserts on the muscular process and outer surface of arytenoid; may be subdivided into *thyrovocalis* or *internal thyroarytenoid*, which forms the medial edge of the vocal fold, and *thyromuscularis* or *external thyroarytenoid*, which is laterally placed; functions to regulate internal longitudinal tension of the vocal folds.

thyroepiglottic ligament ligament which attaches the epiglottis to the angle of the thyroid cartilage.

thyrohyoid muscle a paired muscle originating from the thyroid lamina which courses vertically upward inserting into the lower border of the greater horn of the hyoid bone; contraction decreases the distance between the thyroid cartilage and hyoid bone.

thyromuscularis see *thyroarytenoid muscle*.

thyropharyngeus muscle see *inferior pharyngeal constrictor muscle*.

torus palatinus a bony protuberance sometimes found where the intermaxillary and transverse palatine sutures join.

torus tubarius a ridge in the nasopharyngeal wall posterior to the opening of the auditory (eustachian) tube, caused by the projection of the cartilaginous portion of this tube.

total glossectomy complete removal of the tongue.

total laryngectomy the surgical removal of the entire larynx including the cricoid cartilage, thyroid cartilage, epiglottis, hyoid bone, arytenoid cartilages, true vocal folds, and ventricular folds.

tracheostomy a surgically created opening into the trachea through the neck with the tracheal mucosa attached to the skin.

tracheotomy a surgical incision into the trachea.

translational uniform motion of all points on a body in a straight line; when referring to mandibular movement it explains jaw protrusion and retraction when movement is bilateral and lateral jaw swing when unilaterally activated.

transport to convey from one place to another.

transverse muscle of the tongue intrinsic tongue muscle; fibers arise from the tongue septum, course laterally and insert in the lateral tongue margins; contraction narrows and elongates the tongue.

trismus persistent contraction of the masseter muscles (muscles of mastication) resulting from failure of central inhibition.

true vocal folds see *thyoarytenoid muscle*.

unilateral occurring on, performed on, or affecting one side of the body.

upper cervical esophagus portion of the esophagus beginning at the UES and extending distally to the region of the suprasternal notch; consisting of striated muscle fibers.

upper esophageal sphincter (UES) also known as the *pharyngoesophageal* or *cricopharyngeal sphincter*; an area of higher muscular tone at the junction of the pharynx and esophagus.

upper motor neuron conducting cell of the central nervous system; neurons in the cortex that conduct impulses to the motor nuclei of the cerebral nerves or to the spinal ventral gray columns.

uvula a pendent, fleshy mass; when used alone, it refers to the *uvula palatina*, a small, fleshy mass of glands and muscular fibers hanging from the soft palate; also known as the palatine uvula.

vagus nerve cranial nerve X; mixed motor and sensory nerve with wide distribution throughout the body; serves the pharynx, larynx, trachea, lungs, heart, and gastrointestinal tract.

valleculae a shallow groove or depression; indentations between the lateral and median glossoepiglottic folds.

velopharyngeal port region between the oropharyngeal and nasopharyngeal cavities; closed during the pharyngeal stage of swallow.

velum a thin, veil-like covering or partition; the soft palate.

ventricular folds also referred to as *false vocal folds*; mucosal tissue superior to true vocal folds in larynx that attaches anterolaterally to the arytenoid cartilages.

vermilion border edge of red tissue that distinguishes between face and lip tissue.

vertebral vein vessel that arises from the suboccipital venous plexus and serves the upper six cervical vertebrae; drains blood from the cervical esophagus.

vertical muscle intrinsic tongue muscle; fibers originate from tongue dorsum mucous membrane, course downward and laterally to insert on the sides and under surface of the tongue; contraction flattens out the tongue.

videofluoroscopy in the study of swallow function, a radiographic study in which information regarding bolus transport time, motility problems, amount, and etiology of aspiration can be obtained.

viscosity resistance of liquid to flow resulting from a shear force.

vocalis muscle also known as the *thyroarytenoid* muscle; the muscle which constitutes the main body of the vocal folds.

xerostomia dry mouth.

yield stress amount of force required to propel a fluid.

Zenker's diverticulum also known as a *pharyngoesophageal diverticulum*; a protrusion of mucosa and submucosa through the posterior muscle layers of the pharynx.

zygomatic muscle muscle arising from the zygomatic bone, coursing downward and medialward to insert into the orbicularis oris; contraction draws the corner of the mouth upward and outward.

zygomatic process the massive projection of the frontal bone that joins the zygomatic bone to form the lateral margin of the orbit.

INDEX

accidental trauma, 188
achalasia, 160, 161
adaptive seating devices, 138
Addington, W. R., 157
aging, 101–102
    effects of on swallowing parameters, 103, 247
    versus pathology, 102
airway protection mechanism, 56–57, 59, 98–99
    maximal protection parameters, 63
amyotrophic lateral sclerosis (ALS), 167
anatomical planes of view
    anterior-posterior (A-P) plane, 110, 118–119, 247
    axial (cross-sectional) plane, 110–111, 113
    lateral plane, 110, 113–114, 117–118
    oblique plane, 110, 121
    superior plane, 110, 119–121
anatomical slice, 111, 113
aspiration, 63, 157, 158, 189–190, 193
    behavioral therapy for, 179
    following endotracheal intubation, 189
    and inflatable tracheostomy tube cuffs, 193
    in the laryngectomy patient, 218, 219
    mechanical causes of, 248
    medical therapy for, 179
    neurological causes of, 248

tests used to detect, 198
    See also silent aspiration
aspiration pneumonia, 59, 157, 204
    diagnosis of, 117, 119
autoimmune disease, 164, 167–168, 168, 169–170, 170
autonomic nervous system (ANS), 22, 74–75

barium, 131, 132, 247
    aspiration of, 142
    barium bread, 142–143
    double contrast use, 132
    single contrast use, 132
    See also contrast radiography
Baron, E. M., 198–199
blepharospasm, 159
bolus, 2
    characteristics of, 99, 247
        and contrast radiography, 136
        effects of on swallowing, 100, 101, 247
    difficulty manipulating, 146
        behavioral therapy for, 178
        medical therapy for, 178
    importance of sensory information in transport, 245
    loss of control of, 156
        behavioral therapy for, 178

Botox, 159, 160, 222, 226
Botulinum toxin. *See* Botox
botulism, 201
bougies, 222
bradykinesia, 166
brainstem lesions, 163–164

cancer, 153
    esophageal cancer, 223–224
    laryngeal cancer, 217–223
    metastasis of, 80
    nonsurgical treatment for
    chemotherapy, 224
    intraoral prosthetics, 214
    oral-motor exercises, 213–214
    polite yawn exercise, 220–221
    radiation therapy, 213, 224–226, 249
    sensory stimulation, 214
    pharyngeal cancer, 217
    pre-cancerous tissue changes, 205
    surgical procedures for, 210–213, 224
        glossectomy, 211–212, 249
        hemilaryngectomy (vertical laryngectomy),
            218–219
        lip resection, 211
        mandibulectomy, 211
        near-total laryngectomy, 219
        palate resection, 213
        pharyngolaryngoesophagectomy, 223
        supraglottic (horizontal) laryngectomy, 217–218,
            249
        total laryngectomy, 219–223
candidiasis, 200–201
carotid endarterectomy, 199–200
central nervous system (CNS), 74
cerebrovascular accident (CVA), 153, 162–163, 248
cervical spine surgery, 198–199
cheeks, 28
    muscles of, 28, 245
chemical agents, ingestion of, 202
chewing, 2, 95
    chewing difficulties, 156
        behavioral therapy for, 178
    movements associated with, 35–36
    muscles used during, 245
    as stereotyped behavior, 36
Chi-Fishman, G., 31, 55–56, 98–99
chorea, 165
collagen vascular diseases, 153
computed tomography (CT scan), 113, 122, 143–144
connective tissue diseases. *See* collagen vascular dis-
    eases

conscious sedation, 127
contrast radiography, 122, 130–131
    barium swallow, 131, 247
    esophagram, 131
    modified barium swallow, 133, 136–138, 141–142,
        247
    pharyngoesophagram, 131, 133, 247
    protocols, 134–135
    spot films, 131
    upper gastrointestinal series, 131, 247
    videofluoroscopic swallow study (VSS). *See* contrast
        radiography, modified barium swallow
cough reflex, 59, 157
cranial nerve examination, 241–244
cranial nerves, 74
    CN V (trigeminal nerve), 32, 34, 49, 52, 55, 163,
        211, 245
    CN VII (facial nerve), 15, 22, 24, 25, 28, 38, 49, 55,
        76, 155, 245
    CN IX (glossopharyngeal nerve), 23, 31, 38, 47, 49,
        76, 163, 199, 245
    CN X (vagus nerve), 31, 47, 49, 51, 56, 59, 75–76,
        77–78, 84, 158, 163, 199
        branches of, 75–76
        types of fibers in, 77
    CN XI (spinal accessory), 47, 49, 76, 163
    CN XII (hypoglossal nerve), 29, 31, 35, 49, 55, 155,
        199, 245
cranium, anatomy of, 3–4
    temporal bones, 3
        mastoid process, 3–4
        styloid process, 4
        zygomatic process, 4
    sphenoid bone, 4
cricopharyngeal dysfunction, 161
cricopharyngeal myotomy, 82, 83, 221, 222
cricopharyngeal sphincter (CS). *See* upper esophageal
    sphincter

Daniels, S. K., 97–98, 163
deep pharyngeal neuromuscular stimulation
    (DPNS/DPNMS), 50, 237
degenerative diseases, 153
deglutition. *See* swallowing
delay in triggering the pharyngeal swallow, 158
    behavioral therapy for, 179
dentition, 18–19, 245
    deciduous teeth, 19
    malocclusion, 19
    permanent teeth, 19
dentures, 20
dermatomyositis (DM), 169–170

Dettelbach, M., 197
diffuse idiopathic skeletal hyperostosis (DISH), 202–203
diverticula, 204–205, 222. *See also* Zenker's diverticulum
Donzeli, J., 198
drooling, 156, 248
    behavioral therapy for, 178
    medical therapy for, 178
Du Mond, C. E., 213
Dua, K., 95
dyspepsia, 205
dysphagia, 152, 155
    esophageal symptoms, 160–161
    neurological etiologies associated with, 153–155, 248
    oral stage symptoms, 155
    pharyngeal stage symptoms, 155–158, 248
dystonias, 159

edema, 225–226
electrocoagulation, 128
electroglottography, 56
electromyography (EMG), 20, 27, 36, 56, 84, 199–200
    surface electromyography (sEMG), 164, 213–214
electropalatography, 31
endoscopy, 122, 124–126
    limitations of, 56
    upper gastrointestinal endoscopy, 126–128
    See also fiberoptic endoscopic examination of swallow; fiberoptic endoscopic examination of swallow with sensory testing
endotracheal intubation, 188–189, 248
Ensrud, E., 61
enteral feeding, 84
enteric nervous system, 74, 78
epiglottis, 42, 47, 56, 59
    epiglottitis, 201–202
    as trigger site of the swallow response, 97
esophagus
    anatomy of, 68, 70–73, 110
    Barrett's esophagus, 205, 207
    blood supply to, 78–80, 246
    cancer of, 223–224
    diffuse esophageal spasm, 160–161
    esophageal manometry, 87–88
    esophageal pressure, 87–88
        age and gender effects on, 88
    esophagitis, 207–208
    esophagoglottal closure reflex, 77
    innervation of, 73–74
        enteric nervous system, 78
        peripheral nervous system, 74–78
    motility disorders of, 70
    nutcracker esophagus, 161
    physiology of, 80–87
    See also lower esophageal sphincter; upper esophageal sphincter
EZ-EM, 137

faucial arches/pillars
    anatomy of, 15
    as trigger points for the pharyngeal swallow response, 49–50
fiberoptic endoscopic examination of swallow (FEES), 110, 125, 126, 128–129
fiberoptic endoscopic examination of swallow with sensory testing (FEESST), 126, 129–130
fibrosis, 213, 226, 249
Filntisis, G. A., 225
fistulas, 221, 224
fluoroscopy, 113–114, 129
focal laryngeal dystonia. *See* spasmodic dysphonia
Forrestier's disease. *See* diffuse idiopathic skeletal hyperostosis
Foundas, A. L., 97–98, 163

gag reflex, 238
gagging, 156
    behavioral therapy for, 178
gastric pull-up procedure, 223
gastroesophageal reflux disease (GERD), 205–207
gastrostomy, 84
gender, effects on swallowing variables, 102, 104
Guillaine-Barre syndrome (GBS), 167–168

Hamdy, S., 163
Hamlet, G. S., 52
herpes simplex, 201
hiatal hernia, 128, 209
Hiiemae, K. M., 55
Hilgers, F. J., 221
Horowitz, J. B., 222
Huntington's disease (HD), 165
hyolaryngeal complex, 53–56
hyperbaric oxygen therapy, 225

infection, 153, 201–202
intraoral prosthetics, 214
    palatal lift prosthesis, 214
    palatal obturator, 214, 217
    palatal reshaping prosthesis, 217
Ishida, I., 55

jaw exercises, 215

Kendall, K. A., 62, 102, 99

Lambert-Eaton myasthenia syndrome (LEMS), 168
Langmore, S. E., 128
Larson, C. R., 27
larynx, 1
    anatomy/muscles of, 56–57, 59
    cancer of, 217–223
laryngeal penetration, 158
    behavioral therapy for, 179
lateral medullary syndrome. *See* Wallenberg's syndrome
Leder, S. B., 189, 197
Leonard, R. J., 62, 102
lips
    anatomy of, 11, 13
    lip exercises, 215
    lip strength, 27
    muscles of, 25–27, 245
Logemann, J. A., 27, 49, 94, 171, 237–238
Lou Gehrig's disease. *See* amyotrophic lateral sclerosis
lower esophageal sphincter (LES), 70, 71, 81, 84–85, 246
    anatomy and physiology of, 85, 87
Ludwig's angina, 201
Luschei, E. S., 213
lymphatic system, 80

macroglossia, 169
magnetic resonance imaging (MRI), 113, 122, 143–144
mandible, 4–5, 9
    anatomy of, 6–6
    angle of the mandible as a radiographic landmark, 7
    muscles of
        for mandibular closing, 32–34
        for mandibular opening, 34–35
manofluorography, 123, 144–145
manometry, 122–123, 144, 145–146, 161
Manual of Dysphagia Assessment in Adults, The (Murray), 128
mastication. *See* chewing
maxillae, 4–5
    anatomy of, 5–6
McCall, G. N., 31
McKenzie, S. W., 62
metabolic disorders, 153
Mioche, L., 20
modified Evan's blue dye test (MEBDT), 198
Momiyama, Y., 52
motor equivalence, 94–95, 97–99, 247
mouthfeel, 137
mucositis, 225–226

multiple sclerosis (MS), 164–165
Murray, K. A., 27
muscle fibers, types of
    cardiac, 73
    smooth, 73
    striated, 73
muscles of facial expression, 25
muscular dystrophy (MD), 169
    Duchenne's muscular dystrophy (DMD), 169
    oculopharyngeal muscular dystrophy (OPMD), 169
myasthenia gravis (MG), 168
myopathy, 169

nasal regurgitation, 158
    behavioral therapy for, 179
    medical therapy for, 179
nasogastric tube, 84, 218
neoplasm. *See* cancer
neurological pathology, *See* dysphagia, neurological etiologies associated with
nuclear medicine, 122, 143
nucleus tractus solitarius (NST), 49, 50

odynophagia, 160, 201
Olsson, R., 61
oral cavity, 9–11
oral preparation time, prolonged, 156
    behavioral therapy for, 178
osteophytes, 202, 248–249

palate, hard, 5, 6
    anatomy of, 6, 16
    clefts and defects of, 16
palate, soft. *See* velum
Palmer, J. B., 55, 61
parenteral feeding, 84
Parkinson's disease (PD), 165–166
Passavant's pad, 53
percutaneous endoscopic gastrostomy (PEG), 84
peripheral nervous system (PNS), 74–78. *See also* cranial nerves
peristalsis, 60, 73, 80
    primary peristaltic waves, 73, 81, 246
    secondary peristaltic waves, 73, 81, 246
    as stripping action, 80
    tertiary peristaltic waves, 73
Perlmann, A. J., 213
pH studies, 146–147
    ambulatory 24-hour testing, 147, 247
    Bernstein examination, 146–147
pharyngoesophageal (PE) segment. *See* upper esophageal sphincter

pharynx
 anatomy of, 44–45, 47–48, 60
 cancer of, 217
 pharyngeal phase of swallowing, 42–44, 245–246
  delay in triggering, 248
  hypolaryngeal elevation, 53–56
  laryngeal protection during, 56–57, 59
  opening of the upper esophageal sphincter, 61–62
  progressive pharyngeal contraction, 60–61
  trigger points of, 48–51
  velopharyngeal closure, 51–53
 pharyngeal stasis, 158
  behavioral therapy for, 179
 pharyngeal swallow response, 49
 pharyngitis, 202
 pharyngoglottal closure reflex, 95, 97, 99
 and pressure differentials, 42–44, 246
 sections of
  laryngopharynx, 45
  nasopharynx, 45
  oropharynx, 10, 21, 45
Plummer-Vinson syndrome, 208
pocketing, 13, 15, 28, 156, 165, 247–248
 behavioral therapy for, 178
polymyositis (PM), 169–170
positron emission tomography (PET), 113
progressive systemic sclerosis (PSS). *See* scleroderma
pseudobulbar palsy, 166
pseudoepiglottis, 222–223
pulse oximetry, 237
pyriform sinus stasis, 158
 behavioral therapy for, 179
 medical therapy for, 179

radionecrosis, 225, 249
Rasley, A., 171
reduced hyolaryngeal elevation, 158
 behavioral therapy for, 179
reflux, 87, 205, 208
 laryngopharyngeal reflux, 205
rheology, 136–137
Robbins, J., 94

saliva, 21, 224–225
 composition of, 22
salivary glands, 21–22
 parotid salivary glands, 22–23, 245
 sublingual salivary glands, 22, 23–24, 245
 submandibular salivary glands, 22, 24, 245
 See saliva
Sasaki, C. T., 222
Schatzki's ring, 208

scintigraphy. *See* nuclear medicine
scleroderma, 170
sclerotherapy, 128
sensory receptors, 37
 chemoreceptors, 38
 mechanoreceptors, 37
 nociceptors, 38
 proprioceptors, 37–38
 thermoreceptors, 38
sensory stimulation techniques, 50
sicca syndrome, 21
Sihler's stain, 84
silent aspiration, 133, 156, 189
 identification of, 157
 neurophysiology of, 157
Sjögren's syndrome, 170, 201
Sonies, B. C., 55–56, 98–99
spasmodic dysphonia (SD), 159
 types of, 159
squirreling. *See* pocketing
Stachler, R. J., 197
Stemple, J., 200
Stoeckli, S. J., 136
Stone, M., 31
strictures, 209–209, 221–222, 249
stroke. *See* cerebrovascular accident
Suiter, D. M., 197
sulci, anatomy of, 13
swallow control, 154
swallow event
 muscle activity related to
  bolus containment, 96
  bolus control, 96
  hyolaryngeal elevation, 97
  mastication, 96
  oral bolus propulsion, 96
  pharyngeal elevation and constriction, 97
  velopharyngeal closure, 96
 terms associated with
  duration of hyoid movement, 44
  duration of laryngeal closure, 44
  duration of laryngeal elevation, 44
  duration of UES opening, 44
  duration of velopharyngeal closure, 44
  oral transit time (OTT), 44
  pharyngeal delay time (PDT), 44
  pharyngeal response time (PRT), 44
  pharyngeal transit time (PTT), 44
swallowing
 continuous swallows, 31–32, 98–99
 discrete swallows, 31–32, 95, 97
 methods of evaluating, 247

swallowing (*continued*)
   neural regulation of, 152
   normal swallow, 94–102
   and respiration, 62–63, 246
   stages of, 2, 94
     1. oral preparatory, 2, 25–37
     2. oral, 2, 25–37
     3. pharyngeal, 2, 42–63
     4. esophageal, 2, 68–88
   swallower variables, 101–102
   See also swallow control; swallow event
swallowing center. <I>See<P> nucleus tractus solitarius
syncope, 205

tachyphagia, 165
Tanaka, E. 61
taste, 38
temporomandibular joint (TMJ), 5, 9, 245
movement in, 35–36
   rotation, 36
   rotation/translation, 36
   translation, 36
Terrell, J. E., 224
thermal gustatory treatment, 50
thermal tactile application (TTA), 50, 176
thrush. *See* candidiasis
tongue
   anatomy of, 16–17
   muscles of, 28
     extrinsic, 28, 29–32
     intrinsic, 28–29, 245
   taste buds on, 17
   tongue exercises, 216
tonsils, 15
torticollis, 159
toxins, 153
trachea, 59
tracheostomy, 189–190
tracheostomy tube
   cuffed, 190, 193
   cuffless, 190
   decannulation, 195
   effect on aspiration, 193, 197
   fenestrated, 193, 195
   non-fenestrated, 195
   with one-way speaking valve, 195, 197–198
tracheotomy, 189
   symptoms associated with induced dysphagia, 190
traumatic brain injury (TBI), 153, 164
treatment strategies, 171, 176–177
   carbonated thin liquids, 174
   chin tuck, 172

cold, textured, and/or flavored bolus, 173
decision-making process for controversial practices, 237–238
effortful swallow, 174
electrical stimulation of the thyrohyoid musculature, 175
head back, 172
head tilt to the stronger side, 173
head rotation to the weak side, 172, 248
mechanical soft diet, 176
Mendelsohn maneuver, 175
oral-motor exercises, 175
order in which they should be introduced, 171, 248
pureed diet, 176
Shaker exercises, 175
side lying, 173
super-supraglottic swallow, 174, 176
supraglottic swallow, 174, 176
thermal tactile application (TTA), 173
thick diet, 176
thin liquid diet, 176
variables that help determine course of treatment, 171
trismus, 226
twilight condition. <I>See<P> conscious sedation

ultrasonography, 31, 55
upper esophageal sphincter (UES), 2, 42, 70–71, 81, 246
   anatomy and physiology of, 82–83, 85, 87
   innervation of, 83–84
   opening of, 61–62, 246
   pressure generated at, 87–88
   spasms in, 222
   treatment of dysfunction of, 159
uvula, 16
   bifid, 16

vagus nerve. *See* cranial nerves, CN X
vallecular stasis, 158
   behavioral therapy for, 179
velum 6, 245
   anatomy of, 6, 16
   clefts and defects of, 16
   muscles of, 36–37
Veyrune, J. L., 20
videoendoscopy, 157
videofluroroscopy, 157, 222
videomanometry, 144
vocal folds
   false, 57, 59
   true, 4, 56–57
Vocal Function Exercises, 200

Wallenberg's syndrome, 163
webs, 208–209

xerostomia, 21, 201, 224–225, 248, 249
X-ray equipment, 130

Zenker's diverticulum, 82, 204, 249
    symptoms of, 204
zygomatic bones, 6